THE OTHER SIDE OF THE CLOSET

THE COMING-OUT CRISIS FOR STRAIGHT SPOUSES AND FAMILIES

Revised and Expanded

by

Amity Pierce Buxton, Ph.D.

John Wiley & Sons, Inc.
New York • Chichester • Brisbane • Toronto • Singapore

Copyright © 1991, 1994 by Amity Pierce Buxton, Ph.D.
Published by John Wiley & Sons, Inc.

Author's Note: The real life stories in this book, selected to illustrate common issues rather than private lives, are told in the spouses' and children's own voices, with some alterations made for literary and privacy purposes. Every effort has been made, to the best of the author's ability, to keep the privacy interest intact (except for the stories by Jane and Jim, who choose to come out publicly from their side of the closet). The effort to protect individuals' privacy may inadvertently result in a description of a real person unknown to the author. Any such resemblance is purely coincidental.

Publisher's Note: This book is designed to provide ideas and information about the subject matter. The ideas, procedures, and suggestions contained in this book are not intended to replace the services of a professional counselor or trained health-care professional. A professional counselor or trained health-care professional should be consulted regarding the use of any of the ideas, procedures, or suggestions in this book. The names and identities of the individuals in this book have been disguised. Any similarities to other individuals is coincidental.
The author and the publisher hereby specifically disclaim any and all liability arising directly or indirectly from the use of application of any of the ideas, procedures or suggestions contained in this book and any errors, omission, and inaccuracies in the information contained in this book.

This Publication is designed to provide accurate and authoritative information in regard to the subject matter covered. It is sold with the understanding that the publisher is not engaged in rendering professional services. If legal, accounting, medical, psychological, or any other expert assistance is required, the services of a competent professional person should be sought.

Library of Congress Cataloging-in-Publication Data:
Buxton, Amity.
    The other side of the closet : the coming-out crisis for straight
spouses and families / Amity Pierce Buxton.—Rev. and expanded.
      p. cm.
    Includes bibliographical references.
    ISBN 0-471-02152-0 (alk. paper)
    1. Bisexuality in marriage—United States. 2. Coming out (Sexual
orientation)—United States. 3. Homosexuality—United States.
4. Married people—United States—Psychology. I. Title.
HQ74.B89 1994
306-76'5—dc20   94-9325

Printed in the United States of America.

10 9 8 7

dedication

To my children...
whose love sustained me in my journey
from trauma to transformation,
after my husband came out in 1983

the few friends who knew...
and dared support me,
without knowing what it really means
to be on the other side of the closet

the two million other straight spouses and their children...
whose stories aren't here,
yet who could tell similar tales of pain and
increased strength and understanding

and the readers of this book...
with hope for spouses facing a partner's coming out
for mixed-orientation couples trying to stay together,
and for their children coping with grown-up issues;

with compassion for homosexual and bisexual persons
coping with the intolerance of society;

and with encouragement to those who view gay and lesbian
issues from extreme positions to consider the middle ground,
where the human condition common to us all plays
out its uneven course in individual lives.

acknowledgments

The professionals and hundreds of
spouses whose assistance was crucial to
the completion of this project are too
numerous to list. Special mention goes
to Sandra Auerback, M.S.A.,
George Deabill, Ph.D.,
Ronald C. Fox, Ph.D.,
Bill Jones,
Webster Lithgow,
Kathy McMahon, Psy.D.,
BettyClare Moffatt, M.A.,
Charles Moser, Ph.D.,
Sharon Nathan, Ph.D.,
Jay P. Paul, Ph.D.,
Aurele Samuels,
Riette Smith, M.S.,
Bryan Strong, Ph.D.,
Jane E. Vennard, M. Div.,
Claire Ortalda, my editor, whose
challenging mind helped me clarify the
confounding issues straight spouses
and children face, and PJ Dempsey, at
John Wiley, who quickly discerned
the social import of this
growing phenomenon.

PREFACE TO THE REVISED EDITION

In 1986, the San Francisco Gay Fathers asked me to research what happens to spouses when their partners come out as gay, lesbian or bisexual. For five years, I talked with four hundred and fifty spouses and partners across the country. Thirty-one (twenty-nine straight spouses, a gay husband and a lesbian wife) agreed to tell their stories in depth. This core group was representative of all respondents: in age (twenty-two to fifty-seven), in education (high school through graduate school), in occupation (wife/mother to domestic cleaner to administrator) and in length of marriage (from three to twenty-six years). Only one spouse of color from the total respondent group, however, consented to tell her story.

Analysis of the narratives, using a phenomenological approach (rather than a priori hypotheses) and content analysis of self-reports of the total group revealed common issues and typical recovery stages. Some findings were validated by the literature and discussions with therapists. Most of the data, however, exposed unexplored areas of the straight spouse's experience, notably their isolation and diversity of resolutions. The most important findings appeared in the first edition of *The Other Side of the Closet*.

In the three years since the first edition went to press, the pace of social and political changes relating to homosexual and bisexual persons escalated. More married lesbians came out, the bisexual community grew and gay issues gained media attention and entered the political process.

During the same period, I talked at length with six hundred more individuals including children and grandparents from forty-six states and several foreign countries. Gradually, an initial hunch grew stronger: the coming out is a family matter and, to understand it better, children's reactions need to be examined directly. To fill a gap in the literature regarding children's experience over time as well as to reflect current trends, it was decided to reissue *The Other Side of the Closet* in an expanded edition.

As in the original study, a representative group of children, aged from eleven to thirty-two, agreed to tell their stories. The narratives were analyzed and then examined in light of the literature and interviews with therapists who work with similar children. In addition, two spouses, who experiences mirrored recent developments, shared their tales.

This new edition, based now on accounts from more than one thousand spouses and family members over eight years, broadens our understanding of what the coming-out crisis means to the family and to the larger community. The Introduction is updated as are discussions of bi-straight and lesbian-straight couples. Two stories in the first edition have been replaced. One, in Part Two, is told by a wife in a bi-straight marriage of thirty-two years. In Part Four, a husband relates his struggle after his lesbian wife came out just as the 1992 anti-gay rights campaign erupted in Colorado. The new Part Six gives voice to children's long-term concerns.

As a parent and spouse, as well as researcher, I feel that a closer look at such families is needed at this turning point in the nineties. The intensity of the debate over gay rights, from Congress to church pulpits, drowns out legitimate concerns raised on both sides about social justice and community stability. As with any societal change, the future of our children will be built only after the debate quiets down. Do we leave its design to whoever wins the shouting battle? Or do we look seriously now at damage already incurred and call for a society that promises personal security and full community participation for everyone regardless of orientation? To do so may require questioning long-held beliefs. Not to act will perpetuate coming-out tragedies for thousands of families, year after year.

It is my hope that this new edition may open a window on a neglected aspect of the controversy. It reveals the problems with which families are forced to deal because of the domino effect of homophobia. The very pressures that made many gay, lesbian and bisexual persons marry as "the right thing to do" have led instead to family breakups and suffering.

A book containing pain and anger is not easy to read. But tracing the transforming process that families undergo to resolve profound dilemmas can be rewarding as well as enlightening. May this book be read as it was written—with humility to look candidly at real life events, with sensitivity toward everyone impacted and with hope that we might learn from our mistakes to create a better world for our children.

Amity Pierce Buxton
San Francisco

contents

introduction

COMING OUT
IN MARRIAGE

THE UNTOLD STORY

So they sit and watch me
they wonder, they whisper...
and still I lay pinned under the load.
—Hanna, 35, mother of three, 1988

Hanna is a cheerful and capable woman who tried to hold her marriage together for two years while caring for her three children under the age of twelve and keeping secret her husband's two arrests for sex acts in men's public restrooms. The night before she finally sought therapy, she wrote the lines above.

What Hanna didn't know was that she is only one of about two million women and men across the country who are or were married to a homosexual or bisexual partner[1] and that her children are among about 3,500,000 youngsters born to such families.[2] Only a few spouses are aware of their partner's sexual orientation when they marry. In some cases the partners are not sure. In time, the truth comes out with painful consequences for all involved.

What happens when a husband or wife comes out of the closet has been hidden too long from public view. It is a profound crisis that cuts across race, socioeconomic class, religion and age. Interviews with hundreds of women and men from coast to coast attest to the devastation that uttering the three words, "I am gay," can have on a straight spouse. The coming out thrusts the spouse into the closet as well.

The way out is a long, wrenching struggle marked by, guilt, anger, grief, illness and sometimes suicide attempts. In the end most issues are resolved with positive results. *The Other Side of the Closet* presents the untold story of the struggle—not to cast stones at gay partners, but rather to reveal an integral chapter of gay, lesbian and bisexual history.

The Closet

Behind the married partner's coming out lies his or her own traumatic tale. Most homosexual or bisexual persons don't want to be rejected for belonging to a minority which Judeo-Christian society historically has stigmatized as unnatural, immoral or criminal. Therefore, many people who are attracted to the same sex deny or repress these feelings. Fearing rejection, job loss, social status or self-respect, some adopt a straight lifestyle entirely and others only publicly. Because the same-sex drive is both compelling and stigmatizing, becoming comfortable with it may take a long time. Keeping it hidden consumes much psychic energy but the sacrifice to offset guilt or to meet life goals in an anti-gay climate seems worth it.

According to most research studies homosexuality and bisexuality seem to result from the interplay of many biochemical, environmental and psychosocial factors operating from conception through adolescence. No definitive cause has been found.

At any given time, there exists a small minority of homosexual persons in society. Exact figures are due to varying definitions and research methods. Until recently, the commonly accepted estimate came from Alfred Kinsey's studies of the sexual behavior of adult white males (1948) and adult white females (1953). Using a zero-to-six point continuum of sexual behavior from exclusively heterosexual through bisexual to exclusively homosexual, Kinsey reported that eight percent of the men, aged sixteen to fifty-five, had been exclusively gay for at least three years, including four percent who reported only gay experiences. From two to six percent of the women, aged twenty to thirty-five, were more or less exclusively lesbian. Studies as recent as 1993 suggest much lower percentages.[3]

Bisexuality presents a less definitive picture, but it is clearly a distinct orientation in which a person is turned on by both genders. Bisexuals include not only men and women who report somewhat equal homosexual and heterosexual experiences but also those who engage in mainly same-sex or almost exclusively heterosexual activities. In any one person, the mix over time can be fluid. Research suggests that at least twice as many bisexual as homosexual persons exist,[4] and estimates rise when identity, fantasies and other dimensions are considered.[5]

Many homosexuals sense an attraction to others of the same gender in childhood or adolescence; bisexuals usually do so somewhat later. Others, including a number of lesbians, do not experience homosexual feelings until mid-life. Once same-sex yearnings are honestly acknowledged, a conscious choice can be made as to how to handle them.

About twenty percent of gay men marry.[6] Whether their homosexuality is latent, denied or consciously hidden, they desire children and seek the security that marriage affords in a society that values the family. While they may genuinely love the women they marry, Michael Ross suggests that internalized homophobia and social pressure are major factors in their decision to seek marriage.[7] In contrast to gay men, most women who are sure of their lesbian orientation rarely consider marriage. Bisexual men and women who marry—the exact percentage is unknown—are, of course, sexually attracted to their mates.

The majority of married gay and bisexual men say they sensed being different from other men or realized their same-sex preference when marrying, but most decided to live a straight lifestyle, remaining gay only in self-identity, feelings or fantasies. Many believed their love was strong enough to make them forget or overcome their sexual attraction. This assumption was often supported by psychiatrists who counseled that homosexuality was a phase that could be overcome by having a good wife.

Once married, whether uncertain about their orientation or hiding it, many husbands gradually heed latent or repressed feelings and begin secret gay contacts. Clandestine gay sex can be quick and anonymous without the possible consequences of affairs with women—yet with the risk of arrest. Laud Humphreys' study of anonymous sex in men's restrooms suggests that married men who comprised fifty-four percent of his sample compartmentalize this "tea room trade" from married life.[8] Husbands who begin secret affairs do suffer increasing guilt.

Most homosexual and bisexual men who are not yet comfortable with their sexual orientation continue to hide their secret lives. After stressful soul-searching some tell their wives, privately or with the mediation of a therapist, for the sake of honesty or relief from inner turmoil. Others admit the truth when a suspicious wife confronts them or when outside evidence, like an arrest or AIDS diagnosis, reveals their secret.

Many men remain closeted, some keeping their wives satisfied and fulfilling parental responsibilities and others neglecting or criticizing their confused spouses. The need to conceal sexual orientation can be so overpowering that some keep silent even after being diagnosed with AIDS.

Lesbian and bi wives, rather than seek isolated anonymous sex, typically develop close relationships to one woman at a time. Once they realize and admit their sexual orientation, some keep it secret and others tell their husbands fairly quickly.

Liberation

The increased incidence of husbands and wives coming out over the past thirty years reflects major changes in our society. Following the gay-baiting tactics of the repressive McCarthy Senate hearings in the fifties that aroused fear of homosexual men, the sixties brought a sweeping reversal of social attitudes that affected homosexuals, along with other minorities.

The civil rights movement of African-Americans and the sexual revolution liberalized views held by the majority of society toward minority groups and sexuality. By the late sixties, African-Americans were participating in many levels of society from which they had been excluded. Human sexuality began to be a respectable subject for academic study, trade publications and individual therapy.

These liberalizing movements boosted the confidence of the homosexual minority in cities across the nation to lead more openly gay lives. The 1969 successful stand of gays and lesbians against a police raid of Stonewall Inn in Greenwich Village established a model of gay power strong enough to fight for and win their civil rights as an oppressed minority. Within a short time, gay baths, bars, tea rooms and a variety of designated meeting spots mushroomed coast to coast.

Meanwhile, lesbians, having developed group identity during and after World War II, formed a separate strand of the growing feminist movement sparked by Betty Friedan's *The Feminine Mystique*. Soon, they were a powerful minority, with lesbian publications, public meeting places and bars appearing across the country.

The seventies saw gay liberation stabilize and expand. In 1974, the American Psychiatric Association voted to remove homosexuality from the list of pathological diseases, lessening the stigma attached to gay persons and activities. The American Psychological Association followed suit. By the decade's end, bisexual persons, erroneously labeled gay by society and classified as such in most studies and the media, had formed their own network to celebrate their unique orientation. Expanding the sexual revolution, books and media publicized non-traditional relationships such as open marriages, ménages à trois, communes and group sex.

In the eighties, openly gay and lesbian individuals were seen in mainstream activities from business to politics. Gay and lesbian organizations created public identity and gained political clout for homosexual persons nationwide. Gay therapists and support groups were available for counseling men how to come out. More gay and bisexual husbands, gaining self-esteem, told their wives. More lesbian and bisexual wives, having easier access to other lesbian and bi women, acknowledged their orientation and came out to their husbands.

In the midst of this ground swell of gay, lesbian and bisexual pride, three events rekindled negative attitudes against homosexuality. First, the rising death toll from AIDS made many people fear gay men as potential carriers of death—even though the disease is not limited to high-risk homosexual men. Second, the 1986 Supreme Court decision to uphold Georgia's law criminalizing sodomy reinforced such laws in some thirty other states. Third, the Vatican reaffirmed that active homosexuality is a sin in the eyes of the Catholic Church. The resulting resurgence of anti-gay sentiment prompted homosexual and bisexual groups to increase political action toward securing rights long denied to them.

In the early nineties, the conflict intensified. Gay and lesbian topics filled the media as campaigns to overturn gay rights laws were waged in Oregon and Colorado. In the nation's capitol, debates on lifting the ban on gays in the military filled Congress and a lesbian lawyer was confirmed as undersecretary for the Department of Housing and Urban Development. Surveys that reported lower percentages of gay persons in the population than previously estimated made headlines along with studies that suggested possible genetic factors linked to homosexuality. Spokespersons for the religious right were elected to school boards nationwide, and thousands of gay, lesbian and bisexual citizens marched on Washington in April 1993 to assert their rights.

Over these three decades, the growing momentum of the sexual revolution, gay liberation and the feminist movement impacted the lives of many mixed-orientation couples. As gay and bisexual husbands acted on their orientation, their wives, empowered by feminist pride and new sexual expertise, tried to exert equal power in the couple's sex life. The men's resulting feelings of being further trapped in marriage added fuel to their drive to come out to their wives.

The impact was more abrupt in lesbian-straight marriages, since both feminism and gay liberation encouraged lesbian wives to lessen the power husbands exerted over their lives. As they pursued women's rights and independence, more discovered their homosexuality, came out and left their husbands.

No one foresaw the negative effects that the long overdue recognition of gay and lesbian rights would have on marriages and families. The liberation cry of gay, lesbian and bisexual marriage partners became a sword that sundered the world of their spouses and children.

The Other Side of the Closet

The devastating impact of gay and women's liberation on the lives of straight wives and husbands whose partners come out cannot be minimized. Most spouses endure their pain in silence on their side of the closet, while their gay, lesbian and bisexual partners find support from their respective communities. The coming out—a cause of celebration for the partners—unintentionally creates profound trauma for their spouses. Shocked, they feel rejected sexually and bereft of the mates that they thought they had. Whether twenty-three years old with toddlers or sixty-eight with grandchildren, spouses are typically too traumatized at first to realize how their partners' disclosure will affect them. Some spouses leave the marriage at once or ask their partners to leave, while others find that their mates plan to leave immediately. Still other spouses stay, unsure of what will happen and hoping the marriage might still work.

Only as shock subsides can straight spouses begin to understand homosexuality and homophobia and how those realities affect them and their children. Though relieved to know the reason behind prior changes in the partners' behavior or problems in marital sex, most feel hurt, angry and helpless. The partners' closet seems as much a prison for them as it was for their mates. More spouses leave the marriage at this point. Some stay.

Whatever action is taken, spouses slowly realize that they face seven major issues. These include damage to their sexuality; negation of their concept of marriage; conflicting spousal and parental roles; destruction of their own self-concept; breakdown of trust and integrity; possible family break-up and disintegration of their belief system.

The magnitude of these challenges overwhelms most spouses. Yet, at the nadir of despair, what seems like rock bottom can serve as a stepping stone to new possibilities. Just as mythical heroes and heroines undergo seemingly impossible trials to reach their goal and in the process discover their true worth, so spouses can direct their lives toward positive change as they work through the painful consequences of the coming out.

Although some coping strategies are more constructive than others, there is no single, correct resolution. Depression, illness and breakdown may occur, but the struggle need not continue in that direction. Many alternative routes lead to understanding and transformation within the marriage or upon divorce. By seeking therapy, Hanna took such a route, becoming more capable and confident than before the coming-out crisis.

Because the trauma is so profound, the process of recovery and transformation is long and arduous, requiring courage, patience and persistence. It typically takes at least a year to resolve the pragmatic issues of damaged sexuality, changed relationship and conflicting parent-spouse roles. Two or more years are generally needed to resolve the more complex issues of fragmented identity, integrity, family configuration and belief system. All told, it usually takes more than three years to construct a new life and far longer to look dispassionately at the experience.

Individual timetables vary, depending on what the partner and children do, competing demands of family and work, number of years married, length of time the sexual orientation was hidden, quality of the relationship, number and ages of children, degree of family and outside support, outside interests, job skills, community attitudes, physical health, age and personal style. Straight husbands tend to suffer more traumatically at first but then recover more quickly than straight wives.

The stories and analyses that follow present a collective portrait of how spouses and their families come to terms with the disclosures. The stories are told in the voices of straight wives and husbands, a gay husband, a lesbian wife and children. Representative of common perceptions, feelings and coping strategies, each anonymous tale could have been told by others struggling with this situation.

The spouses' stories are grouped into six sections according to the most pressing issue that individual spouses faced. The children's stories form their own section. The seven parts are presented in the order of emotional stages through which straight spouses typically progress. Each part concludes with a discussion of major implications of the highlighted issue and constructive coping strategies that spouses and their families have used successfully.

Together, the stories and commentaries expose the closeted struggle of spouses and their families, the unintended victims of victims of a homophobic society. However inadvertent, the painful consequences of a partner's coming-out on his or her spouse and children cannot be ignored. At the same time, the crisis is often the beginning of healing for all concerned.

<u>one</u>

SEXUAL MISMATCH

DAMAGED SEXUALITY
OF THE STRAIGHT SPOUSE

When the initial shock subsides, straight spouses are typically devastated by what seems like a rejection of their sexuality. How to adapt to their partners' sexual attraction to someone of the same sex is the major concern for most spouses. They have suddenly become the non-preferred sex partners and often feel rejected as women or men. As partners celebrate their true sexual orientation and their courageous honesty in disclosing it, spouses feel bereft of their marital mates—causing confusion and anger.

Even though the partner may not have known, accepted or dared to reveal his or her homosexuality or bisexuality, the fact that the different sexual orientation existed at all makes the spouse typically suspect some dysfunctioning in the couple's lovemaking and some damage to his or her own sexuality.

For many spouses, the partner's revealed homosexuality or bisexuality alone prompts immediate divorce. Others try to work through it to preserve the marriage, as the stories in Part Two show. Whether they stay or leave, most spouses gradually realize that the hidden sexual disparity has already harmed their sexual functioning and self-image. This is particularly true for spouses of gay or lesbian partners who have little or no erotic attraction to them. The rage many feel can persist for years.

The following stories told by two wives and a husband of homosexual partners illustrate how unknown sexual incompatibility can profoundly affect the marriage and the straight spouse's sexual identity. The concluding section highlights major problems related to the sexuality issue and outlines several effective strategies that spouses have used for healing sexual damage.

Personal Stories

Brainwashed
Moira

I'm no longer that freckle-faced redhead who won the Good Samaritan prize and got engaged to Tim Conally shortly after high school in Brooklyn. That was someone else, who never made a decision and wanted to be cared for the rest of her life.

One memory stands out from that period, when Tim was on a construction crew and I was a clerk in an office near his job site. One evening we were to meet after work. After an hour's wait, I called him from a pay phone.

"Why are you so stupid, Moira?" Tim shouted. "Use your head. Don't stand around waiting, for God's sake! Get a bus and go home if I don't show."

A few weeks later, we were to rendezvous again. When he didn't come within twenty minutes, I caught the bus home. Just as I opened my door, the phone rang. It was Tim, asking, "Are you dumb or what? When I say I'll pick you up, you be there."

"Tim, a couple of weeks ago you said...."

The wedding took place as planned because I cared and would do anything to keep that handsome, black-haired man loving me.

For the next twenty years until the early eighties, I tried to comply with his confusing demands. "If only you were thin like our neighbor," he'd say or "Why aren't you a better cook like my sister?" Then, once I'd lose weight or try new recipes, he wouldn't like my figure or my food. In our sex life it was, "If only you did this, Moira...or felt like that."

After six months of not having sex very often, I asked him why, figuring I could do something to meet his wishes better.

"I like women to be aggressors once in a while."

That night, I took the initiative and he turned over to sleep.

"Hmm, I'm doing something wrong," I thought.

The following night, I tried again, laughing a little and showing enthusiasm. The same negative response. "What I'm doing really must be wrong," I told myself. "Maybe my intentions should be clearer."

A few nights later, announcing my desire for sex, I acted highly seductive.

"No, not tonight," he said and rolled over.

Humiliated, I vowed never to try again.

Shortly thereafter, Tim asked me one morning, "Why aren't you pregnant yet, Moira? Go see a doctor."

Though I was furious, my sense of humor came to the rescue. "I'm not the Virgin Mary, Tim. You've got to have sex with me if I'm going to get pregnant."

I got pregnant by the end of the year, when Tim was working two jobs to make ends meet. Six months later, looking through one of the magazines he often brought home, I came upon several photos of naked men. Puzzled, I asked about them at dinner.

"God, you're dumb! It's normal for us men to be curious about other nude men."

Having led a sheltered life in a parochial school system and a Catholic family, I bought his answer. Being ignorant about homosexuality, I was scared not to accept what he said.

In bed that night, Tim asked, "Do you think I'm gay?"

"Of course not." What did I know? A wife doesn't think that about the husband she loves. Besides, he'd made me pregnant.

Three months later Beth arrived. Tim was crushed it wasn't a son. Two years later when Vicky was born, he was disappointed again. His letdown was so intense that the hospital staff talked about it. When Vicky and I got home, he ignored her. Never touched her. Within six weeks he started drinking heavily and blamed it on being trapped with the first daughter and super-trapped with the second.

By then I was trapped too, a twenty-four-year-old woman taking care of a two-year-old, a baby and an alcoholic husband.

Tim drank for fourteen years, mostly in bars. He got through the day on a quart of vodka, staying drunk most of the time even at work, where they covered for him.

At home I wondered how much longer living with an alcoholic was possible. I decided that when the girls went off to school I would look for a job and get out of the house.

During the next six years we moved twice. Because sex with a drunk is not good, I avoided it except for one night after Vicky was finally old enough to go to school full time. A month later my doctor discovered that I was pregnant, sending me into total depression. A new baby would keep me home another five years.

When I told the doctor how Tim's drinking frustrated me, he said, "You're wrong, Moira. Count how many drinks he has. That'll prove that he isn't alcoholic."

In my low state, there wasn't much to fall back on. Then a friend said he'd seen Tim go into a gay bar one night when Tim had said he'd been someplace else.

That evening, when I brought it up, Tim said, "Oh, yeah. When I found out it was a gay bar I left." Then he added, "If you threaten to throw me out for this, Moira, you'll go first, bag and baggage."

By then I was totally out of control. Subconsciously I felt that if I found out that Tim was homosexual it would break me completely. "Let it go, Moira," I told myself.

Meanwhile I was losing my temper with the kids, screaming at them all the time—a real pain to live with—while Tim made it clear that was why he drank.

The few times we had sex during these months were more trouble than pleasure. Finally Tim asked, "What will we do about it?"

"I frankly don't know and frankly don't care," I sighed.

From then on Tim slept on the living room couch. Four months later Amanda was born. For the next five years until she went off to kindergarten, my depression and complaining tirades gradually became worse and I grieved for Tim as I watched him kill himself with alcohol. Day after day I asked myself, "What am I doing here?" I realized that I was really just an unemployed single parent of three kids.

Once Amanda started school a job became imperative. It would provide an outlet for my frustration, extra spending money and a way to support myself in the event of divorce. Yet seeing myself as lazy and stupid, incapable of performing—everything Tim said—I was frightened. Since I hadn't worked for so long, my talents were an unknown quantity. The part-time receptionist job that came up seemed like a good compromise.

A year later we moved to a four-bedroom house so everyone would have a bedroom. When the girls first saw it, Vicky asked, "Which bedroom is Daddy's?" "Of course," I thought, "all she's seen is Tim sleeping on the couch!"

The next year, seven years after Tim's retreat to the couch and no sex, his supervisor told him he'd be fired if he didn't quit drinking. In April 1980 he attempted sobriety for the first time.

A few weeks later, a friend I'd run into at the market said he'd seen Tim going into some gay hangout.

When I mentioned it after dinner, Tim said "Oh! That had nothing to do with me. It was just because I was drinking."

"O.K., forget it! It's behind us. You're sober now."

In this time of sobriety, Tim tried very hard to be nice to me, although he still blamed me as the cause of his drinking.

One night that summer, we were watching television with Amanda in the family room. Sitting on the hearth, she looked over at us on the lounge chair, where Tim had his arm around me and I was lying against him.

"Are you two going to get married?" she asked suddenly.

I looked at her, wide-eyed. "Amanda, we are married. We're your mom and dad,"

"No, you're not."

I laughed a little. "Why would you say that?"

"Because married people hug and kiss and hold each other and say nice things to each other. All you two do is fight and argue and scream." Then she smiled. "Are you going to get married?"

One night, a few weeks later, after finishing the dishes, I popped into the living room where Tim was reading the paper. Feeling light-hearted, I said, "Hey! The kids are watching TV. Why don't we go up to the bedroom and fool around a little."

"They're watching TV."

"Tim, did you hear me? I'm not kidding."

"No, Moira. I just want to read."

And that was it.

So in my nineteenth year of marriage, I called up a man who had been pursuing me at work and started an affair, petrified he'd say, "My God! It's no wonder your husband doesn't want to have anything to do with you. You are horrible."

That was not the case. There was nothing wrong with me except for being totally inexperienced, fearful and very naive for a woman who'd been married for nineteen years. After eight months, though still frightened and unsure of sex, I realized that the relationship was only sexual and stopped seeing him.

With only Tim in my life again, my suspicions about him could no longer be ignored. Everything began to fall into place. Then one night when the kids and he were watching a TV show about gays, I heard him say, "Oh, those fags! Those queers! Ugh!"

In a rage, but waiting until the kids left the room, I accused him of being a gay.

"Yes," he screamed, spinning around to face me, "I occasionally get off on sex with a man."

Shocked, I began to look for evidence. Over the next few days, proof was everywhere—telephone numbers on scratch pads, reports from friends who'd seen him in gay places. Again I accused him. I needed him to confirm what I wanted to deny.

"Sure," he shouted, "a man's body turns me on."

I still couldn't believe it and we didn't discuss it further. By fall, all we did was argue.

Finally, Tim asked, "Just what do you want, Moira? Write it to me. I'm tired of talking."

My letter was very nice. It reflected the way I was raised. "If you're gay," I began,

> I want to know so you can get on with your life and I with mine. This isn't any good for the kids or us. We're miserable and the kids will be too. I want an answer soon because the holidays are coming.

When he hadn't answered by December, I asked him outright, "Are you gay, Tim? Are you?"

He started shouting. "Only you and your vicious, accusatory mind would suggest such a thing!" Starting out the door, he turned. "Try to kick me out and you'll see who's thrown out."

Come March, Tim still hadn't answered the letter. By mid-March, on my return from a weekend company retreat, he acted strange and the girls reported he'd been away most of the time.

At breakfast on Monday I asked, "So, are you planning on leaving?" "No," he said and went off to work.

That night I said, "Look, Tim, I wasn't kidding. Are you planning on moving out?"

Silence.

"What is going on? You haven't answered my letter. I can't live like this any more."

When he still gave no reply I yelled, "Don't tell me nothing!"

"Yeah, I'm gay," he said matter-of-factly, "and I want a divorce."

No discussion. He was gay and the marriage was ending. I'd been married to him for twenty years and he'd never discussed it with me. As I found out later, he'd talked to gay men about it at a two-day gay conference that weekend.

When we told the kids about the divorce, they didn't understand. They blamed me for it, since I'd been such a grouse, yelling at them all those years. Within a few days we knew that they had to be told the real reason.

Tim drove them down to the park on Sunday afternoon to tell them alone. In ten minutes they were back.

"What!" I cried, as they walked in the door.

"I told 'em I was gay," Tim said, "and asked if they had any questions. They didn't, so we came home."

The girls' faces were ashen. "Mom?" Vicky said, her eyes asking all the questions that hadn't been voiced.

For the next two hours I talked to them about what it meant to be gay, the social and church pressures Tim had grown up under, the homosexual lifestyle—everything except the hurt and anger I felt. That was carefully concealed under the caring behavior I'd been taught to show, no matter what.

"We're going to help him move and get set up in his new life," I told them. "We've got to make him comfortable."

Caring deeply for Tim's parents, I offered to help him tell them. Since he'd had a year of sobriety, none of them would understand our divorce unless he told them the truth. Reluctantly he agreed.

I called his mother to say we'd be coming down on Saturday. Halfway through dinner, Tim told them we were divorcing. In total shock, everyone let loose a barrage of questions. "Didn't you do this? Didn't you do that?"

Finally, Tim's mother turned to me and asked, "Didn't you love Timothy when you married him?"

"Yes, I did."

Then she turned to Tim, asking, "And you loved Moira?"

"No."

Time stopped. My face turned scarlet. My stomach twisted. Never had I sat through such humiliation. "I wish I hadn't come!" beat like a drum in my head.

Over the next tormented weeks, Tim told me how he'd fooled around before we married, and how the first year we were married, he'd started looking for gay men and going to gay baths, theatres and bookstores. He was so fearful somebody would find out he was gay that he wouldn't hug our male friends. He had sex with me just enough to legitimize the marriage, "and," I thought, "to have three kids."

Seeing my dismay, he said, "I really want to help you, Moira. You've got to remember when we married, the Catholic Church, family, schools, everybody, said you weren't supposed to be gay. It was evil, vicious, dirty. So you had to try to be something you weren't—straight and married."

"Oh, I see," I thought. "You want to help me understand you. I've got news for you. I want to understand *me*."

The next night, I met Tim at the door, crying and screaming,

"You didn't love me! You married me just to look straight. You brainwashed me!"

"I refuse to deal with you, Moira," he called over his shoulder as he went to the kitchen, "since you can't act like an adult. When you decide to grow up and talk like an adult, we can discuss it." With that, he left for the evening.

A few weeks later we talked. "Consciously or unconsciously," he acknowledged, "I tried to make you kick me out of the marriage."

"And when I tried to kick you out, you threatened to throw me out! You had me either way, didn't you? If I had pushed you out or I'd left, you'd never have had to admit the truth to anybody. You'd have been the victim." My rage was mounting.

During this time Tim still went out cruising and had the support of gay organizations, activities and psychiatrists, while I stayed home with nothing to do and no one to talk to. Tim didn't want me to tell anyone.

"I'm dying," I thought, "and nobody knows why."

Then he moved out with our help. Once he was gone I never missed him. My crying came out of grief for the twenty years I had put into the marriage, not over the man who left. The fact that I no longer cared for the man I'd been married to for so long made me sadder.

One night shortly after he left, Tim gave me the book, *I'm O.K.—You're O.K.*. Inside it he'd written, "You really are O.K."

He meant it nicely but I laughed to myself, thinking, "Now that I know you're gay, nothing's wrong with me. You jerk, now that you've gone, you think that you can eradicate all the pain you caused and get on with your life?"

Then I paused, appalled at what his legacy to me was. "How can I ever undo all the brainwashing that made me believe everything was my fault?" I asked myself. "You're not O.K., Tim, and I'm not either." Outraged, I closed the book, never to open it again.

Tim's brainwashing left me scared to get out on my own full time. Believing I was stupid, I went to see a counselor, someone to take care of me. "I don't know who I am," I began. "I kept changing myself to be so many things for Tim. It's what kept me in the marriage."

For five sessions I talked about the damage done to me and our marriage by Tim's behavior as a gay and an alcoholic. "I'm afraid of sex and question the motives of any man who wants to get close," I explained. "I don't believe in love or marriage. That makes me sad because I was raised to be married and have kids." Then feeling wistful, I added, "It would be great to get married again. But marriage has no value now."

With each outburst over what Tim had done to me, I said, "He did it because he was an alcoholic...because he was gay."

The sixth session the counselor asked, "Why can't you simply say, 'Tim did this to me.' Why do you have to excuse him because he's gay or alcoholic?"

"Because if I say, 'Tim did this to me and that to me,' without explaining his behavior, that makes him the most calculating and cruel human being I've ever known."

"So?"

That was the breakthrough. It finally dawned on me how terribly used I'd been. Tim needed the marriage and the kids for his respectability and then set out to make me divorce him. He'd used me the entire marriage—half of my life, my adult youth! My anger came pouring out.

"He didn't think twice about using me, a woman—the very type he didn't want around—as a shield," I screamed. "He has no right to take a woman as a wife and mother for his children just so he can look straight!"

My deep rage persists to this day, five years later. Anger is my only connection to Tim's gayness, though he's never felt it directly. He knows it's there when it comes out over concerns for the kids. Some day if the occasion arises, he'll receive my wrath. When he does, the issue won't be the Catholic Church's homophobia, which made him do what he did. The issue will be what he did to me—not asking me, not telling me before we married, not giving me a choice.

Because I'm a Man
Dan

We came from traditional backgrounds. We had a traditional marriage. We looked the traditional couple—I, tall, dark and fairly handsome, and Sally, just a little shorter and blonde. While I worked she took care of the house. Bringing in the money, I had the power. Sally felt powerless but learned how to get power by dispensing or withholding sex, almost like prostitution. If she wanted something we'd have sex. When she wanted to punish me we couldn't. Too naive to catch on, I thought we had a good sex life.

After we married in the early seventies, my salary as a pilot for a commercial airline put Sally through college. In the first ten years my job took us to three different cities. During our years in New York and St. Louis, Sally was always the first to try new things, always ahead of me, looking over her shoulder and saying, "Come on, Dan." Setting up activities, she brought me into them—natural childbirth, home delivery, breast feeding, child care. We delivered our two daughters, Ginnie and Sue, at home. Sally got involved in La Leche League and took parent effectiveness courses. She also hired as many women tradespeople as possible. Our gardener, our painter and even the car mechanic were women.

Our circle of friends was made up of her friends. Dear to her, they were her emotional support. That worked out well since I didn't have the skills then to express my feelings openly. When she lost those friendships each time we moved, depression set in. She became so close to one woman in St. Louis that when we left after two years to go to Boston, she was immobile for a long time. "I love her so," she told me, "but not in a sexual way," she added quickly.

Once we settled in Boston I became the one who tried new things while Sally stayed stuck in her depression. Through work I started some personal growth classes that were very helpful. Feeling I'd discovered a path of awareness, I kept telling Sally, "Hey! Here's a new way to think, to live."

The second year there I joined a men's support group, an off-shoot from one of my classes. Walking into my first meeting and seeing the nine men sitting there, I thought to myself, "Oh boy, a bunch of queers," just because it was a group of men. Like all the men I knew, my feeling was, "You don't touch men. You don't talk to men about anything but sports or finances." I soon found out that the other males in the group came from all walks of life and only one was gay. Gradually they became my emotional support.

About this time I took a weekend workshop on extrasensory perception. In one of the first ESP activities, a good-looking woman stood up to introduce herself to the group. "My name is Nanette," she began. "I'm bisexual. I've been bisexual for seventeen years."

Her words caught my attention. I was amazed that she had the courage to stand up before a room full of people and come right out about her sexuality. I listened hard to what she had to say.

Nanette had been married for sixteen years and had four kids. Throughout the marriage she'd brought home women to her husband and herself for threesomes—sometimes for a night, other times for months of living together.

The next workshop activity was to pick out the person we were most attracted to and go tell her or him. Right away I went over to Nanette. As we talked, her dynamic power attracted me. But it was a dark charisma.

Sunday night I told Sally all about the workshop and suggested, "Why not come to the next one in the series?" Since she'd finally shaken off her depression, I wanted her to share the high I was feeling from personal growth. Our marriage had never seemed better. We'd never been happier.

"O.K. Sounds interesting," she said and arranged for a sitter to take care of the girls.

When we arrived at the next workshop, there was Nanette. I introduced her to Sally. Immediately the two women connected. For the rest of the workshop, they were the only two people in the class who were in sync all of the time. Everyone expressed amazement at how they seemed to be in tune with each other—classic soul mates.

Ten days afterwards Sally ran off with Nanette.

I was completely floored, though not completely surprised. Sally had told me she was attracted to Nanette the night they met. "I'd like to experiment with someone of the same sex," she'd said.

Thinking "Gee, that's rather cool," I'd encouraged her to do it.

Once Sally announced she was leaving, feelings of guilt began to arise. "Did I subconsciously arrange for this to happen by introducing her to Nanette, figuring she'd be swept off her feet and run away?" The question agonized me for the next two years.

After Sally left, my first move was to try to win her back, to get her to come home and talk, to make love. Within a month I stopped trying. "I can't compete with this woman," I decided. "It's obviously some tricky technique in lovemaking she has that I can't duplicate because I'm a man." Again there was this sense of an evil force.

What a terrible blow to my ego it was! I'd rather Sally had run off with a man than a woman, a hundred times more. I'd have understood that and been able to combat it. "Sally," I would've said, "I can earn more money. I'm stronger. I'm faster." This way I felt I was not an adequate man. It completely destroyed my self-image.

It also destroyed my confidence in Sally as Ginnie and Sue's mother. "Their mother's a lesbian," I thought. "Therefore she's not a good mother so I'll keep the kids."

Sally's leaving came out of the blue to Ginnie and Sue. It wasn't as if it had been a bad marriage and everybody knew there'd be a divorce eventually. Their first reaction was, "Who's going to take care of us?"

The answer wasn't terribly clear for five months. My hurt wiped me out. At first I felt sorry for myself, moaning, "Oh I'll never find another woman to have such good sex with!" Then it was a rapid downhill course that lasted a year. I withdrew into myself, barely able to take care of myself, my children or my house. My neighbor kept sending me notes saying, "Your yard's a mess! Why don't you pull your weeds?" All I could do was eat until I was up over two hundred pounds.

Within weeks of Sally's running off, I had to go to a flight check course. It was bizarre. Every night I was on the phone calling my brothers and sisters to see who could watch my kids. Every day I was taking the course, which was taught by the only woman instructor the airline had. And, by God, it turned out to be the only time in my career that I flunked the final check flight—under the supervision of a woman. It seemed like there was a conspiracy of women against me.

So I operated as a flight engineer for the time being. In that capacity, there was nothing unsafe I could do. Had I been flying the controls, I would have grounded myself. As upset as I was, a crash could have been highly probable.

Soon my condition was so bad I arranged my flying schedule to have Wednesday nights free to meet with the men's support group. I needed people to tell my woes to. I didn't know how to unload to my male friends. Family counseling helped too. Each week Sally and I and the girls went alternately to a counseling center and to Family Services.

Ginnie and Sue, aged nine and five, didn't know what was going on. They had their mother coming in and out of the house to watch them while I flew, and me coming in and out of the house to and from flights. At other times they were farmed out to different aunts and uncles. Soon it was clear that a nanny was needed to watch them when I was flying.

A few months after the nanny came, I realized that a stranger watching them couldn't do as good a job as their mother. "Wait a minute!" I told myself. "There's no connection between Sally's sex life and whether she's a good mother." It had taken me a year to figure that out.

By then divorce proceedings had begun. Nanette filed for divorce too and left her husband, whereupon Sally and she moved into our house with two of her kids. Little Sue, by then six, immediately hooked onto Nanette and thought she was wonderful. I too still found her a special woman—a dark force, but special.

A month after Nanette and Sally moved in, our family counselor said in a session with just Sally and me, "The children want to know why their mother's in the bedroom all the time with Nanette. I suggest you tell them or they're going to hear it on the street corner from other kids."

Sally did the telling that night. "I'm lesbian," she said. "I'm in love with Nanette and we spend lots of time together doing lots of things."

The girls showed no negative reactions then, but it added to Sue's emotional upheaval from the divorce. She was so upset that one night she ran down the hall, through the dining room and out the window.

Five months later Sally and Nanette and all the kids moved into a house they rented together. When both divorces were final a few months after that, they each received enough money between them without having to work. So there were the two women and four kids in what was quite a nice household.

To come up with the money needed for alimony and child support, I rented out the girls' bedrooms. The first renter was a woman who told me she'd been a lesbian. The following week, there was trouble with the car. When I brought it to our woman car mechanic, I discovered that she was an active lesbian. "God!" I thought, "it seems like the world is filled with lesbians!"

After many months of feeling lonely, I wanted to date. "But it's been years since I've pursued women," I realized with surprise.

My men's support group seemed like an obvious source of help. At the end of our next session, I announced looking around the circle, "I'd like to go out on a blind date. Could any of you give me a phone number?"

"No!" Eight guys faced me saying, "No, Dan, we won't give you any phone numbers. You're pathetic-acting and pathetic-looking."

I went out to my car and cried. The next day I joined the local gym and began exercising. It was the start of an uphill climb still in progress six years later.

The men were right. I was a pathetic jerk responsible for Sally's leaving. The next few days were spent mulling over the question, "Why else would a woman leave me other than that I was short-changing her?" That weekend I sat down and, with my logical mind, listed the areas where I fell short as far as women were concerned—touching, feelings, sensuality, sexuality, giving and receiving. "Building these up may not make your life work, Dan," I told myself, "but it's the way to satisfy a woman."

One by one I tackled those areas. I took workshops on massage and bought my own table. I took a course on sensuality and then began classes on human sexuality. Sexuality was a big issue for me because of Sally's rejection of me as a man on top of all the guilt about sex I'd grown up with.

Slowly healing began. In the process I was able to expand beyond the focus on my inner growth. I pulled out all the weeds in the garden and bought house plants which I tended with a real green thumb.

Four years after Sally left me, Nanette left her. Sue saw it as a second divorce. For weeks she wouldn't go to school, not wanting Sally out of her sight. Gradually, an hour at a time, she went back until she was there full time.

Soon my circle encompassed Sue and Ginnie. No longer heating up TV dinners, I began cooking for them. This spread to cooking classes and teaching them to cook. They got massaged on my table; we went together into our hot tub, naked, as a family and ran around without clothes on, as a matter of course.

One day the family counselor told me, "You've got to cut down on the girls' sexual exposure, Dan. They're too agitated right now and too young to have an outlet. It's too much on top of Sally's lifestyle."

"That's a shame," I said. "It's important that my children see me nude. It's positive and healthy. I saw my parents nude."

About this time I took a course on "Surviving Divorce." In the third session the women and men separated to list characteristics of "the perfect person" of the opposite sex. When we compared our lists they were the same. "I didn't know we want the same thing," I said to the instructor, thinking, "Gosh! Many women enjoy sex!"

Inspired, I placed an ad in the local paper that weekend.

Forty-two-year-old male working on touching, feelings, sensuality, sexuality, giving and receiving. Looking for a woman to help me grow in these areas.

To my surprise six nice women answered the ad. One became a permanent friend. My dating had begun. Not wanting to be in another unequal relationship, I chose only working women.

That autumn a flyer for an Outward Bound program caught my eye—three weeks of winter mountaineering, the toughest of their challenges. "Aha!" I told myself, "this will be my test." I'd never hiked in winter. I'd never done ice climbing. I'd never been through any survival experiences but I needed to prove I was manly.

In January fifteen men—the other fourteen all twenty years younger than I—were ice climbing, making igloos in blizzards and sleeping in the snow on pads with little canvas covers in twenty-below-zero weather. For three weeks I held my own.

Success made me feel proud. But the feeling of being okay didn't last. I needed to prove myself over and over. Getting strokes from others was great but my own were needed. Before long, I started training for triathalons and completed the "Iron Man" race in Hawaii—a two-and-a-half mile swim, 112-mile bike ride, and 26.6-mile marathon—making me very proud of myself.

From then on triathalon training was my primary hobby. Every day, I swam, bicycled and ran. It became a way to maintain my weight, my self-esteem and my emotions. Over the next two years I did three more "Iron Man" courses.

Now six years after Sally ran away, my health and life are all together. I'm a much better person than I ever was and feel better about myself. If we were still married I'd probably be soft, fat and out of shape and never would have done any of these things.

My work towards personal growth was triggered by pain I wouldn't wish on anyone. Sally's running away was the most painful thing that ever happened to me. It was rejection of me as a person and as a man, the failure of our marriage and consequent divorce. Sally's being lesbian was only a minor part of it.

Sometimes I wonder whether, if I'd had strong self-esteem at the time, I could have said, "Well, it's her loss. She's giving up a good marriage." Then I laugh. "It is her loss. I am a special person."

Proof of Womanhood *
Jane

This is the first time I've ever told my story publicly and I am afraid. I feel shaky and vulnerable and alone. Just as you felt alone and vulnerable and afraid when you found out your husband, wife, son or daughter was gay; or when you first risked telling someone you were gay and a look of horror flickered in his or her eyes; or when you first spoke publicly for gay rights. In facing the fear to speak openly, I experience a deep strength and power, a great sense of freedom out of doing and being what I must.

I met John in Taipei, Taiwan, in the early sixties. I was teaching and John was in the military. We were both twenty-three and we fell quickly and passionately in love. When our tours were up we returned to this country and decided to marry and settle in the San Francisco Bay Area where my family lived. Both families were thrilled. John's parents from Indiana called me the "pretty little wife from California." We had a family wedding, bought a Victorian house to renovate and pursued our careers. Our marriage was good. We loved each other and felt secure. We did the things our parents

---

*Adapted from a speech, first convention of Parents and Friends of Lesbians and Gays, Denver, May 5, 1982.

approved of and what we had grown up expecting to do. We were productive and we saved money. We had friends and had fun. Our sexual relationship was mutually satisfying. It was a safe, comfortable and well-programmed marriage. Life was the way it was supposed to be, just the way we'd always dreamed.

And then it changed.

Seven years after we married, Martin entered our lives. John met him through business and started spending a lot of time with him. He found Martin fascinating, a man with a wealth of experiences. As the weeks went by and the friendship grew, Martin told John he was gay.

John shared that information with me within two weeks, crying many tears about Martin's difficult life. "He's felt such prejudice! He had so much pain growing up gay," he told me. "He was alienated from his parents."

Five nights later John came home crying again, this time for himself. "I've fallen in love with Martin and I don't know what to do." Then he cried for us.

At that moment our lives turned upside down. The unimaginable had happened. Thirty years of dearly held assumptions blew apart. It was like trying to stand on water. Everything was in waves. There was no solid ground anywhere. "If this is real and all the former rules are untrue," I thought, "then everything might be false and then again, anything might be true."

It was terrifying and exhilarating! There was a sense of breathing free, of shattering old patterns, of opening up to limitless possibilities with no more boundaries to our lives.

Once John brought Martin home to meet me, the three of us began spending time together, trying to figure out what was happening. Martin didn't know what to do any more than John or I. John was the first straight man he'd fallen in love with and he didn't want to break up a marriage. So we spent hours and days and weeks talking and talking, discussing possibilities, exploring options.

I loved that period! New things were happening. A zest and liveliness entered our lives. John and I grew closer; Martin and I grew to love each other. Wonder surrounded us. I felt that on some very deep level nothing really had changed, that John and I were still a couple and we'd just opened up our marriage a little bit to include another person.

Then Martin left and I realized nothing would ever be the same. John began to face his own questions and his agony. "Was this just Martin or is it me? Am I really gay or not? What will this mean to our marriage? Who am I anyway?" As John went in search of his own identity, his exploration excluded me. I was left to face my own fears, my own pain and my own questions of identity.

The most painful part of this period was our isolation. We told no one about what was happening or the turmoil we felt. We had nowhere to go, no information, no support. Pulling away from our friends and families, we isolated ourselves in our questions and hurt.

My pain, isolation and confusion about my own worth led me to decide that all of our trouble must be my fault. I decided that I had caused John's homosexuality, that none of this would have happened if I'd somehow done something differently or been a better person. "Why wasn't I enough of a woman?" I wondered, and began to view myself as incomplete, worthless, bad, wrong.

After years of not smoking, I began smoking. I started drinking too much. Sometimes I'd leave the house, get halfway through San Francisco, panic, and have to go home. I was beginning to shatter and didn't know how to stop myself.

Then I discovered I was pregnant, making me sink deeper and deeper into despair. For several months questions hounded me. "Should I have this baby? Could I bring a baby into this marriage? Am I capable of facing an abortion?"

I decided to seek therapy. My first choice was a group in which the participants already knew each other. When I arrived, they asked, "What's your issue?"

"I've just found out my husband is gay and I'm pregnant. I don't know what to do. I guess I need support."

The leader then turned to me and said, "I think you'll have to examine your part in creating this situation."

Then a woman in the group said, "Well, that's not much of a problem. I've got this problem and that problem...."

I felt attacked, invisible, unheard. I never went back.

Next I tried my family doctor who had told me I was pregnant.

When he heard the whole story, he wasn't unkind, but had no idea what to do other than recommend a therapist.

Happily the therapist was a woman but she was a Freudian analyst. I was in crisis and she wanted me to come three times a week to free associate. I was trying to make decisions about the life of my baby and she wanted me to talk about my relationship with my father! Six months pregnant, I slid further and further into despair.

The next month the baby was lost in natural miscarriage. While there was a great sense of relief on one level, on another the loss was the final blow. I was losing my husband, yet that baby was going to show me and everyone else in the world that I was a woman. Now I had lost the proof of my womanhood. Little of the following months remains in my memory. I was functioning but in deep, deep depression.

That spring I visited my gynecologist for a checkup after the miscarriage. Though I didn't know him well, I hysterically poured out my fears that I wasn't a complete woman, that I couldn't carry a baby, that there was something fundamentally wrong with me.

He sat listening until I stopped. Then looking directly at me, he said very slowly and clearly, "Jane, there is nothing wrong with you."

His words penetrated my darkness.

He repeated, "There is nothing wrong with you." Then he added, "Your head made the wrong decision to have this baby and your body made the right one. There's nothing wrong with you."

His words were my first glimmer of hope. Someone from the outside world heard me. Someone was validating me.

The next week, I wrote my sister about everything that had happened. Since we weren't close, telling her was a big risk. "I'm desperate," I concluded, "and have nowhere else to turn."

She wrote back immediately with love and support, telling me she'd get Mother to talk with me somehow. After years of closeness, my mother and I were now barely speaking. She had noticed my despair and withdrawal. Yet because of the need for secrecy I'd pushed away her questions, her concern, her love. Both of us felt sad and angry and guilty about it.

My sister put Mother on a plane to visit her in Denver. "I can't tell you everything that's going on," she told Mother when she arrived, "but it's Jane's issue and her life. There's nothing you can do but wait. No one's to blame."

When Mother came back to San Francisco, she called me right away. The tension between us eased.

Within weeks I called the office of my analyst. "Please inform Dr. Blum I'm not coming back." Five minutes later Dr. Blum called. "Don't you think you ought to come in and talk about it?"

"No," I told her, "I'm never stepping foot in your office again." What an incredible feeling of power and freedom! I was taking charge of my life for the first time in months.

Then I found myself a lover. This wonderful man let me know in no uncertain terms that I was a woman. Through his love and caring and passion, my shattered identity began to heal. I was going to live after all.

John and I stabilized emotionally at that point, although we didn't know what to do next. Knowing the old marriage was gone and our sexual relationship was over, we looked for a new direction. We'd gone through so much together we didn't want to part.

Our decision was to invite lovers to live with us communally. So he had his lovers in the house and I had mine. We had large family meals together. People drifted in and out.

John still hadn't come out to anyone else but me. Our family and friends didn't know what was happening or what we were doing. We avoided the issue when we couldn't avoid friends and lied outright when necessary. The secrecy became extremely distressing the summer we visited John's folks in Indiana.

On our return I said, "We've got to stop pretending everything's fine. We've got to begin telling people the truth."

But we didn't.

That fall, a year after Martin entered our lives, I realized I wanted a divorce. I told John one noon while we were eating in a restaurant in the city during his lunch hour.

Pain covered his face. Then he looked at me and said, "I'm afraid you're going to mess up your life if you leave."

That was the last response I expected, but his words released my rage and removed any doubts about my decision. "My God!" I shouted. "What do you think my life is now?"

Once the decision was made I wanted to move quickly. Knowing nothing about divorce, I called my sister. Her husband, a lawyer, gave me the information and advice I needed. Together they let me know that I had their love and support. "My family is beside me," kept going through my head. "I don't have to face this alone."

When divorce proceedings began, we had to tell people why. I told my mother first—the whole story. She was less concerned about John's homosexuality than about my "promiscuous behavior." Though upset, she was relieved that she and I were talking after a year of silent hostility.

John told his parents about the divorce but not that he was gay. Deciding that the failure of the marriage was my fault, they wanted nothing more to do with me and asked me to give back the family ring. The wrench of that final exchange has not gone away.

On January first we started living separate lives financially, but I couldn't separate emotionally. John didn't want me to go. Many friends wanted me to stay. The temptation was strong. The gay world seemed wonderfully nurturing. There was a place for me there. But John and I knew that for the sake of both of us I needed to leave.

Once I felt some hope of finding life outside my secure but hurtful path with John, I moved to Big Sur, a mountain retreat along the California coast. All summer I lived there by myself, camping, hiking, wandering the beaches, sleeping—very much alone. By fall I had decided to remain in that healing place. There was much to put to rest and to put together. I felt like a fawn—newly born, dependent, insecure, trembling—yet filled with the potential of growth.

That first autumn I enrolled in a women's workshop, "Liberation from Within." Remembering my negative experiences with therapy, I went to the first meeting with all my defenses up. Though I acted carefree and self-assured, I was trembling inside. The group was small, seven or eight women, with two leaders who were kind, gentle and intelligent. As they made me feel safe, I relaxed my guard.

One of our first exercises was, "Who Are You?" Separated into pairs, we were to ask our partner gently, over and over, "Who are you?" The idea was to uncover the richness and diversity of our identity. My partner began. "Who are you?"

"Jane."

"Who are you?" she asked again.

I had no answer.

"Who are you?" she prodded gently.

"I don't know," I whispered and began to cry.

This experience and the following workshop activities helped me understand it was all right not to know who I was, that when we let go of pretending to know who we are, true self-knowledge can begin. Saying honestly, "I don't know who I am," had begun the exciting journey of self-discovery which I have continued—with rests, backslides, and detours—ever since.

For the next three years I lived in Big Sur. John and I stayed in contact, dealing with our anger, guilt and grief individually and together. Sometimes months passed with no communication and then we'd come together to talk and cry, yell and laugh. As we shared times of need and joy, we each grew stronger. Gradually our friendship deepened, based on our independence, individuality and honesty.

While we lied to others, we never lied to each other. John's courage the night he told me he loved Martin was the single most important factor in my discovery of what truth is. His courage to speak his truth was his greatest gift to me.

Eighteen years earlier we had vowed to love each other until death do us part. Although the marriage is dissolved, we continue to hold the vows sacred.

ভ   ভ   ভ   ভ   ভ

Seven years later, Jane is an ordained minister, counseling and teaching in Denver. She has remarried and become a mother to two stepchildren. John and she remain friends.

Healing Sexual Damage

Possibly the most devastating issue confronting a straight spouse is how their partner's newly revealed sexual orientation has affected marital sex and the spouse's own sexuality.

In the confusion of the coming out, straight spouses typically wonder, "What am I up against? What does homosexuality or bisexuality mean for me?" Whether their partners are bisexual or homosexual, the fact that there is any degree of same-sex orientation or behavior at all results in the spouses feeling rejected as sex partners. They must then contend with the ensuing pain and sexual difficulties.

Healing sexual damage entails five major steps:

- Identifying how the same-sex orientation affected marital sex
- Recognizing the damage to sexual identity
- Expressing pain from sexual damage
- Understanding homosexuality and bisexuality
- Restoring a healthy sexuality.

Identifying How the Same-Sex Orientation Affected Marital Sex

Determining how the partner's same-sex attraction has affected the couple's sex life is the first step toward healing sexual damage. It depends on how long the partner actually knew he or she had homosexual feelings and concealed the information from the spouse.

Many of the couples studied for this book enjoyed satisfactory and for some passionate sex during the first years of marriage. Others always felt something was missing. Still others, as time went on, were falsely accused of being undersexed, frigid or oversexed. "Some gay husbands are terrified by their wives' sexual desire and interest in sexual exploration," says Jane Vennard, founder of the National Task Force on Spouses of Gays and Lesbians. "That's why they criticize the women's sexuality, making them feel 'wrong' to want sex."[1]

In many cases lovemaking decreases as the partner's criticism increases. Many straight wives, assuming that men have the greater sex drive, believe the criticism. The wives' false self-images are reinforced every time they desire sex with and then fail to seduce their husbands. Seeing themselves as sexually inadequate, they then repress sexual desire. Moira epitomizes women who, viewing themselves as sexless, give up wanting or trying to make love.

Straight men married to lesbians often develop a similar pattern, as their wives accuse them of not understanding women's needs and of not knowing how to give them sexual pleasure. One husband in New Orleans, for instance, blamed himself when his wife said she could reach orgasm only by herself. From such rebuffs, many straight husbands believe they lack the sexual prowess men are assumed to have and feel incompetent.

After the partner comes out, most spouses begin to realize that the partner's sexual orientation, not their own sexual deficiencies, is the real reason that sexual tension was missing or limited in lovemaking. Looking back, many begin to see how the sexual mismatch plagued the relationship from the start. Full sexual intimacy may never have been achieved. Without intimacy and sexual desire, all the emotional, physiological and spiritual responses that comprise human sexuality couldn't be fully experienced in the marriage.

While many partners who are aware of their different sexual orientations find others to satisfy their sexual needs, their spouses generally do not. In retrospect, many spouses see their incomplete sexual experiences as a violation of their right to sexual pleasure. As one angry wife said, "I was just a way for my husband to masturbate!"

Outsiders often raise questions about the sexuality of people who marry homosexuals in the first place. Yet there don't appear to be any traits they share that distinguish them from their peers who marry heterosexuals.[2] Though a number of spouses of gays are sexually inexperienced, ignorant or insecure, so too are many spouses in heterosexual marriages.

The fundamental problem is that straight spouses are the wrong sex for their gay partners. Though learning better communication skills or sexual techniques may help, they can never totally bridge the gap. Without knowledge of the actual sexual incompatibility, straight spouses' efforts to attract their partners are futile and their images of themselves as sexually incompetent are constantly reinforced.

Recognizing the Damage to Sexual Identity

The discovery of the partner's same-sex orientation often seems to spouses like a confirmation of their own sexual inadequacy. More troubling, the coming out causes many spouses to doubt their manhood or womanhood. Such a devaluation of sexuality and sexual role deals a double blow to sexual identity. Unraveling the twofold damage, primarily the concern of spouses of homosexuals, is the second step of sexual recovery.

Rejection of spouses' core identities by the persons they are intimately involved with is one of the most painful aspects of the coming out. Since self-image is closely linked with sexual role, the rejected spouse may feel like less of a woman or man. This reasoning explains why Jane rejoiced after she got pregnant. Now she had proof of womanhood. And why Dan fretted that he was not enough of a man to win Sally back from her lover.

Some spouses begin to doubt their own orientation. According to sex therapist Sharon Nathan, Ph.D., wives who seek sex therapy often ask, "What does it say about me that I married a gay male? Am I *really* interested in sex (with men)? What was I getting out of it?"[3] One man wondered why he was attracted to his wife's female lover before she was and why he was drawn to two lesbians.

Similarly, Martha, a thirty-five-year-old actress who had always sensed something was missing from her marriage felt attracted to a woman artist who came on to her. Martha's husband's subsequent coming out increased her suspicion that she, too, must be homosexual until she took a Sexual Attitude Restructuring (S.A.R.) workshop to settle the issue. She found that she was not lesbian, simply attracted to the woman's body because of her sensual artistic nature at a period when she was starved for physical intimacy.

It would seem that the discovering of the hidden reason for sexual problems in the marriage would erase the spouse's doubts of sexual inadequacy. It doesn't. Guilt and self-doubt automatically resurface for many spouses. They typically wonder, "What did I do to cause the problem?" A more constructive response would be something like, "His (or her) homosexuality helps to explain our difficulties. Where do we go from here?"

The habit of self-blame is hard to break. Many wives relive every day of the marriage trying to see how they might have caused their husband's lack of response. By making themselves the culprit, they don't have to blame their husbands, an acknowledgement too painful for many at first. Supporting their husbands is top priority, even if it compromises the wife's sexuality.

Many gay husbands contribute to their wives' low self-esteem by blaming the wives' sexual inadequacies for driving them to men. Family and friends, too, sometimes compound the situation through uninformed accusations or denials of the partner's homosexuality.

As spouses gradually understand how the sexual incompatibility affected marital sex, they usually stop blaming themselves. Instead most begin to feel that their sexuality has been damaged as a result of the sexual mismatch itself and, in some cases, their partner's unjustified criticism. Many feel that these factors prevented full exercise of their sexuality. They fear, because of years of limited sexual activity, that they may no longer be able to function sexually.

The longer the sexual disparity has operated undetected in the marriage, the greater the damage to spouses and the greater their anger. This is more an issue for wives of gay and bisexual men than for husbands of lesbians, since lesbians tend not to conceal their orientation once discovered. Many straight wives feel cheated and robbed of their birthright. Those married for more than a few years often believe that their injured sexuality is as irreversible as their husband's gayness. They fear that the damage can't be repaired any faster than it took to be inflicted and never completely.

Wives whose husbands have hidden their active gay life for several years often come to believe that their sexuality was sacrificed for their husband's need for protective cover. Some feel exploited, used as a sex machine for childbearing until it no longer served that purpose. Moira called it being Tim's "shield" from society.

Even the most sympathetic wife may erupt in anger at being used as her husband's protection from social discrimination. As unintentional as his behavior may have been, the sexual harm she experienced seems unforgivable. Outrage may begin to outweigh compassion felt for his plight in an anti-gay society. Many then feel an urge to fight back. This is a natural reaction and a positive step towards recovery.

Expressing Pain from Sexual Damage

Anger and pain from damaged sexuality need to be released before such feelings grow out of proportion and provoke self-destructive or counterproductive actions. Sharing feelings is the third strategy for healing damaged sexuality and one that is crucial in every stage of recovery until the coming-out trauma has been resolved.

It is critical to find a friend or family member with whom to share emotions. The spouse needs to hear, "It's okay!" from people who care. A man, no less than a woman, needs a shoulder on which to cry without shame.

Yet many spouses don't tell anyone what is now "our secret" out of loyalty or embarrassment. Some are asked by their partners not to tell because of fear of anti-gay reactions in the community or loss of job. Others feel uneasy about broaching the sensitive subject, fearing "rejection, disapproval or ostracism, because of the stigma attached to homosexuality," report Dorothea Hays and Aurele Samuels in their 1986 study of twenty-one straight wives.[4] Locked into the husband's closet by the secret, wives feel the impact of homophobia without having an escape valve. This isolation increases their distress.

Friends or family sometimes suspect what's happened from their own observation, like Moira's friend who saw Tim at a gay bar. Or they guess there is some kind of a problem from the spouse's haggard appearance, weight change or hypersensitivity, or in a couple's constant bickering. While friends tend to keep quiet out of respect, denial or avoidance of the problem, their expression of concern can be a great relief to the spouse. By gently asking, "Is there something wrong that you'd like to talk about?" or "Do you think he's gay or might be leaning that way?" friends can let the spouse know that they are willing to listen and aren't repelled by gayness.

When the spouse finally shares the secret, it should be with someone who is a supportive listener. Friends often try to calm or discourage the spouse's anguish and anger. But what the spouse needs is someone to listen with empathy and respect for his or her feelings.

In many cases, spouses receive uninformed, stereotypical or moral judgments when sharing the secret. Many of the women in Hays and Samuels' study met disbelief or ignorance.[5] Some friends, feeling uncomfortable with the situation, may drop away. Anticipating such reactions, spouses need to choose carefully who they confide in and be ready to correct misinformation.

The most helpful support usually comes from those in the same situation—individuals or support groups. Other spouses understand the anger resulting from sexual rejection. They can suggest from their own experience effective ways of coping. A support group, run by a counselor or straight spouse, provides a common perspective by which spouses can handle trauma more realistically.

Other straight spouses can be found through the partner's contacts, counselors, churches, public health agencies, personal ads in the newspaper, gay and lesbian organizations and resources for spouses listed in Appendix B.

Anger and the feeling of being victimized may last for months until spouses understand more about homosexuality, the pain of hiding it and ways of tapping into their own resources to overcome the damage.

Understanding Homosexuality and Bisexuality

As spouses try to sort out angry, hurt and confused feelings, it becomes critical to find out what homosexuality really means on a practical level to them as straight spouses. Many wonder if the partner is lost forever or if their own sexuality is permanently damaged.

A factual understanding of bisexuality and homosexuality, the fourth task of restoring sexuality, helps spouses relieve anxiety and gain a more accurate perspective of their own sexuality. It is also necessary in accurately assessing the likelihood of continuing or reviving marital sex.

The partners of the spouses are a primary source of information about same-sex attraction and behavior. Ideally they can provide firsthand experience as well as intimate support that their spouses need during this difficult stage. In turn, the spouses' interest may help ease the partners' feelings of guilt and defensiveness, making the sharing of information easier.

Often support form the partner is not forthcoming. Preoccupied with their own problems, many partners don't understand the pain and confusion on the other side of the closet, which, in many ways, is similar to the agony they have experienced. Responding to their concerns would be tantamount to admitting that they have hurt their spouses. Yet this lack of support only increases the stress.

If the partner is not supportive, it may help to point out, "Look, I'm going through what you did before you could accept your gayness and come out. I need the same kind of support and information for my coming out as you needed then." Although being assertive is hard during a period of devastation, the urgency of the need for help may require it.

Ways for couples to bridge the gap of understanding are discussed in *When Husbands Come Out of the Closet*, by therapist Jean Schaar Gochros, Ph.D.[6] What spouses need most from their partners is loving support while they work through the coming out, an approach outlined in *Coming Out: An Act of Love*, by Rob Eichberg, Ph.D., co-founder of Coming Out Day.[7]

Up-to-date factual books on homosexuality and bisexuality are also key resources. Researching the topic is usually a more reliable way of getting information than asking the partner or friends who may be ill-informed or biased. Through reading, spouses can gradually digest the facts and apply them to their individual situations, without the distortion of stereotypical notions about homosexual or mixed-orientation relationships. (See Appendix A.)

It is often embarrassing for many spouses to enter libraries and bookstores on such a quest. They feel stigmatized along with their partners, guilty by association. To deflect possible raised eyebrows, statements like "I'm doing a research paper" are effective.

Since much printed material about homosexual and bisexual orientations is inaccurate, it's advisable to check facts with a credible professional or support organization. Available by phone or letter to provide reliable information and counsel are many organizations devoted to gay, lesbian and bisexual issues such as the Institute for Advanced Study of Human Sexuality in San Francisco, the Bisexual Information and Counseling Services in New York City, the Gay Switchboard in most large cities, and the Parents, Families and Friends of Lesbians and Gays (P–FLAG) listed in Appendix B. Such professional help is crucial for spouses in communities where little about homosexuality is known or accepted.

Getting to know other gay, lesbian or bisexual persons, such as the partner's friends, is another common and effective way to gain an understanding of homosexuality. Face-to-face encounters also help desensitize anti-gay feelings and correct misconceptions. Gay activities and meeting places abound in large cities, such as gay and lesbian bookstores, bars and public events like the Gay Men's Chorus. Though some women enjoy participating in such activities with their husbands, others find it too painful to see physical displays of affection between them and other men.

Through reading and direct experience, the spouse may be surprised by the diversity of homosexual and bisexual behaviors and lifestyles. At the same time, the distinction between the partner's sexual orientation and the spouse's heterosexuality becomes painfully clear. Dan, in looking back, finally recognized lesbian feelings in Sally's extreme devotion to women friends. Although each realization causes more pain, the spouse is one step closer to recovery.

When a spouse accepts that homosexuality and bisexuality gradually develop through the interaction of many factors beginning with conception, hopes of "changing" the partner or restoring the old relationship fade. Now the spouse sees that the partner has little say about his or her same-sex attraction except how to handle it. No magic wand can turn the mate into an exclusively heterosexual person.

The difference between the partner's and spouse's sexual orientations can seem like an uncrossable chasm. During the time it takes to accept the stark reality of this sexual disparity, it helps to remember that many other women and men have weathered its pain.

Restoring a Healthy Sexuality

Because of the emotional upheaval caused by the realization of the sexual mismatch, many months may pass before the spouse can ask, "What can I do about the damage?" Restoring a healthy sexuality, the fifth step of recovery, usually doesn't begin until the second year after the coming out, or when the couple's sexual disparity has been completely accepted. Typically it takes at least another year to achieve sexual confidence and even longer to feel fully restored.

Healing sexual damage can be facilitated through study of human sexuality, therapy and dating. Courage, patience and faith in regenerative powers are indispensable factors in recovery. Spouses who remain with their partners will need their cooperation, too, to restore a healthy sexuality within the marriage, a relationship issue to be discussed in Part Two and most often affecting bi-straight couples.

Since a healthy sexuality hinges on a sense of self-worth, it's critical to address self-esteem issues at this point. Many spouses find counseling, self-help books and introspection helpful in this process. Jane, for example, didn't come to terms with how John's gayness had affected her sexuality until she went to the mountains to sort out the truth about herself.

Once the spouse begins to regain self-esteem, a realistic view of his or her sexuality can be formed. There are many helpful books available on human sexuality, ranging from *Joy of Sex*, edited by Alex Comfort, M.B., Ph.D.,[8] to *Radical Love: An Approach to Sexual Spirituality*, by Dody H. Donnelly, Ph.D., Th.D.[9] Other books recommended by straight spouses are listed in Appendix A.

Many spouses work through their sexual identity crisis with the help of counseling or therapy. Marriage and family counselors, social workers, psychotherapists, sex therapists and doctors can be found through other straight spouses, the yellow pages of the telephone directory, the Department of Human Services and gay, lesbian and bisexual organizations.

Because of the closeted nature of homosexuality, there is a dearth of knowledgeable counselors outside of metropolitan areas. For this reason, spouses should determine, before making an appointment, how much experience the professional has had with straight spouses or mixed-orientation couples and whether he or she addresses the unique sexual concerns of straight spouses in the actual sessions.

Once in counseling, spouses should be wary of advice that emphasizes marital, psychological or moral problems to the exclusion of sexual problems in a mixed-orientation marriage. If the sexuality issue is not addressed, spouses may need to supply factual information clarifying sexual problems that mixed-orientation couples encounter. If that doesn't prompt appropriate guidance, they may consider relying on supportive friends and family until other reputable professional help can be found.

Course work in human sexuality can provide fresh insight to spouses struggling with sexuality issues. Workshops on human sexuality, such as the Sexual Attitude Restructuring course sponsored by the National Sex Forum, are given in many metropolitan areas. More formal courses, like those Dan took to strengthen his understanding of human sexuality, are offered by many colleges, universities or institutes.

Alongside reading, counseling and classes, exploration of ways in which spouses can give themselves sexual pleasure, such as self-caressing, may help to revive moribund sexuality.

As the spouse gradually regains sexual confidence, he or she may feel ready to start dating. It's best not to begin too soon or wait too long. Dan felt so desperate that he asked his men's group for blind dates before he was ready, while many wives over thirty fear there is little time left to regenerate their sex life. Impediments women foresee in finding a lover or remarrying include age, few available single men and their own sexual insecurities. Those with school-age children often believe no one will want to marry a gay man's ex-wife with children. These apparent blocks to meeting eligible mates may seem more forbidding than the reality, as many wives discover once they take the plunge.

Whether dating begins during the marriage or after divorce, straight husbands, compared to straight wives, generally find it easier to meet the opposite sex largely because more unattached women are available.

For some spouses, feelings of sexual inadequacy may persist even after they begin dating. "Why in the world would a man want to love me?" is a common question of former wives, reports a thirty-six-year-old administrative secretary who started a support group for former spouses after her husband of eighteen years came out.

Spouses' marital history may cast a shadow on their dating experiences, too. Many women learn not to mention that their husbands or ex-husbands are gay until dating becomes more serious because dates often jump to one of two conclusions—either "She must have had a problem with sex" or "She's starved for sex." Rejection or pressured sex may result, increasing the women's apprehension and insecurity about dating.

The threat of AIDS also poses a problem. As will be discussed in Part Two, HIV-antibody testing is imperative for everyone, including the spouses' and the partners' lovers, and should be done before engaging in sexual activities. When spouses are on the verge of entering a serious relationship, they have a moral obligation to inform their lovers that their partners or ex-partners are gay. Through the information may make dates pause, most will respect the honesty.

Because of AIDS, it's crucial to go slowly and to find out about a date's sexual background before consummating the relationship, tempting as it seems. Shared laughter and gestures of affection and caring—touching, kissing, hugging, or holding—can be immensely satisfying as a temporary replacement for sexual intercourse and can help the spouse prepare emotionally for the more complex sexual experience. For wives for whom infidelity may be out of the question, sheer affection and caring experiences alone are enormously helpful.

Gradually spouses begin to see themselves as normally functioning sexual beings. In time they may even be able to look back at the sexual mismatch with irony. As an ex-wife in Sacramento said with a half-smile, several years after her husband left her for a gay lover, "I had to seduce him every four months when I couldn't stand it any longer, enough so we had three children in five years."

Martha, the actress described earlier, blossomed with a heterosexual lover. "My sexual awakening at forty-five," she wrote, "was an extraordinary spiritual experience. Incredible beauty was in everything around me, inspired by my renewed sexuality. I felt competent in everything. People saw me as a different person."

Despite seemingly overwhelming obstacles, a number of spouses, old and young, men and women, develop long-term heterosexual relationships including marriage. Six of the thirty straight spouses studied in depth for this book have remarried. While some spouses remarry soon after the coming out, it may be better to wait until all major emotional issues have been resolved and recovery is well under way.

For spouses who choose to stay with their partners, sexual damage may be healed within the marriage through various non-traditional arrangements, therapy and joint commitment to make the sexual relationship mutually satisfying. The stories in Part Two show how three women, along with their husbands, developed alternative ways to satisfy their sexual and other marital needs.

two

TRIAL AND ERROR

CHALLENGE TO TRADITIONAL MARRIAGE STYLES

While some spouses are left by their partners after they come out and other spouses leave because of the sexual incompatibility, infidelity or existing marital problems, many spouses question whether the marriage needs to end just because the partner is gay or bisexual.

Usually it is straight wives, not straight husbands, who pose such a question, since often homosexual and bisexual men wish to stay married. Many gay or bisexual husbands don't want to leave because they still love their wives, give the marriage top priority or want its "cover," and desire continued contact with the children. Most lesbian wives, on the other hand, leave soon after coming out to their husbands, some because of negative views of sex with men as well as a sexual attraction to women or a particular lover. Though less is known about bisexual wives, a number like Nanette in Part One stay married.

Many gay-straight couples have an unusually strong bond of friendship based on shared interests. The coming out threatens that bond as much as the marriage. Wives in such marriages often feel driven to try to preserve the bond and make the marriage work at whatever cost, despite disparate sexual needs. Typically they love their husbands too much to leave or fear the consequences of ending the marriage. Divorce would destroy both the bond and the family unit and, in the case of spouses bound by financial or emotional dependence, severely affect the quality of their lives.

Few models of successful mixed-orientation marriages are available. As couples forge their own paths between the exigencies of their individual situations and conventional mores, the straight spouse generally makes the most adjustments to accommodate the same-sex needs of the partner. Rarely does a gay husband decide not to pursue his gay interests in deference to his wife's needs. Some bi wives and husbands do.

Working out a viable alternative to the conventional marriage is a process of trial and error that takes several years. Along the way, many couples discover that the marriage no longer serves their best interests. Yet working through the relationship crisis often results in a new and lasting bond.

The following stories illustrate alternative marital arrangements and ways of relating developed by three couples after the coming out. The concluding section highlights major problems mixed-orientation couples face and strategies by which many have developed new relationship patterns that have endured whether or not they stayed married.

Personal Stories

Our Own Timetable
Carol

The day of reckoning was July 25, 1986. Dave and I, in our early twenties, had been married three years. Our second daughter, Deidre, had arrived six days before and Mom was visiting to help with two-year-old May. Dave got home late after seeing his therapist, Roger.

"How did it go?" I asked. "Want to talk about it?

"Yes, but later, Carol, in private."

Finally in bed, Deidre asleep in her bassinet beside us, Dave began, as my heart beat faster and my palms became sweaty.

"Well, first, Roger isn't just a therapist. He counsels gay people." Dave paused and then he said, "I'm gay, Carol."

I waited for him to say it was a joke but he didn't. All he said over and over was, "This is the worst day in my life."

I wanted to cry out, "Just what does being gay mean, anyway?" But Mom was there and the girls asleep so my cries were muffled.

When I saw the anguish in Dave's face, being the mothering type that I am, I tried to console him. We tried to console each other.

"I accept your being gay," I finally said, "but does it mean we have to divorce or we can't make love anymore?"

"I don't know," Dave said, "but I think it's best if you and the girls go back to Oregon when your mother goes next week."

All the next day I wondered, "How can I organize a cross-country move with two small children in less than a week?" That night I told him, "I need time for this to sink in before I move anywhere."

From then on I kept track of what happened in my journal as the meaning of Dave's words sunk in.

🍎　　🍎　　🍎　　🍎　　🍎

August 11, 1986. Well, Mother is leaving Baltimore tomorrow and I'm packing a box of our things for her to take, going through all our possessions, trying to decide what to keep and what to toss. I even have to divide up the junk drawer!

I'm going to sell my wedding dress. It's just collecting dust. Besides it doesn't mean what it once did.

I'm resigned to the fact that life will never be the same again. It will be completely different from how I envisioned it, but that's not so terrible. I'm not naive. I'll be a single mother, support or not, and will have to work and put the kids in day care. That makes me sad, but there's no choice. Some people will think my life is forever ruined, but I don't. It's just changing, drastically maybe, but with these changes I'll grow.

August 30. I feel excited about my new relationship with Dave. Many people, especially women, can't believe how understanding and accepting I am of him. That says a lot about how they feel about their husbands! I seem to have a better relationship with my gay husband than they do with their straight husbands.

(Later) Maybe I have it together, but some days I feel as if I'm going to fall apart with sadness. When I move back home to Oregon, I'll be alone and so will Dave. I'll have two children to care for by myself, but he won't have the chance to care for them at all. When I feel sad like this, it shows and makes Dave sad too. Though he tries to console me, it doesn't help.

August 31. Sometimes I feel I'm the only person who has any compassion for Dave and what he's going through. Too many people think, no matter what I tell them, that he's found a new life and is sending me and the kids home so he can live unrestricted. But it's not like that!

His parents should know what a compassionate, thoughtful, generous, loving son they have. Instead they say that he's a "stranger" and, because he's planning to stay in Baltimore, that he's selfish. I know what they're going through, but they shouldn't lay that guilt on him. This is not easy to handle so why can't they think about what their son's going through?

September 5. Joy of joys, I'm not going back to Oregon after all! Dave's been a wreck all week. He finally realized what our splitting up would mean and it hurt too much. There wasn't a good reason to separate. We only thought we had to. We need each other. Who says we have to split up?

I've already sold the crib, so I guess I'll have to buy another.

September 10. Dave and our neighbor Curt went out to gay bars Friday night. Dave said it felt good to finally be a part of the gay life.

Saturday Curt and his wife Pat came over and as usual these days, the subject turned to sex. After a few beers it was obvious that Dave and Curt wanted each other sexually. Pat and I decided that if our husbands are going to sleep with men, it might as well be with people we know and like. So I went to bed alone and Dave went next door with Curt and Pat after I made it clear that I wanted to know if anything happened.

The reasons behind Dave sleeping with a man versus a woman are completely different. My reactions are, too. I cannot, try as I may, compete with another man. I can be gorgeous and intelligent, but if Dave wants a man, nothing I do can change that. I might as well be a frog. It's not easy, but I know he loves me as much as ever and I love him. We *will* be happy.

(Later) Dave did sleep with Curt, but didn't tell me until today, after we talked about the importance of openness and honesty.

September 17. It's so hard for me to face my insecurity. I never realized how emotionally dependent I am on Dave. I was basically insecure when I met him. Then I lost weight, became more confident and assertive. But now? I guess it was false security. Now I have to find real security within me.

September 26. I need to get a night job or something! Dave has this meeting on Tuesdays and that meeting on Thursdays and here I sit, telling myself I'm content.

October 3. Dave is coming out in more ways than one. He's having more aches and pains or actually finally acknowledging them. The real Dave gets headaches after all.

October 10. Well, he's not wearing his wedding band anymore. I guess he thinks that he can't be totally gay if he wears a symbol of heterosexual marriage. But it hurts!

It's ironic how I've been feeling so insecure just when Dave is feeling more secure about himself. For the most part, the changes in my life are good, but why does it have to be so different?

October 11. Dave had his hair cut and, boy, does he look gay! He's going through an adolescence of sorts, "boy crazy" and more than ever caring how he looks. I feel threatened, not as needed. I thought I could always satisfy him in every way, but it's clear that I can't.

October 29. Dave is depressed, mourning the "best little boy in the world" that he used to be. He always assumed that he'd be happy, not sad.

November 11. I resent the fact that if I want our marriage to work, I have to do all the accepting. Can I continue to accept all the changes I never bargained for? Or will I have to leave him—another change? I'm scared.

I don't give a damn if my situation isn't unique. As far as I'm concerned, no one knows how I feel. I'll never have all that I hoped for. Oh, I still hope, but not with the eternal optimism I once had. It's no one's fault, reality just slapped me in the face. Sometimes I want to slap it back. Is this why people become so cynical?

November 16. God, what was I going through on Sunday? It must have been the group therapy I went to Saturday. There are eight women including myself, the youngest. About half are trying to keep their marriages together and half are divorced or separated. I talked about fifteen minutes. Compared to the other women's problems, mine seemed trivial. Yet today I realized that if my problems make me cry and feel depressed, they aren't so trivial.

Sometimes I'm afraid I won't always be a strong person.

November 17. The Sunday paper had an article on gay husbands and a couple of them were on a talk show. They seemed to be doing a fine job of making their relationships work. Finally, role models!

December 12. Well, I just made a major decision on my own! The girls and I are going to move back to Oregon a year from now. Hopefully Dave will want to come with us.

December 15. Although Dave isn't wild about the idea, he said that he'd come with us. But he suggested that we move back sooner—this summer. If he has to leave his favorite city, he doesn't want to prolong the agony. I'm thrilled.

January 6, 1987. Dave now thinks it's inevitable we'll grow apart because we were brought up in totally different worlds. The "proletarian" Dave that he pretended to be isn't really him. It was a rebellion. He's actually more like his parents who are always doing this or that—busy all of the time. He thinks we're dull since we never do anything. He has cabin fever.

We may not be the socialites his parents are, but we're certainly not dull. So he's more frivolous and I'm more practical. Can't we complement each other?

Now I know there's no such thing as "forever." I always thought we were forever. That's why I left college after freshman year to marry Dave while he finished. What a fantasy! I guess no one's certain what their future will be. Nothing's guaranteed. Did I really think that once I got married I'd be immune? The sooner I can accept reality, the sooner I won't hurt so much. If there's any way I can prevent it, I'll never get hurt again.

January 7. We'll be O.K. Dave loves me, likes, appreciates and respects me. We've decided that if we ever show signs of growing apart, we'll do whatever it takes to keep our relationship alive, even if it means living apart.

January 14. I can't believe it's good or right to feel so much pain. After group therapy I came home and Dave did me a "favor" by trying to make me see reality. He said that there's a fine line between optimism and delusion and that I don't see the difference. But my optimism gives me strength. I know that Dave and I might live apart one day but why dwell on it?

January 21. Sometimes I think Dave wishes he had never married me or had kids, although he loves us all very much. Things would have been much less complicated. Sometimes I think it might almost have been easier, but not better, if Dave had died. Then there would be one grieving period, not something new each month.

January 28. For a while whenever Dave and I made love, I thought it was because he couldn't get it elsewhere. After finally talking to him about it, I now know that isn't true. We make love because he wants to and I want to. Meanwhile, when he goes out, he always practices safe sex.

January 29. I quit group therapy. My problems didn't seem bad enough to share and I felt stifled.

I know Dave may fall in love and move out one day. I'm not looking forward to that, but I'm determined not to be standing in the doorway wondering what to do next. I am going to be happy!

April 12. Now Dave is undecided about whether or not to move back to Oregon. Maybe he should stay here, not because I want him to, but because it's something he has to do. On the other hand, I think he should give Portland another chance.

April 16. Well, Dave has decided to stay here with the option to change his mind at any time. I'm relieved because the tension of wondering whether he will or won't go is gone. Now I can get on with the move.

April 22. Once again Dave has changed his mind! He will be coming with us after all! After he made the decision to stay, he never felt good about it. We're leaving at the end of May.

June 22. We're in Portland, renting a big house with a garden from my brother's sister-in-law. Sometimes I wonder if it was the right decision to come back. Would I have if Dave weren't gay? I don't think so.

Strange as it sounds, I'm happy he's gay. I've grown so much and become more open-minded. Our children are likely to be more open-minded also. One very important thing is that other people know I'm not ashamed. Maybe I'll write a book one day!

September 3. What a roller-coaster year it's been! Dave and I are in a sort of limbo as individuals as well as partners. He's trying to balance his gay life with his family life, but the two don't seem to be blending well. I never did think of him as a husband. The term doesn't fit. He's more like a "life partner."

January 24, 1988. I know I can handle Dave having an affair and am entitled to affairs of my own. But what will happen if he falls in love with someone? He assures me that he wouldn't drop me for another. Does that mean sharing him? What will that be like?

I really miss the romance in our life. When I met and fell in love with Dave in high school, I finally understood all the love songs. But now that I know he's gay, those same songs are hard to listen to. It doesn't seem fair. I feel a great loss.

Dave says his feelings for me haven't changed and he still feels romantic. When I feel the least bit romantic, I wonder if I'm a fool for caring and a fool for staying. But how foolish is it to love and care for someone who loves and cares for me? I want to be important to him. Is that so foolish?

January 26. It's been eighteen months and sometimes I feel I haven't gotten too far. Other times I'm amazed. When I reread my journal and realize the emotions that I've grappled with, it's clear that I've grown.

May 26. Despite our obvious contentedness, a lot of people have trouble understanding why I still live with Dave. Some think I should divorce him and move out just because he's gay. They don't think a gay-straight relationship can work. Others don't care to know about our lifestyle as long as we stay married and act like a couple.

Sometimes I wonder why I don't divorce him or at least move out? But we like living together, not to mention the financial benefits. For now this is what works for us. Without guidelines for a situation like ours, we have to create our own timetable.

One definition of marriage is "any close union, i.e., marriage of the minds." Our minds have been "married" for almost five years.

September 22. Dave read my journal today and said that it was too sugarcoated, that I wasn't being totally honest with myself. Maybe he's right. I always refer to his moving out as something that might happen in the future. Because it seems years away, I don't want to think about it until I have to.

But it will happen sooner than I think. We have an eventual plan to move into a flat his parents own in a nice neighborhood with good schools. Then, we'll save money so Dave can move out in a year. My logical side thinks it would be best for us both. My emotional side thinks Dave wants to leave because I stifle him. Maybe we're stifling each other.

It's exciting and scary all at once, but I'm grateful that there's time to truly prepare myself, not that it will be easy.

October 10. Two of our good women friends debated with Dave all afternoon and evening about our relationship. They were on the verge of outrage, telling him he couldn't be in love with me. Seeing him so upset, I reassured him.

January 22, 1989. Our friends were right. Dave can't be in love with me. I know he loves, cares for and respects me, but "in love" means deep devotion, passion and sole attraction, which isn't what he feels for me. And I'm feeling less of that for him. We haven't made love for two months and our kisses aren't much different from how I kiss my brother. Sometimes I hurt as much as I did when he told me two and a half years ago.

February 4. After rereading my last journal entry, I don't feel as bad. Dave and I have talked since then. It's clear that our relationship is still new to us. We're the only couple I know in this situation.

April 6. Having put on ten pounds and finding myself yelling at the children, I finally started seeing a therapist today.

July 2. There's never a perfect time, but now's the time to separate. The resentment between Dave and me has been building. Today in therapy I realized I had to get it over with. Dave's uncle, meanwhile, called us chicken for putting it off. We'll separate after our vacation, before the girls start school, so they won't have too much to cope with all at once.

November 10. It's working out as well as any separation. The vacation eased the hurt a bit. In a way I'm excited to be in total charge of the house and have more time to myself when Dave is with the kids. We have a joint checking account and pool our money. Since we can't afford to get Dave an apartment even with my waitressing, cleaning houses and baby-sitting, he's at his parents' house. Hopefully that will help them accept his being gay.

With the kids' school, my jobs and home projects, I'm very busy. I need to be because the nights are lonely. I'm not ready for a new relationship and now with the risk of AIDS, flings are out of the question. It is so lonely, but not forever. It makes me feel better to remember that I still have my bond with Dave which we vowed was forever.

The Best Solution
Audrey

It was the mid-sixties when a friend wrenched me out of my family home to move in with her and another friend in Los Angeles. "What are you going to do, Audrey?" she teased. "Spend the rest of your life with your mother?"

Mama protested. Not particularly progressive, she frowned upon my leaving home without being married. She was anxious that I wasn't married or dating much at all.

My friends and I were twenty year olds playing at being adults. Soon after I moved in, someone fixed me up with a law student named Scott. When he walked in, attractive and dark-haired, he smiled a beautiful smile. I liked him instantly, the first man I'd felt that way toward. "So friendly and open and sensitive!" I thought, thrilled by how comfortable I felt with him.

I'd always been concerned about my sexuality. From an early age, I'd felt different from other little girls, not knowing how to act with them as they talked about boys and flirted. Although I was fairly attractive with black hair and olive skin, thinking I wasn't like them put a stigma on me.

On my first date with Scott we went to the movies. As he guided me to my seat, his hand felt comfortable, big and warm and dry. That hand meant I'd be taken care of, unprepared as I was to get out into the world on my own. "This is the man I'm going to marry!" I exclaimed silently.

At home that night I thought, "It's perfect. Mama would die to have a Jewish lawyer for a son-in-law." Also some fears were dispelled. "Maybe I *am* okay!"

With Scott away at law school, our relationship was a long distance one. One weekend I went up to be with this prince, feeling insecure about the little sexual experience I'd had. Then when we slept together, everything that could go wrong did. But he continued to write and called me for a date when he returned to town.

"I don't understand," I thought to myself, "but I'll go for it."

We dated on and off for a year, during which time he got a job teaching like all the guys who wanted to beat the Vietnam draft.

He came over often and we began sleeping together each visit. It was much better now and I felt comfortable with sex for the first time.

Soon he was calling every day at noon. His predictability was a little confining, but I got used to it. Since he was a man I could be with, I wanted to safeguard this relationship.

We began to see each other every Saturday night and one evening sitting in my room one of us said, "Why don't we marry?"and we both agreed.

No rockets or fireworks, just the appropriate thing to do.

His family and mine were hoping for it. Both were Jewish, his from the old country and mine protective and conservative.

Since the next day was Mother's Day, we told Mama first before making the engagement official.

We didn't want rings or a big wedding. But Mama, who was dying of cancer, wanted a wedding. She won out. We were married in Palm Springs, California that winter.

We moved to a nice, neat community in Orange County where we set up a little apartment. We did everything expected of young married couples except join in the social activities of the apartment complex. We felt separate from all the other couples we saw going up and down the elevator. They seemed to be making friends with each other. Neither of us knew why we weren't. Though Scott was adaptable, I felt like an outsider, uncomfortable in my body and my identity which didn't seem to fit.

The first two years of our marriage were great. We laughed at the same things and shared lots of interests. We both worked, I at a part-time sales job and Scott as an intern in a law firm. He was wonderful around the house and taught me, who had never even had a fresh vegetable before, about everything. He didn't mind mothering me and we had wonderful times together.

Our sex life was easy. Scott wasn't demanding nor interested in a lot of sex. We made love once a week at the most, which was comfortable for me.

Scott masturbated a lot, but that wasn't a problem for me, having no reference point of how often married men do it. I was pleased he could relieve himself without making a lot of sexual demands on me.

Scott wanted children. Whenever he brought it up, I tried to put it off. Part of me didn't want to commit to children because I wasn't absolutely sure I'd be with this person all that long.

By the second year we'd made friends with two couples outside the complex. Weekends with them and working during the week was our life. Mama had died by then, as well as her expectations of me to be more like other women.

The wives of the couples were friends I'd known before I met Scott. Lil had been at camp with me and Mary was one of her friends.

The first time I'd met Mary was awkward. Lil had warned me that I wouldn't like her. When I picked them up to go for a drive that day, Mary acted strange. Looking at her in the back seat through the rear view mirror, we made eye contact and from that moment on, I felt off kilter. I couldn't handle it.

Mary couldn't either. We picked a fight and stopped speaking. A year or so later, I found out that she and Lil had been lovers. In a panic, I knew that it was absolutely necessary to stay away from them. I certainly didn't want to know a lesbian, much less be one.

Once Scott and I were safely married in our little nest, Mary made contact again. She was dating a lovely fellow named Don that Scott and I both liked. We began doing things with them and we four became close friends. Then they became engaged.

Tuesday before the wedding Mary and I went shopping. When she drove me home, we talked in the car and agreed to continue our conversation the following day at her place. She wanted help in lining her kitchen shelves. I called work to take the day off and told Scott where I'd be.

The next day changed my life totally and radically forever. When I got to Mary's apartment, there was no shelf paper. Instead she propositioned me.

I was scared to death. It wasn't because I was married and this would be cheating. It was, "Oh my God! Here it is. It's going to happen any second." Instantly I knew what had been suppressed all those years.

While Mary had had sex with other women, she was my first. It was unbelievable. It somehow seemed more reasonable that I was married than that she was about to be while coming on to me like this.

Watching Mary act the happy bride at her reception that Sunday, I was mesmerized. "How's she doing this?" I wondered.

Halfway through the party she came by our table and tapped me on the shoulder. I followed her into the ladies room. In a stall, in her bridal costume, she seduced me again. I couldn't believe it, thinking, "She's outrageous!"

After their honeymoon Mary and Don continued to get together with us on weekends. While Scott and Don watched old Twilight Zone shows on late night television in the bedroom, Mary and I messed around in the living room.

I had no thought about Scott or what he was doing or what he knew. All I felt was that it was great that he and Don were such buddies. It made life a little easier.

On July Fourth we two couples and Lil and her husband rented a house for a week. As the week progressed, something seemed changed in Mary's regard for me. Panicked I thought, "If she leaves, I have no other way of getting into the lesbian world."

Sunday morning Mary told me she'd met another woman and was leaving Don and me to be with her. She didn't tell Don why she was leaving him, but she told Scott, not mentioning her ten-month affair with his wife.

I was a wreck, not so much from heartbreak as from despair. "She's leaving Don in the marriage, but she's really leaving me and I have to go on living in this sham marriage," I thought.

All summer I didn't know what to do. I wondered whether I was sick or just thought I was. I was scared to death to tell anybody and get help. Then somewhere along the line a solution flashed in my mind: "Leave Scott and be on your own." It would be a first step toward telling the family my lifelong secret.

My gayness frightened me. Seeing women or men walking together holding hands or kissing, revolted me. Being so homophobic, I was afraid of Scott's judgment of me. "But I have to leave him and tell him why," I kept telling myself.

One night I finally got up enough courage. Scott was studying for the bar in bed as he'd done for weeks. Scared and feeling great pain, I entered the bedroom and sat down on the bed. "I've got something very serious to talk to you about, but I don't know how to begin." I was like a child, head hung low. I started stammering. "I-I-I have this problem...Mary's leaving Don has something to do with..."

"I know what your problem is," Scott interrupted.

"You couldn't possibly know what my problem is!" I said, feeling affronted. "How could you?"

Tears welled up in his eyes. "Because I have the same one."

"What do you mean?"

Tears were streaming down his face. "I have the same problem with men that you have with women."

"What!" I exclaimed, not very compassionately. I was flabbergasted and angry that he was stealing my thunder. "How could he be doing this?" I thought. Then I asked, "What are you talking about?"

Scott poured out his heart. He'd known about and acted upon his homosexuality since his teens. "Having had experiences with men, I was frightened to marry. I knew what might have to be given up. Then I met you and liked you. Meeting you was my first chance to have a normal life. It helped me be willing to give up the other."

As he spoke I was thinking, "Here I was crawling in here mustering up enough guts to say this thing and he's now telling me his story. I've been blind to everything about this person!"

We stayed up all night talking. At first I couldn't believe he'd given up gay sex when he'd married me. As he shared more of his past, I no longer doubted him. He wanted so much for the marriage to work.

Then it was my turn to speak. First I told him about my decision to leave and then about my feelings and Mary.

"My God!" he said when I finished. "I sensed something going on but had no idea it'd gone that far. You were in love with our best friend!"

The next night I said, "I've got to leave you, Scott."

"Oh no, please don't," he cried. "Stay, Audrey, I beg of you. I don't know what form the marriage can take, but stay."

"No, I must go."

I told my father about my leaving the following day. This sent the family into shock. We had been married for three years and seemed like the perfect couple.

I found an apartment in the city but was so incapable of taking care of myself that I ended up at my father's place. I also kept checking in with Scott.

Each time I stopped by Scott fainted. Coming to, he implored me, "Please come back. I can't handle it."

The desperation in his voice made me realize how afraid he was of living the gay lifestyle openly. "If I leave," I thought," his cover will be blown, especially with his parents."

Our separation was too hard for me to handle also. One evening I went to see him. "O.K., I'll come back. It's the best solution, but let's get out of this suffocating community and move to the city. We'll have to have an open marriage with a twist. You go out with men and I'll go out with women."

"Absolutely fine." He smiled, the first in a long time.

Once we found an apartment we drew up a contract with one rule of the house: "Our house is not to be tainted in any way. We'll never do it here."

Living in Los Angeles, my life became more confused. Scott and I seemed the same to any outsider. But Scott, not interested in having a relationship, instead was having anonymous and bathroom sex, feeling a lot happier not knowing their names. And I was falling in love with a woman every other month, a kid let loose in a toy store.

Each time Scott came home I asked, "Where did you go? What did you do? How did you do it?" Hearing the drama of his activities excited me since my contacts were very different. His stories were fascinating. He told me of making eye contact and walking past the other man and then turning around to arrange to meet. "You know, the *Gayellow Pages* lists meeting places," he said one night.

"They're published?" I exclaimed.

"Sure," he said and brought out the book.

Reading it the next two hours, I burst out laughing. "I can't believe it! Pots and pans, fifth floor, of the department store in the mall and third floor stacks, west, of the main library. Where have I been?"

Experienced in gay affairs, Scott waited out each of my relationships until it had run its course. He never showed jealousy, although he acted irritable if I saw a woman for more than two months. I was the one who got upset, feeling pressured to be with Scott whenever I was distracted with my lover.

When I acted petulant like this Scott would say, "Now be a big girl with big girl responsibilities," putting us back into the child-parent roles we had established when we'd first married. Even though he supported everything I was doing to grow, he controlled my "allowance" and acted miserly about tuition money when I went back to college.

By then I had begun therapy to grow up emotionally as well as sexually, toward the ultimate goal of being on my own. After many of the sessions I would exclaim to Scott, "Oh, the world's so big! There's so much I don't know! And I want to know it all!"

Sometimes Scott would pat my head, saying, "Yes, dear, you'll find out," in the old-worldly way his parents had. Other times he made fun of my therapist.

"He thinks it's nice that I learn about myself," I thought, "but not too much."

For four and a half years I went in and out of relationships and Scott ran around with whatever men he could find. Gradually I got to know myself, building identity and confidence. Yet though part of me was alive another part was miserable.

All this time Scott and I had good times together, often traveling in the States and Europe. On one trip abroad we were laid up in New York. I was miserable but Scott went to a bar. When I finally joined him we made friends with another couple from California, Ben and Marge, also en route to Europe. Once on the Continent we four got together a few times.

Six months later Ben and Marge returned to Los Angeles and found an apartment near the new duplex we'd just bought. We saw them often, partying together until we passed out. Ben and I had a bantering relationship of one-liners. He seemed gay to me but Scott didn't know or care. As time went on it became clear that Ben wasn't in love with Marge and that she was absolutely mad for him.

One night when Ben and I were drinking, I told him about Scott's and my situation.

"Oh," he said. "I knew something was unusual about you two."

"Well," I thought, when nothing more was said, "I guess he's not going to admit to his homosexuality."

A month or so later when Marge was away on business, Ben hung out with us one night. Scott went up to bed at eleven, while Ben and I polished off whatever we were drinking. I began talking about gay bars, where he should go, what he should do and how he should do it.

By then Ben was drunk. "Maybe I'd be interested," he said.

"Scott's got a list of bars in the *Gayellow Pages*. It's up in the bedroom. Go on up and get it." With that, I passed out.

When I awakened several hours later, the lights were still on. "Where is everybody?" I mumbled, going upstairs to bed.

As I neared the bedroom I blinked from all the lights on there too. "That's odd," I thought. "Scott went to sleep way before Ben left."

When I looked in the doorway, they were both nude—Ben sitting at the edge of the bed looking the other way and Scott lying down, his head on the pillow.

"My God!" I gasped and stumbled downstairs, feeling betrayed and very angry.

A couple of minutes later Ben appeared dressed. We talked till dawn. "We had no idea how much we meant to each other," he said, "until we had sex tonight. We couldn't stop." Then he added, with a serious undertone, "You know who sent me up there."

Scott showed his head a few hours later. "Listen Audrey, we had no rule saying I couldn't have a relationship. I just didn't have one. But that wasn't how we set up this contract."

So our life changed again. As Ben and Scott continued to see each other over the next year and a half, I felt jealousy I'd never felt before and fury that I couldn't have my way any more.

It was a taste of my own medicine. Though Scott and Ben kept saying that I had pushed them together, I felt betrayed by them both. Before long being with Ben was no longer enjoyable. There was a cutting edge to our relationship.

Scott got Ben and Marge an apartment connected to ours by the roof, over which he and Ben ran back and forth to have their affair. Marge didn't know. They tried to stop for two months but it didn't work. When they resumed, Ben told Scott not to tell me. He did anyway.

Just as it got to be too much for me, a new woman friend captivated me. One night she called me on being married.

"It hasn't bothered anyone else."

"Well, it bothers me. Find someone it doesn't bother."

That was fuel enough to tell Scott that our arrangement was over. "You have your love affair that you can't give up and I've met someone who won't play this game. It's time we ended this."

Once again Scott fainted. When he revived he begged, "Don't leave me, Audrey," and began to cry.

Somehow I got myself together and moved to an apartment across town. It might as well have been another planet, I was so scared. It meant I had to take care of my entire life, including face up to who I really was—a thirty-one-year-old lesbian in her second year of graduate work in psychology.

For weeks Scott was a wreck. He lost weight. He took to his bed for several days until Ben came over and made him get up and go to work. He began to roam the city and bring people back to his house, living the single gay man's lifestyle. Ben stayed in his life but refused to leave Marge.

For two years, although we lived across town from each other, we double-dated and met each others' friends. The third year we went to New York together and I stayed on to visit a childhood friend.

On my return I announced, "I'm moving to New York."

It didn't happen, but it was a turning point. Scott went away with Ben that Thanksgiving, the first holiday we weren't together. From then on taking holidays without him wasn't a concern. Our social times together became less enjoyable and tapered off. Finally we separated legally.

It was another three years before divorce proceedings began, which didn't require much discussion. Only then, six years after I'd left, did we stop seeing each other socially and separate our friends and interests totally.

Over the next six years I had two lesbian partners and am still with the second. Ben and Scott developed a wide circle of friends and traveled together, a real gay lifestyle with lots of money between them.

Scott still calls every noon for a brief exchange, something about his mother, something about my work. He's my lawyer for whatever I need. I'm his psychologist. His call feels absolutely right.

My life would have been different if gays and lesbians were allowed to play the flirtation and mating games of adolescence. Part of me feels that would have been terrible because I wouldn't have met Scott, as dear to me as any of my close friends. I can't imagine marrying anyone but him. The feel of his hand nineteen years ago made him an immediate choice, absolutely normal.

On another level, where I am today and who I am is the right choice for me.

Fine Tuning
Siri

Jerry and I became inseparable that summer, working at the resort—both blondes, both the same height and age. He was in charge of campground activities, and I waited tables. At night, he helped me clean up; days, I helped him prepare songs.

When my mother met Jerry, she loved him. "He's brought out the young Siri, the outgoing little girl that withdrew in her teen years."

We got together frequently after we returned to our colleges. Two years later, after graduation, we married and went to Chicago. Jerry began seminary and I taught school until I got pregnant with our first son Lou. Thus began a twenty-one year saga, as we moved from an inner-city parish to a series of parishes and university towns for four or five year stints. A second son, Mike, was born along the way. Gradually, Jerry changed his profession to teaching literature, preached on the side, and got his doctorate. I baby-sat to make ends meet and, when the boys started school, began to teach violin.

At first, everywhere Jerry went, I went too, scared to be alone at night, especially when we were in the inner city. Gradually, being alone wasn't bothersome until Jerry was offered a year's teaching position in Arizona. This meant that I and the boys would have to stay in Ohio so Lou wouldn't have to change schools. Jerry kept saying he wouldn't go if I didn't want him to.

When I finally said, "I don't want you to leave us," Jerry said, "Sorry, it's all settled."

Really mad, I jumped in the car and drove until midnight, feeling hurt and hoping Jerry would worry. He was asleep when I returned. It was morning before I could say how overwhelming his going away would be for me. "I don't know how I can handle it!" I wailed.

He went.

Our sixth move was to Charlotte. Jerry taught college and gave sermons in our little parish church, while I taught violin at our home.

The third summer there, things didn't feel right. Our sex activity dwindled to nothing until Jerry said, "You know, Siri, I think I could be celibate the rest of my life."

"Oh..." I murmured, feeling great sadness.

That fall, Jerry got a part-time job in Raleigh and, to avoid driving back and forth, made plans to find an apartment.

"When shall we go pick out your place?" I asked one night.

"Oh, there's no need for you to come."

Sunday, October 31, was Jerry's day to preach. As I listened to his sermon, I thought, "He's saying something to me." I didn't know what exactly, but I felt apprehensive.

When we arrived home, Jerry said, "Let's have lunch and then I want to tell you something."

"No," I said, hardly breathing, "Tell me now."

We sat right down in the kitchen, but before Jerry spoke a word, I knew what he'd say. "Are you gay?" I asked.

Crestfallen, he said, "I had this little speech prepared about what a good person and how wonderful you are, but, that I am gay."

It was like a fist to the gut. Everything seemed to drain to my feet. "What are you going to do?" I asked, shivering.

"I'll get out whenever you want me to."

I gasped, "I don't want you to leave until it's absolutely necessary."

"Well, there's someone I'm going to be living with."

"Who?"

When Jerry didn't answer, I asked, "Don't you think I'll have to know who this person is?" The words were barely out of my mouth when I remembered the conference Jerry had attended with some man, when I'd thought he'd gone alone. I'd overheard him laughing about it afterward, talking on the phone with this fellow. Now the implications clicked. "Is it Chuck?"

"Yes."

I burst into tears and went upstairs. All I could think through the sobs was, "He's leaving me to go live with Chuck." Then I began calling my family and my closest friend. It never entered my head they shouldn't know.

They all were supportive and understanding, though my brother expressed disappointment in Jerry. Then I called Lou and Mike, all this in the same day.

Lou, at a local college, asked, "Want me to come over?"

"Oh, yes."

When I called Mike, he said, "Kick Dad out! You believe in monogamy. He can't give you what you want. I couldn't stand my girl friend telling me she was leaving me for another woman."

"Oh, no!" I gasped. "I don't want him to leave me."

Jerry had set up an appointment for us to see a counselor. After the man heard our story, he turned to me. "We all deserve love," he said. "Let Jerry have his. You go your way."

"Hmmpf!" I said silently. "Where's *my* love?"

The counselor was still talking. "Jerry doesn't have an intimate or an emotional tie with you, or a commitment. Let him go."

As Jerry nodded, all the anger I had at him went right to the counselor. "I want help for me and us, not help to break up," I thought. "It isn't fair." I was getting madder and madder, but, as usual, pushed it down and vowed never to see that man again.

Mike moved back home and commuted to college. Confused and torn, he supported both of us. When I couldn't sleep and went downstairs to cry, he sat and talked with me.

Mostly, I was numb even though Jerry's and my sex life resumed with a flourish. "Whoa," I thought, "who is this person I've known for twenty-seven years?"

He didn't fit the stereotypes of gays though there had been hints about his sexuality over the years. Once another minister's wife came by one day when Jerry was in Arizona. "I want to talk about our husbands," she'd said, sitting in our living room. At some point, she mentioned gay men and asked, "How do you and Jerry work this out?"

"He doesn't talk to me about problems other people have." Startled, she got up. "Oh, I'm sorry. I've got to go."

As the door closed, I telephoned Jerry. "What's she telling me? Are you gay?"

"No, I'm not gay."

The next day, I mentioned the incident to my sister. After a pause she asked, "Do you think Jerry is gay and, if he is, would you stop loving him?"

"No and no," I'd replied.

That was when my heart palpitations started and I began to lose weight.

Now my answer to my sister was being tested. The hardest thing was knowing that Jerry was excited about living with Chuck and leaving me behind. One night I asked, "Jerry, do you want to divorce me?"

"Oh no, I plan to come back and see you on weekends, since Chuck will be coming back to see his grandmother," he said, and then added, "I don't want our sexual relations to stop either."

I wasn't so sure I'd allow that. "I'm willing to share," I thought, "but I want to be the first person in his life."

Since Jerry was taking our car, I bought an old VW from friends who were divorcing. When I brought over the check the wife said, "If you want a counselor, try mine. Ann is good."

I started seeing Ann right away, and then Jerry joined me. She'd never worked with a couple like us, but she was perfect. She never berated Jerry for who he was or what he'd done, and she never got upset with me for whatever feelings I had, nor did she ever tell me what I should or shouldn't do.

At home, Jerry and I talked a lot. He answered any questions—and I had tons—mostly about things he'd done in the past but denied.

Like the Saturday he'd gone to play tennis with Chuck and I'd ridden my bike over to watch. On the way, I fell and scraped my leg. I couldn't find him on the courts so I went home, bleeding and fuming.

"So, Pinhead," I asked, when he came home, "Where were you? I went to the trouble to go watch you play and got hurt on the way, and you weren't even there!"

"Oh, well, we went around to the other courts."

That made no sense since those were his favorite courts and they weren't even full.

One night, after I brought up the umpteenth incident, Jerry said, "Some of these things wouldn't have happened, Siri, if I'd known you wouldn't throw me out. But the world was telling me, 'You can't have both a woman and a man in your life'."

In my grief that the marriage was over, I had to talk a lot, as long as someone would listen. My closest friend, a Baptist, was totally against what Jerry did but supported me and often played the devil's advocate to help me see reality. "God's planted you in my life!" I said one day, realizing that without her support I couldn't handle the strain.

Other friends were angry that Jerry hurt me, and many said, "He wants to have his cake and eat it, too." But no one turned against him; everyone continued to invite both of us to events.

Jerry commuted between Charlotte and Raleigh through December and located an apartment in Raleigh where he and Chuck would live. Their move was set for after Christmas.

The day they were moving his first load over, Chuck told Jerry, "I can't go through with it. I'm not going with you."

That Friday, Jerry was to come back for his second load. He arrived for dinner, later than he'd promised.

As he walked in the back door, I yelled, "Why are you late?" and began to pound his chest.

Jerry turned right around and walked back out the door.

"Oh, please," I called out and ran after him into the back yard. "I'm sorry. Come back in."

Jerry moved to Raleigh that week and his job became full time. He didn't come back weekends after all, because he was busy teaching Sunday evenings, being on call at his church and going to gay community activities. Finally one weekend he said, "Siri, come over here and stay in my apartment."

So I began spending weekends in Raleigh. Other people stayed there during the week which didn't sit well with me, but I felt it wasn't my right to ask him not to invite them. It was his apartment.

It was hard to wait patiently for Jerry to decide where he wanted the relationship to go. I so wanted him to say, "Siri, I'd like you to come live over here."

One night Mike called me in Charlotte. "Mom, you're always in Raleigh with Dad," he said. "You might as well move over."

All this time Jerry was having a relationship with Russ, who didn't like my being in the picture.

"Siri is part of my life," Jerry told him, "and will continue to be a part of my life. We need to share."

"That's demeaning," Russ insisted.

That June I began to wonder whether or not to plan my fall teaching schedule in Charlotte and take on new students.

Ann said, "Go ahead as if you were going to stay here."

I did, but, scared that something might make Jerry say "Good-bye" forever, I was careful what I said to him about it.

Over in Raleigh, Jerry began to look at houses haphazardly, without saying why. We were looking together by midsummer. The idea that maybe we'd be getting back together excited me, but, afraid to push, I continued to wait.

Then Jerry located a house down the street from Russ.

"No, Jer. This won't work," I said, without hesitation. "I cannot live knowing you're going down the block to your friend."

So he left me to look on my own. In August, I found a house close to his job, just as Russ broke up with him. We moved in just before Thanksgiving; and by then, Jerry had met someone else.

He told me about Win during our counseling session with Ann.

"I can't handle this," I said, standing up abruptly. "I'm out of here," I shouted and stormed toward the door.

"Siri, come sit down," Ann said quietly.

So I did. There was nothing to do. "It was all in the works," I thought, "out of my control."

For the next year, I drove back and forth to Charlotte, three times a week, to teach a load of forty students. It exhausted me but kept me busy. Just living in Raleigh was difficult—having the new person in Jerry's life and being away from friends upon whom I depended for support. All I could do at home was to curl up on the sofa in a deep depression.

"Siri," Jerry kept saying, "it's only recreational sex with Win. The only time I was involved intimately was with Chuck."

We continued to see Ann weekly in her Raleigh office. During each session she suggested ways to help us forge a new path for our relationship. Some I couldn't handle, like separate bedrooms or a place for Jerry and one for me. Then she asked, "What would you do if Jerry brought people to your house?"

In my heart, that was out. "I can't have that in my home," I said.

Jerry had lied so much about his activities before, it was hard for him to be honest with me now. But I needed him to be truthful and told him my need in a counseling session.

When Jerry pledged he'd never lie again, Ann warned, "You're not going to be able to tell the truth all the time."

"Sure I am," he said.

But he often felt I'd be hurt less if I didn't know certain things. Something always happened, though, and I found out, which hurt worse than his telling me himself beforehand.

As my loneliness persisted, I toyed with the idea of joining Jerry in his gay social activities. "It would be too hard," I told Ann. "I've never been comfortable around men, except Jerry, who made me forget my adolescent withdrawal."

"Do it when you're ready," she said.

A few months later, seeing I was still hesitant, she counseled, "Just say, 'O.K., I'll try' and go, feeling nervous."

So, scared, I went with Jerry to his gay parents group. The minute I walked into the room, the president came up and threw his arms around me, saying, "Siri, I wish my wife was as understanding."

All the men accepted me. From then on I went to Pride Day, to gay and lesbian picnics, all around, with Jerry. Each new step was difficult, but a help, because I got to know the people he was meeting. It no longer was "This is Jerry's lifestyle and this is mine or ours over here." We'd met in the middle. I was part of it. It was also great to hear them say, "We love to see your two smiling faces."

Until then, two years after Jerry's announcement, whatever he gave, I took, fearing he'd leave if I didn't. Now I was ready to start asking something from him. Ann suggested we write separate lists of what we wanted out of the relationship. "Whatever you both agree on will go in the final contract."

"Weekends are important to me as family times," I wrote, "even if it's just you and me. So I'd rather you go out week nights."

The final contract read, "Jerry can be out two weekend nights a month, but one weekend night will be with Siri for at least four hours. Jerry can have six outside sexual activities a month, no more than two a week and these need to be with different partners. Be home by midnight, call if late, no overnights and no surprises."

We were supposed to look at the contract weekly and ask, "How is it working for you or do we need to fine tune it?" We never did, but it stayed in the back of our minds as I discovered which gay activities I could take and which were difficult. Jerry's going to the baths turned out to be easier to take than his seeing a special friend. Fast sex was better than the other.

Our own sex life stayed good. Jerry always made the first move but often asked, "What would you like from me?" Occasionally he added, "I wish you'd initiate it more." I never did, partly from insecurity but also from wanting to know for sure he desired me.

All this time, Jerry didn't think of himself as gay and didn't like labels. But whenever he told his story at gay parent meetings, he started with, "I'm gay and this is my wife."

One night I took exception. "If you have sex with me and I'm not a man, how can you be gay?" So he began to call himself a bisexual.

About the same time, it dawned on me that Jerry really wasn't different from who he was before. "He's the same person I've known all these years with this one added dimension."

That fall I hurt my back and wasn't mobile, so Jerry went to buy me a cordless phone. He planned to go to the baths afterwards, but on the way decided, "Gee, instead of going to the baths, I'll get home sooner if I just stop at this restroom."

That was where he was arrested. Boiling with resentment, I had to get up and get myself dressed to go bail him out and then sit a while with my back hurting. By the time he was released I'd put my anger down inside, doing more harm to my stomach.

In a few weeks the case was dismissed and he was put on a year's probation.

For the Mardi Gras ball that year, Jerry decided to go as a Dallas cheerleader. Together we picked out a skirt and top, and, as usual, I got ready to do his nails.

"No, no," he said quickly. "I'll do it myself downtown."

He called me later that night. "Guess who I ran into? Rick is in town. We're going to the baths."

I was furious. "Jerk! He knew all along Rick was coming," I muttered, "but wouldn't tell me up front 'cause I'd get mad. He'd rather have the fun first."

After that, I questioned Jerry whenever I really wanted to know the answer. "Are you telling me the truth?" I'd ask and try to believe whatever he said even if it didn't click.

By then I was feeling better about myself. I was taking classes for a masters, going to Ann's women's group, teaching my students, and helping other straight spouses in the area.

A few months after Jerry's probation year was up, he was riding his bike home from work and saw some guy on the side of the road, beckoning him. "I'll just go see what he wants," he said to himself, braking. It was a policeman.

An hour later, a car pulled into our drive. The driver, a woman, came up the walk, carrying a bicycle helmet. As I opened the door, I'm thinking, "He's been hurt," as she's saying, "He's O.K. Don't worry."

The woman, a vice cop, said, "Your husband has been arrested. He asked that you be told."

My stomach turning, I said, "I don't believe this. He promised it would never happen again. Why he would do this?"

"It's not your fault," she interrupted with genuine sweetness. "He's the way he is. You mustn't feel like that."

I finally got to pick up Jerry hours later, and for once there was anger in my voice. "I'm disappointed in you. You weren't going to do this anymore. I don't understand." That was it, none of my usual belaboring.

"I don't understand either."

Since it was Jerry's second arrest, the lawyer charged more and the sentence was harder. Jerry chose the option of a sex offender course. When it was over he made it very clear he did not plan to repeat the incident.

That was a year ago. Over the ensuing months, we did more fine tuning. On Tuesday nights, if there was free pool at his favorite bar, I didn't need to do something as a distraction. But if he went to the baths or someone special invited him over, I worked on some project and made him go to a neutral place like the supermarket before coming home.

When Jerry did something that made me really mad, I no longer hopped in the car and drove into the night. I just turned cool, not saying anything. He now knew what that meant. Whenever he got home past midnight and found me in a different bed, he came in and whispered, "Oh, don't be in here. Come get in bed with me."

Halfway through the probation year, Lou called to tell us he had broken up with his longtime girl friend because of another woman. I began yelling at him, enraged. All the anger I should have had at Jerry when he came out was going to my son because he had hurt the girl in his life—just as Jerry had done. I felt her pain.

The next morning I called Lou back. "I've got to explain. I am angry with you, but it's really at your dad through you for what happened three years ago."

We talked a long time. Then he said, "I understand, Mother, but I do want you to meet my new girl friend."

"Some day," I said quietly. I wasn't ready, nor am I yet. There's a lot more processing to be done.

Somehow Jerry and I had lost touch with each other before he came out. Because of the experience, the relationship is better and we're both stronger. I no longer wish he weren't bi. His gay side makes him who he is. It's also how I got to know the gay parents group, the most genuine people I know. We can be ourselves with them. They knew exactly who we are. We don't have to hide.

Redefining a Lasting Mixed-Orientation Relationship

Although the traditional marriage form is shattered as a result of the partner's coming out, many spouses, particularly straight wives, still prefer the security of the broken pieces to an unknown future without partner, marital status or financial support. The need to keep the family together and to be a supportive wife is strong. Many have strong ties of love and friendship to their partners that they wish to preserve above all else. Also, wives who formerly felt estranged find hope in the intimacy of sharing their husbands' secret at last.

When these factors are enhanced by the husband's wish to stay married, a sizeable number of women will go to any length to make the marriage work. Out of blind hope or denial, many don't see the uphill battle ahead. They don't grasp the implications of no longer being their husband's preferred sexual partner even though they may still be their best friend, intellectual soul mate or companion. They often deny the possibility that their husbands might be staying mainly for the security of the family or the facade of "married man."

Even spouses who accept the sexual incompatibility in the relationship often remain undaunted by the challenge. "Now that I know the facts," they reason, "I can make the marriage work." They become what support group leaders Sandra Auerback, M.S.W., and Charles Moser, Ph.D., term, "Superwomen."[1] They juggle marriage, job, home and children, as well as new gay-related tasks undertaken for the partner. In so doing, they may be required to make sacrifices for the marriage they haven't bargained for.

Although a number of couples succeed in preserving the marriage, the majority do not. Despite sincere efforts, the sexual disparity, competition for the partner's attention or unconventional and for some immoral arrangements, eventually become intolerable for most spouses.

Coping with the marriage issue becomes a more constructive process with greater promise of success if the couple, rather than trying to preserve the traditional marriage arrangement, is willing to develop a relationship appropriate to the new circumstances. This goal can be attained, whether or not the marriage itself lasts, through eight key strategies:

- Settling the AIDS issue
- Asserting the straight spouse's sexual needs
- Accommodating to the partner's sexual identity
- Reassessing the mixed-orientation marriage
- Putting the gay factor into perspective
- Rewriting marital rules
- Developing a non-dependent relationship
- Forming a lasting couple bond.

Settling the AIDS Issue

Because of the far greater incidence of AIDS among homosexual and bisexual men than among lesbians and bi women, AIDS is primarily an issue for straight wives and gay or bisexual husbands. HIV-antibody testing, the first task toward reestablishing the relationship, is essential for both husband and wife and, if they engage in extramarital affairs, their lovers. If the partner refuses testing, the spouse's fear of infection may never disappear and it will be much harder to resolve sexual and other marital problems constructively.

Being tested and waiting for results often cause embarrassment and anxiety. Apprehension so obsessed a pregnant woman in Los Angeles that, unable to wait for her partner's test results, she had an abortion one week before the test results came back negative. To lessen fears that might lead to rash actions, it helps to find a trusted friend who can offer support.

HIV-negative test results bring relief, yet anxiety can persist because of the long incubation period of the AIDS virus. If the husband continues to be active, the wife must insist on continued regular testing. An HIV-positive test result for the husband or wife calls for medical and psychological counseling and research into current facts. Wives who face their husband's AIDS diagnosis fear infection and resent being put at risk because of the men's hidden activities. Actually, a low incidence of wives becoming infected has been reported.[2] Helpful advice for handling such concerns about AIDS is offered in *When Husbands Come Out of the Closet*.[3]

Seven of the twenty-six straight wives followed for this study had to cope with their husbands' or ex-husbands' positive test results. Four eventually faced cases of full-blown AIDS, three of whom nursed their husbands until death. Their emotional turmoil was eased by honest talk with the husband and counseling or participation in a support group of similar couples. The experience, though agonizing, brought unexpected rewards of spiritual reconciliation and inner growth. Carol Lynn Pearson's *Good-bye I Love You* describes just such a moving story.[4]

Asserting the Straight Spouse's Sexual Needs

Even with an HIV-positive test result, the couple's sex life need not stop, although it will have to be altered to include safe-sex practices. Many husbands, particularly bisexual men, still feel attracted to their wives. Some men are initially more desirous than before, possibly because of release from repressed homosexuality or sexual arousal from gay contacts. Bi wives, of course, remain attracted.

Given safe-sex protection, it is critical to try to continue or revive lovemaking. Making love is a primary way to affirm and express the union as long as it is a two-way experience. For it to be two-way, the wife needs her sexual needs to be fulfilled by her husband, the second step toward redefining the relationship.

Women who enjoyed marital sex before the coming out have less difficulty asserting their sexual needs. Wives habituated to thinking of themselves as inadequate, however, tend to acquiesce to their husband's disclosed needs without insisting that their own be met. Reminding themselves of the real reason underlying their sexual problems may help them to find the courage to be more assertive. Many find that the very act of specifying wishes reactivates dormant desires. If the husband is reluctant to try alternative ways to give pleasure, the wife will want to find out how committed he is to the relationship, uncomfortable as such probing might be.

Except in those rare cases in which the husband has not been and does not plan to be active with other men, there are but two options for continued lovemaking—safe sex or no sex. Because of the risk of exposing the spouse to AIDS, unprotected sex with a partner who is actively gay should not be considered. In addition, the spouse should insist that the partner limit gay sex to a single lover and only practiced safe sex, so that marital sex won't have to stop because of a deadly risk. Safe sex or no sex means that the wife, in particular, must give up the freely open sexual experience to which she has previously been accustomed because of her partner's lifestyle.

At the same time, the need to express his or her sexual orientation is extremely important to the partner. The 1987 study of twenty-five mixed-orientation couples by sex therapist George Deabill, M.S., Ph.D., suggests that husbands who engage in homosexual sex may feel more satisfaction in the marriage than those who don't.[5]

Maintaining a gay or bisexual identity in the marriage is so important to the husband[6] that if the wife pressures him to limit or abstain from gay sex, he may ultimately feel less commitment to the marriage. The less committed he is, the less satisfied she will be, as in any marriage.[7] The wife's compromise then is to accept her partner's gay activities in exchange for a committed and affectionate relationship with limited or no sex. Not an easy bargain.

Many wives feel resentment about the limitations put on their sex life. Expressing such concerns in a calm manner can reduce tension and may motivate a husband to try other ways to increase his wife's pleasure.

Marriage or sex counseling with a therapist who is knowledgeable about homosexuality, bisexuality and mixed-orientation couples can greatly increase the chances of salvaging the relationship. For bisexual-straight couples, it is crucial that they find a therapist who understands that bisexuality is a distinct orientation from homosexuality and not a transitional state. Without such a therapist, possibilities for the couple to revive sexuality may be bypassed. William Wedin, Ph.D., director of Bisexual Information and Counseling Service in Manhattan, points out that some bi men think they're gay when in actuality they are only suffering from temporary impotence resulting from the stress of the coming out.[8] Some couples think that their problem is gay-related when it is just sexual boredom that can readily be remedied. For others, sexual addiction may be the basic problem. In any case, a good therapist can assign exercises to enhance the couple's lovemaking. Spouses can learn to incorporate what their partners like in their same-sex activity into their lovemaking and partners can learn ways to give their spouses sexual pleasure.

Alternative ways to experience sexual pleasure can reduce the pain of limiting or giving up intercourse. There are some excellent books on expanding sexuality listed in Appendix A. Using their own ingenuity, many couples devise other forms of physical contact that give the women sexual pleasure, such as cuddling, hugging, kissing, caressing and massaging. Most of the wives in Deabill's study experienced sexual and marital satisfaction from such gestures of affection and physical contact from their husbands.[9]

While marital sex may last for bi-straight couples, it does not for the majority of gay-straight couples. Gradually the gay partner's sexual desires may shift as he follows the typical candy store syndrome, seeking varied experiences in gay bars, baths and meeting places. At home, sex becomes infrequent and then stops, despite periodic increases after gay encounters.

Having to give up the sexual core of married life is agonizing for spouses, particularly if their sex lives improved after the coming out. Though love and friendship may compensate for the absence of sex, the feeling of loss is profound. Spouses may try to get along with shared interests and gestures of affection, but this may not be enough to alleviate the hurt.

Spouses who stay in a sexless marriage learn to sublimate, redirect or repress their desire. Many use alcohol, cigarettes, drugs or food as a substitute. More productive and healthy ways to utilize sexual energy include creative pursuits like art, music and dance or physical activities like gardening and sports. Masturbation is an effective way to release sexual energy, but even that doesn't wholly make up for the sexual deprivation.

Respect for the marital bond and strong commitment to husband and family are key reasons why many wives stay in sexless marriages. A Canadian couple married for forty-four years, put it like this, "We have a history, three children, and seven grandchildren keeping us together." Ray, a fundamentalist preacher, struggled with his homosexuality and Winnie agonized over his coming out until they eventually developed a devoted companionship. In the process she formed a close female friendship, a support group and a career. He became a counselor and took a lover, whom he sees weekly, just to hold and be held. They also use the support of several couple groups.

While many wives find the loss of marital sex so painful that they divorce, a number seem satisfied with perquisites like social position, financial security, emotional support or assured companionship. Some continue to live in substantial homes and lead active social lives twenty or more years after the coming out.

Accommodating to the Partner's New Sexual Identity

Even if the wife gets her sexual needs met, nearly every aspect of her life becomes altered by the homosexual or bisexual needs of the husband. Compared to him, she has more drastic changes to make after the coming out. By the time the partner has revealed his orientation, he has already adjusted to it. For her the situation is new. Making necessary adaptations to the partner's revealed sexual identity is the third step toward developing a lasting relationship.

The husband's gay activities may first enter the wife's life as part of their everyday conversations. Some wives are eager to listen to what had been a secret. Curious about their husband's new world, they don't want to feel left out. Other wives don't want to know any details even if silence cuts them off from what their husbands value, because it's too painful or they feel uncomfortable or repelled by their husband's gay lifestyle or mannerisms.

Others may join in their husband's activities, such as Gay Fathers or similar groups, wanting to know what their friends are like and to support their partners openly. Fascinated by a hidden subculture or drawn to support an oppressed group, some like being a part of their husband's secret cause. Some even befriend their husband's lovers, seeing them as "special" because they share the love of the same man. While a few later join gay advocacy groups, many eventually feel isolated and stop all participation.

Most often, the wife is responsible for scheduling her husband's gay activities into the family calendar of child care, household tasks, careers, family excursions and couple activities, reflecting the traditional caretaker role of women. In addition, some wives take on their husband's gay-related needs, such as baking a turkey for a Gay Fathers' party or handling the legal work for a husband's arrest for a sexual violation.

As the wife struggles to cope with all of the demands placed on her, she isn't aware at first of how much she is affected by her husband's double life. For example, she may not see the irony of scheduling quality time previously spent as a couple into the husband's gay agenda.

In the frenzy to keep the marriage going and be "the successful wife," she may think she has the situation in hand. In actuality she has little control. Almost all of her energy is directed toward accommodating her husband's new identity, with little heed paid to her own needs. As she focuses increasingly on supporting her husband's gay lifestyle, she gradually absorbs the gay perspective—becoming the "spouse of a gay (or bisexual)," defined by his identity.

At this point the couple risks developing a destructive co-dependency for the sake of sustaining the marriage.[10] The husband, needing his wife to shore up his self-esteem battered by homophobia, stays in a less-than-satisfying, restrictive relationship. The wife, in order to keep her husband, supports behavior that takes him away from her. In this instance, she may have to consider how much she is willing to sacrifice to make the marriage work.

Reassessing the Mixed-Orientation Marriage

Most spouses cannot sustain the merry-go-round pace required to maintain the semblance of the former marriage. As their energy wanes, it becomes necessary to step back and take an objective look at the marriage and how it is affecting them. This fourth strategy calls for slowing down and expecting to accomplish less than is normally done each day. Time needs to be set aside for introspection and freeing up emotions neglected in the struggle to make the marriage work.

Solitude is most conducive for getting in touch with buried emotions and gaining some insight on the marital situation. To release feelings, it helps to engage in activities that don't require thinking, such as exercise, meditation, music, art, dance, craft projects, day dreams, anything that allows emotions to surface. Tears relieve tension and reveal sources of pain. Laughter helps to create distance from the immediate plight. Each day presents something incongruous to rouse a smile, in the office, at the supermarket, on the bus, with one's children.

Alone and without distractions, spouses can gain the perspective needed to determine how to proceed forward. They may see for the first time how much their partners' "other life" has crept into theirs. Each change of schedule, each missed opportunity for affection, is recognized for what it is after being accepted unthinkingly for months. The relationship may no longer fit their expectations and may seem to be slipping away.

If couples have a contract or an agreed-upon arrangement, it may need to be revised to better serve their needs and to prevent further hurt. Walt and Sara, a young couple in Atlanta, were not able to negotiate a successful agreement. They drew up a contract after he moved out when their baby was three months old. He was to return and be demonstrative to Sara short of intercourse and to spend two nights a week and Saturday with his lover, while Sara was to lower her expectations of complete sexual pleasure. The following year, as Walt spent more than the allotted time with his lover and less time with Sara, she became clinically depressed until the separation she never wanted was the only tolerable option.

The unconventional arrangement itself often becomes the source of discomfort for spouses, arousing unwanted negativity against their partners. Gradually many wives feel jealous or resentful of the time their husbands spend with their lovers and the lovers may begin to appear to be a threat to the marriage. As the wife starts to feel that she has nothing while her partner has his other life, the marriage contract may no longer seem valid. At this point a single incident can seem like a blatant negation of the arrangement. When Scott started to go out with Ben, for example, Audrey, though empathetic with his situation that paralleled hers, felt betrayed. That marked the beginning of the end of their arrangement.

As the partner pursues a gay lifestyle, monogamy often becomes the paramount issue for the spouse whether or not lovemaking has continued. The partner's sexuality, in the totality of its physical, emotional and spiritual aspects, is no longer exclusive to the marriage. Spouses typically feel intense resentment toward this double life, but many are paralyzed and cannot take action because of fear of the future and guilt about failing. For others, their rage often forces the decision of whether to separate, divorce or reconstruct the relationship.

Before stress becomes self-destructive, it is critical to share concerns with a counselor or friend who can help the spouse look objectively at the relationship. A knowledgeable counselor can guide the spouse in resolving conflicting emotions and in sorting out priorities and responsibilities. This includes accepting negative feelings as normal and appropriate reactions to the situation, learning to take care of the spouse's needs first and discouraging wishful thinking or expectations about what "should" be done.

Since partners are going through their own stages of reactions to the coming out, counseling for them, as well as joint counseling, can help to clarify couple issues and raise their awareness of relationship responsibilities.

In such crisis periods when major decisions must be made, intensive couple counseling is very helpful since the partner and spouse often progress simultaneously through similar emotional stages.

William Wedin defines the stages as initial humiliation (the partner's guilt and the spouse's self-blame), a "honeymoon" of feeling mutually valued, rage (the partner feels misunderstood and the spouse duped) and final resolution.[11] Crisis counseling can help the couple get through apparent impasses as they progress through each stage. The goal of crisis counseling is to equip the couple with skills to resolve issues themselves in future crises.

Support groups for straight spouses and for mixed-orientation couples are key resources at this time also. In the growing sense of isolation that the spouse feels, finding just one other person who has been there can make a big difference. Through hearing others' reports of similar problems, such as dwindling commitment from the partner, less couple time and reneged agreements, spouses feel less alone and better able to handle their own crises. By talking with others in the same situation, wives realize that a sexless marriage is a common problem. Support group members also suggest practical options and offer firsthand advice otherwise not readily available.

Support groups can be located through the resources listed in Appendix B. However, because there is a limited number of support groups outside of metropolitan areas, spouses in rural areas may have more success contacting the Straight Spouse Support Network that operates under P–FLAG, listed in Appendix B. Some spouses form their own informal support groups which are often advertised in local newspapers.

Many spouses, in spite of outside emotional support, may be overwhelmed with anger and hurt at the destruction of their monogamous relationships. Often the partner is blamed for all couple problems, diminishing the chances of salvaging the relationship.

Putting the Gay Factor into Perspective

As the spouse struggles with painful marital issues, the partner's gay-ness can assume disproportionate importance. Each time something goes wrong, it's tempting to say, "It's because he or she is gay (or bisexual)." But single-factor answers don't provide much insight into the larger relationship problems. It is therefore essential that spouses disentangle themselves from the polarized "gay-versus-straight" reasoning that they often fall into after the coming out. They can then put the partner's homosexuality into its proper perspective, the fifth strategy of establishing a lasting relationship.

The tendency to view marital problems solely in terms of the gay factor can blind the spouse to other possible causes: physical, psychological, educational, social, financial, work-related, religious, as well as sexual. Failed sexual encounters in any marriage, for example, can be accounted for in part by fatigue, stress, anxiety or alcohol consumption.

The partner's actions should not be judged exclusively on the basis of his or her sexual orientation. Like the straight spouse, the partner is motivated by multiple factors. Sometimes gayness operates; other times, non-gay motives exert a major influence. The newly-revealed sexual orientation doesn't turn the partner into a different person.

As in any marriage, personalities and personal philosophies play a large part in problems mixed-orientation couples face. This is not to diminish the issue of the mixed-orientation and the importance of how couples handle it. However, the spouse may need to reconsider each marriage problem and ask if the partner's gay behavior has contributed to it and if so, how significantly. In some cases, unreliability, irresponsibility, inattention or alcoholism of the partner plays a major part in the couple's problems.

Some estimates indicate that as many as one out of four gay men are alcoholic. Though the disease stems largely from hereditary factors, many men drink to alleviate their pain from the anti-gay social stigma or to engage in gay social activities, from gay bars to private parties, in which alcohol plays a large role.[12]

Clinical psychologist Kathy McMahon, Psy.D., suggests asking the following questions to put the gay factor into perspective. "Does the gayness nullify any reason why we got married? Are positive aspects of the relationship still positive? Does the disclosure enable us to face the new, possibly fearful aspects and become more intimate?"[13]

To answer this, an understanding of the how the couple interacts is required. McMahon raises the important points, "Does his behavior hurt, deny, or affirm me? How much caring and sacrifice is there? How honest is he in admitting mistakes—rather than blaming me or society—and acknowledging any hurt his action may cause?"[14]

Spouses need to consider whether, if the gay factor weren't there, they would still continue to work on the marriage. To come to a satisfactory conclusion, they will need to discern what is needed not only for the partner's sake, but for their own sake and for the health of the relationship. Then they will be able to decide what to reject and what to accept in the marriage.

If the partner agrees to help solve marital problems, the next step is to determine how the couple's needs can be met within the marriage.

Rewriting Marital Rules

To satisfy the needs of both spouse and partner, alternative marriage rules need to be devised, the sixth strategy of this stage. The process is an ongoing one of adjustments and revisions throughout the marriage.

The breakdown of the traditional marriage form forces the couple to reevaluate its basic purpose and their own criteria for a quality relationship. As a wife of a bisexual man said, "We threw out everything we'd learned about the way you're *supposed* to be and figured out what we *were*."

Helpful examples of effective mixed-orientation relationships can be found in the few biographies that have been written, such as *Barry and Alice*[15] and in studies of gay-straight couples in general, notably *The New Couple*, by Rebecca Nahos and Myra Turley[16] and *Uncommon Lives*, by Catherine Whitney.[17]

The most effective straight-gay relationships appear to share non-sexual characteristics such as friendship, honesty and primary commitment to the marriage. The spouse accepts the partner's orientation. In turn the partner is sensitive to the spouse's needs. They each accept the other's need for autonomy. It's a special companionship not available to them in the gay or heterosexual community.[18] The healthiest relationships include physical contact, co-nurturing and commitment to marriage and family.

In working out an alternative marital arrangement, the straight wife usually has to make the greater sacrifices. Each change from the conventional marriage form needs to be considered from the spouse's and the partner's personal, cultural and perhaps religious standards. If there are children, the arrangement must be appropriate to their needs for a stable home environment. Often the husband's gay affairs are considered by the wife to be beyond the purview of the traditional heterosexual marriage contract. Such a woman in Michigan contracted with her bisexual husband that he could continue dating men but not women. His dating women was too threatening to her.

Alternative marital arrangements are as diverse as couples. They range from a Philadelphia wife who invited her husband's lover to live with them; to a professor in San Diego who brings male graduate students home overnight; to a Chicago couple and the husband's lover who live together, by contract, as a ménage à trois; to a socialite couple in Raleigh who each have lovers in another city.

The arrangement that seems to work best for gay-straight couples is allowing the husband to engage in some gay activity while the wife accepts protected or no marital sex and, in some cases, finds an outside lover to compensate for that lack. Among bi-straight couples, some bi husbands elect to be monogamous.

Most couples discover what works best for them through trial-and-error. Often spouses face negative pressure from friends, family or clergy, or they begin to feel uncomfortable with the arrangement for personal reasons, forcing them to rethink their rationale and forge yet another concept of marriage. For the husband of a bi wife in Seattle, it was: "Once I let go of my male ego and realized, physiologically, I couldn't fill all Greta's sexual needs, I was sure of our marriage."

Developing a Non-Dependent Relationship

Just as crucial as reaching an agreeable sexual arrangement is developing a healthy autonomy in the relationship. No alternative arrangement lasts very long without the couple's respect for each other's separate identity. In order to develop a non-dependent relationship, the seventh strategy of this stage, dependent behavior patterns, characteristic of many mixed-orientation couples, need to be replaced with reciprocal ways of interacting.

Three types of dependency patterns; clinging, pupil-teacher and mother-child, are seen among many mixed-orientation couples. Polly and Mike, a childless couple in Buffalo, typify the clinging pattern. They shared a craft business in their home as well as lovers. In several years, a stifling symbiosis began to destroy their closeness.

Audrey and Scott illustrate the pupil-teacher relationship in which the better educated, skilled husband molded her into the perfect wife. This scenario of authority-submission enabled him to create a private world in which to hide.

In the mother-child pattern, as shown by Carol and Dave, typically the husband depends on the wife's nurturing while she ignores her own needs in deference to his.

Such dependency patterns resemble the behavior of couples in which the wife protects her alcoholic husband, denying that there is a problem, therefore enabling the destructive situation to persist. In this kind of co-dependent relationship, both the alcoholic husband and the co-alcoholic wife deny accountability for the harmful effects of their behavior. Similarly, the straight spouse who denies the hurtful effects of the coming out on the marriage is, in effect, helping perpetuate a painful situation.

Couples in dependent relationships need to learn how to relate in mutually constructive ways. Spouses who play the role of "symbiotic dependent," "pupil," or indulgent "parent" need to free themselves from the demands of the controlling counterpart. Realizing this, Polly, the wife in Buffalo, began teaching craft courses in the city, Audrey finished her undergraduate degree and Carol found part-time work and entered therapy.

The spouse who develops autonomy is able to take equal responsibility for the direction the relationship takes. No longer dependent on the partner's needs, the spouse can freely decide if the relationship meets her or his priorities. Spouses, like Siri, who previously repressed their true feelings out of fear of jeopardizing the relationship can now express hurt from their partner's same-sex behavior while still showing empathy. "You have a right to be who you are," an Ohio wife often says to her husband, "but not to hurt others."

As spouses gain equality their partners may think that they've lost control. In response spouses can say to them, "You still have control, only it's equal now." Balance of power allows couples to make sounder decisions about what's best for the relationship in the long run.

Forming a Lasting Couple Bond

Developing a long-term bond is the final challenge for couples who want to stay together. To create an enduring relationship, both husband and wife need to commit themselves to work on it even under forbidding circumstances. The ideal goal is to try as hard as possible together to make it succeed and to keep communication lines open. Even if the marriage ultimately does not last, they will have the satisfaction of knowing that they made a sincere effort and will have gained a better understanding of themselves and the relationship. Many achieve a deeper bond than they had before.

In creating a lasting bond, the goal is not the romantic fantasy with which many couples begin marriage. It is a shared commitment to the concept of a community of two who care for each other's welfare enough to meet any challenge needed to resolve problems. This kind of dedication, psychiatrist M. Scott Peck explains, is necessary for the "security of knowing that the struggle over these issues will not itself destroy the relationship."[19]

Working toward mutual happiness, important in any relationship, is a formidable task for the mixed-orientation couple since the relationship needs are in direct conflict with the personal needs of the liberated partner. Having a shared commitment helps the couple to compromise some individual needs in the interest of the common good.

Deabill's research indicates that a husband's commitment greatly enhances his wife's sexual and marital satisfaction.[20] Miriam and Max, a couple in Denver who have been married for twenty-one years, illustrate this. Since sexual infidelity is unacceptable to Miriam, Max has relinquished gay sex to preserve the marriage and the family. In return he is allowed to engage in gay activities short of active sex.

"My thinking was black and white," Miriam explained. "Max helped me see the gray areas. Now when I get judgmental, I say to myself, 'Look Miriam, that's your husband. Think it through again.'"

Four qualities appear to enhance the development of a long-term relationship: openness, flexibility, candor and humor. Many couples who survive the initial impact of the coming out displayed such traits before the disclosure. Others learn to develop them through deliberate efforts, such as counseling and conscious practice.

Both husband and wife need to be open about themselves, each other and the relationship in order to work through their differences. One way to foster openness is to replace judgmental behavior with acceptance of the other person's differences.

Developing open, honest communication requires that the spouse and partner each take risks, such as rejection of their differing opinions or feelings. For those accustomed to hiding or denying their feelings, this can be extremely frightening or uncomfortable. But ultimately the couple will be rewarded with a deeper sense of intimacy. As psychiatrists Patrick Thomas and Thomas Patrick Malone say, each will "feel and know myself in the presence of another."[21]

Flexibility, the willingness to try alternative ways to interact is also essential. Being flexible includes the ability to be resilient in the face of failure or criticism. A bi-straight couple in London, for instance, survived a public scandal over his arrest in a men's restroom. The wife, by relearning assertiveness, became an equal partner with him in working out with his lover what she calls "a three-point relationship."

Honesty is a third key quality in preserving the couple bond. For example, marriages in which the partner comes out to the spouse early on tend to last longer than those in which the sexual orientation is concealed. Even after a delayed coming out, being honest is crucial in reducing hostility and restoring positive interaction. To express concerns candidly, it helps to concentrate on present feelings and proposed action rather than on past events which tend to arouse blame or excuses. If criticism upsets either person, he or she needs to be reminded that the purpose of the discussion is to solve the problem at hand.

A sense of humor is invaluable, although time may be needed to gain distance from the painful events so that they can be viewed with detachment. Eventually the couple may begin to appreciate the irony of their predicament. One young couple in Virginia, who forbid the word, "straight," in their house, have created a long glossary of synonyms they use with a secret wink.

Through cultivation of these four traits, most couple bonds are enriched and deepened. Reading self-help literature on relationships and talking with other couples, supportive friends and counselors will reinforce the process.

Many couples, especially those with children, desire to preserve their bond whether or not they stay married. As Dave and Carol vowed, "If a problem in the marriage ever threatens our friendship, we'll end the marriage."

Bond-building has been used successfully by separated and divorced couples too, although the physical separation and the hurt from divorce are formidable obstacles. A woman in Phoenix was married for twenty-eight years before her husband came out and two more years while he thought he was bisexual. When he realized he was gay and left, she chose to work through her rage and to develop a platonic friendship with him. Though deeply satisfied when she succeeded, it had taken six stressful years to do so.

Maintaining the bond requires perseverance to work through issue after issue. Will and Betsy, a couple in Boston who have been together three years since the coming out, call the process "mending and tending." Facing their differences openly and honestly with guidance from a priest and support groups of gay professional men and mixed-orientation couples, they have grown in mutual understanding. Will, who stayed in the marriage at first because he loved their children, has developed unconditional love for Betsy.

A small but significant number of couples stay married. While an estimate of fifteen percent is given in several studies, it is not known how many years those couples stayed together nor how many other couples remain closeted and uncounted. When the present research began in 1986, eight of the twenty-six straight wives studied in depth, or thirty-one percent, were still married two to seven years after the coming out, but over half of them had stayed married for at least three years. After five years, four or fifteen percent, were still with their husbands. Three of them would be married still in 1994 were it not for two AIDS' deaths.

The significant finding is that about half of those who tried to make their marriages work succeeded, an important point for couples who are dismayed by the fifteen percent figure to keep in mind. This low percentage is based on all marriages in which the husband came out, not just those in which both husband and wife tried to stay together.

Staying together is not easy, but it can be done. A bi-straight couple in Washington, D.C., still together after nine years, continually renegotiate their relationship. "It all comes back to trust," the straight wife says, echoing the consensus of the couples support group to which she and her husband belong.

It helps to find other couples in the same situation. A gay-straight pair in Des Moines, after meeting another couple still married after fifteen years, exclaimed, "They are an inspiration for us."

Couples who are able to preserve their marriages share the following attitudes: the straight spouse accepts the partner's sexual orientation, the partner values the spouse as the primary relationship and they both hold a non-traditional view of marriage that they have defined together.[22]

When children are involved, other issues come into play that can bring the couple closer together as a family or pit them against each other. Part Three explores common issues and conflicts that parents, particularly straight spouses, face as they try to help their children cope with the consequences of the coming out.

three

GROWING PAINS

CONFLICTING ROLES AS PARENT AND SPOUSE

While the children's needs may be overlooked in the initial trauma of the coming out, they soon demand attention. Of primary concern is how to preserve the bond between the children and the homosexual or bisexual parent. Positive identification with both parents is critical to the children's development of self-esteem, identity and sense of security. At the same time parents need to prepare their children for possible anti-gay attitudes in the community. How to protect them from the hurtful effects of homophobic prejudice without altering their relationship with the gay parent is the third dilemma facing the straight spouse.

Whether or not to tell the children about the partner's sexual orientation is the first concern of many parents. Most parents eventually decide to tell them. While it is important to gear the explanation to the children's age and level of understanding, the spouse's attitude toward the coming out is even more important in how well the children accept the gay or bisexual parent. It is imperative that the straight parent keep her or his personal pain from negatively influencing the children against the gay or bisexual parent.

A second major concern is how to help the children cope with negative effects of the coming out on their lives. Common problems they experience include embarrassment over the non-traditional orientation or stereotypical behavior of the homosexual or bisexual parent; confusion about their own sexual identity; fear of prejudiced reactions of peers; conflicting loyalties to the two parents; and psychological turmoil resulting from separation or divorce.

Trying to maintain a positive relationship with the partner for the children's sake, as well as taking on responsibility for their needs, are among the many demands that prevent spouses from dealing with their own personal issues. Yet in working through the social, moral, sexual and sometimes legal concerns related to the children's well-being, many spouses gain insight into their own issues.

The three stories that follow, told by two straight mothers and a gay father, illustrate typical problems that children encounter after the coming out and the straight parent's conflicts in helping them cope. The final section of Part Three explores major issues that impact the family, especially the children and ways in which both parents can help their children deal with them constructively.

Personal Stories

Dad's Girl and Mom's Boy
Allison

Several years after Peter's mood swings began, when Nicholas was three and Courtney was six, he received a call at home one night. "I told you never to call me here," I heard him say as my heart froze. When Peter brought it up later, I couldn't talk about it.

We'd been married for eight years, after graduating from the University of Nebraska in the early sixties. Tall and dark-haired, Peter was the "boss" as my father had been, which fit right into my pattern of low self-esteem. I loved him dearly.

After the phone call, Peter's drinking became more of a problem. Whenever he was drunk, he accosted me with one of two accusations: "Allison, you're not very bright" or "You're a terrible parent."

"Of all the bad things I am," I thought, "it's not those. I'm a good parent and have above-average intelligence, thank you very much." I'd worked on being intelligent all my life, using books to hide my insecurity, especially with men. Outwardly I was a confident brunette, as tall as Peter.

After months of silence I confronted him one night. "Either you tell me what's going on or I'm leaving. I can't live with your excuses, hostility and verbal abuse when you drink."

"Okay, but later. It's something I need to talk to you about in private."

After the children were in bed I joined him in the living room, where he was sitting in front of the fire crying. Through his tears he told me that a psychologist had just confirmed that he was gay. He also told me that he'd been seeing men for four years. "I'm so frightened," he said. "I'd like to wake up one day and have it be untrue."

"It's as if he's said that he's dying," I thought. "Our marriage will end, but I can't walk away and leave him in such agony."

Before long I realized Peter had never been in love with me and could never love any woman the way I loved him. Though he cared about me as much as he could for a woman, I felt cheated. Feeling rejected as a woman, I resented the fact that he'd had my love but I'd never had his. All of my insecurity surfaced.

For the next four years I talked to no one about what was going on and how bad I felt. It was easier not to say it out loud. I plunged into community activities to distract my thoughts and to boost my self-esteem. Several sessions with a psychologist, plus books on homosexuality, helped me understand what was happening.

In Nebraska where I'd grown up, aberrations like homosexuality were ignored and homosexuals were carefully closeted, but my extensive reading convinced me that gays didn't choose to be gay. The hurt Peter was causing wasn't intentional. Because I loved him he could be excused. Yet the pain was no less profound and couldn't be ignored. To heal I had to learn to unlove him.

"You're on your own now, Allison," I told myself over and over, "without Peter." It took two years before I could tell myself, "I don't love him any more." But deep down I still did.

Peter, meanwhile, was on a roller coaster, acting like a straight family man for periods and then coming home at strange hours, drinking a lot and sinking into suicidal depressions that frightened me.

At home he spent most of the time with Courtney. She'd always been "Dad's girl," but more so when he started gay activities and stopped responding to me. Their closeness made me feel jealous. Our son Nicolas withdrew more. Since he was born just as Peter realized the straight family life wasn't meaningful for him any longer, Peter rejected Nicolas as symbolizing the truth he wanted to deny. So I had to be both Dad and Mom to Nicolas.

The fourth summer after he came out Peter bought me a car out of the blue and we began to remodel the house. Then he was stricken with a viral infection and confined to bed for three months. The constant noise of the workmen and the telephone irritated him. Since his income depended on commissions, this was also a very difficult time financially.

Each day after preparing his meals and leaving instructions with him for the workmen, I'd drive into Milwaukee to supervise preparations for a big fund-raising event. One night after coming home to find the workmen doing what I'd told Peter not to let them do, I blew up and Peter raised a fist at me. By then, I knew the end was near.

Eventually Peter returned to work. Nicholas began first grade and seemed happy with it; Courtney, now in fifth grade, began to feel uncomfortable around boys and their teasing; and I was named president of a prestigious community organization.

For the party honoring me and the new board, Peter promised to come but called halfway through the affair to say, "I'm downtown with the Wallaces. Join us when the party's over."

After bidding everyone good-bye with a frozen smile, I drove to the restaurant in a fury, not believing he was there. "You'll never betray me again," I muttered. "Never, ever."

He was there, but my outrage was so strong that I could barely speak until we were driving home. Then I burst out with increasing volume, "Peter, this is it. I can't take it anymore. I'll never let you do this again." I yelled all the way home and into the house.

When I finally calmed down Peter said, "I understand why you're angry. You've sensed something about Tom. You don't know him but he's been my lover for a year."

It also came out that Peter had bought him a car too, just before getting sick. "So that's why he bought me one," I thought, not pleased.

That night we decided that Peter would go live with Tom during the children's Christmas vacation, giving them time to absorb the news at their own pace. After talking with several counselors about how to tell the children, we agreed to state the facts and then explain what they didn't understand.

The night before we told them we rehearsed what Peter would say to allay any fears they might have. After breakfast the next morning we sat at the kitchen table while Peter told them. He ended with, "I'm moving out today to live with Tom."

"I just knew it!" Courtney said.

Nicolas, who was still distant from his father, accepted the news calmly.

"You'll still live here and go to your school," Peter went on. "I'll be in the city and will see you a lot. I want you to know that this has nothing to do with you and that I love you both very much. I'll talk about whatever you want and answer any questions you have."

Neither child had anything to say then or later that morning when Peter talked with them separately. That afternoon the children and I flew to New York to visit Peter's parents.

Peter called them there later that week. "I want to see you when you get home. There's a fair coming to town. Want to go?"

"Oh yes! We want to meet Tom."

After a successful day at the fair the children began spending weekends with Peter and Tom and went out to dinner with Peter during the week. The four of them also went on long vacations together with as little interference from me as possible.

Once I began talking to friends about Peter, feelings I had repressed for four years started bubbling up. I realized that his rejection of me, not his gayness, was the problem. "Being gay is the same as whether you have green or blue eyes," I explained to the children, friends and family. "There's no choice."

In September I went back to work to keep occupied while the children were in school. Soon my salary was needed to supplement Peter's fluctuating income. Divorce now seemed impossible since the house was collateral for many of his projects.

Every morning I left for the bus before six to be home early enough to drive the children to after-school sports where I cheered them on. They were both straightforward kids, tomboy Courtney and stalwart Nicolas, and they played every sport, every season.

The first year neither of the children wanted to talk about what was happening even when asked what they thought or felt. I told their teachers that we had separated but not why and asked them to call me if they noticed any behavior changes. Since both of them worked diligently at school, their teachers never called. Their grades went up.

When Courtney turned eleven she grew taller and more attractive and became aware of her sexuality. Although she was going through puberty, she remained even-tempered at home and she never fought with her many friends. She was a model child.

Unlike Courtney, Nicolas was angry, usually at me. Every problem was Mom's fault, like the broken shoe laces on his track shoes. "You should have known they might break! Why didn't you have an extra pair?"

Since this was much like Peter's way of relating to me, I had to concentrate on what Nicolas was doing in order not to react to the "Peter buttons" he pushed.

During the first summer after his father left he played with only a few friends. By fall he had withdrawn completely and was angry with all of his friends.

The second month of school his teacher called. "Allison, I don't think Nickie will complete second grade."

We located a psychiatrist and Nicolas went weekly, complaining all the way. He never said what went on but the psychiatrist reported to us every six weeks. Soon he appeared happier and resumed friendships and was promoted to third grade.

Meanwhile Peter was trying to mend his rift with him, but Nicolas no longer wanted to do things with his father no matter how great the activity. For the next two years he didn't even talk about Peter.

Courtney, by then in junior high, did talk about Peter and told a couple of good friends he was gay.

"So what?" they said.

Some months later the son of family friends, mad at Courtney for spurning him, went around telling their friends, "Courtney's father is a homosexual."

Again, the reaction was, "So what?"

By ninth grade Courtney had grown to nearly six feet, a stunning beauty whose slenderness was set off by the stylish clothes Peter bought. She was on the honor roll, all teams and the student council. Yet by February when we three visited Peter's parents, she was a teary-eyed, touchy teenager who snapped at everyone.

"Should I pay attention to this?" I asked myself, "Or quit worrying and let her be fourteen?"

Still anxious on our return, I told Courtney my observations.

"Oh, Mom, I feel so unhappy. But I don't know what about."

For the next few weeks, she would sleep every minute she could for several days and then would be up half the night crying for several days. "School isn't good. Sports aren't good," she said. "It's not Dad. I don't know what it is." She didn't want professional help and I didn't want to force it on her.

That spring she applied to a more demanding academic school in the city with my encouragement, hoping that a change of environment would help.

Two months later Courtney was working at a hot dog stand for a weekend track event. Suddenly her senses started to go, one by one. When her breathing stopped, a friend called 911.

On the way to the emergency room, the paramedics tried to read her vital signs. Courtney remembered floating near the ceiling, watching the scene below. "This girl's going!" one cried. "We're losing her. I can't get a heartbeat or blood pressure."

By the time the hospital called me Courtney had regained consciousness. A co-worker rushed me over to the hospital.

The examining doctor met me and said, "We insisted that Courtney must be on drugs, but she kept denying it. The blood test proved she wasn't lying. What she has is a circulatory problem linked with her menstrual cycle. Nothing can prevent a recurrence, although a high protein diet might help."

When our pediatrician confirmed the diagnosis the next day, he added, "This condition might be psychologically induced."

That Saturday Courtney came into my bedroom before going to sleep. "Mom, if my head's creating this problem, let's do something about it. I'd better see a counselor."

Starting in September she went by bus after school three times a week to a psychologist who specialized in counseling teenagers. Sandy was beautiful, intelligent and married with a young child, a good role model for a teenage girl.

For six months Courtney insisted that she wasn't angry. Then Sandy asked Nicolas and me to come to a session with Courtney. "I don't care that Dad's gay," Courtney explained. "His leaving me is what matters and his drinking. I was so close to him! I was Dad's girl and Nickie was Mom's boy. When Dad left I had nobody. That's why I did everything right at school because I was afraid I would lose Mom too if I screwed up. I kept thinking, 'What if he never calls me again and doesn't even take me to the movies on Sundays?'"

As she talked I thought, "This poor child must have feared offending me too, since our relationship was so tenuous. She lived in terror until she blew up!"

Describing the stereotypical gay mannerisms Peter put on when he was drunk, Courtney said, "I'm so embarrassed. He isn't the same person any more!"

Sandy, the psychologist, asked Peter to meet with her next. He went three times and each time denied his alcoholism.

As Courtney began to face her problem, Nicolas, eleven, developed a volatile personality. His main complaint was that his sister got her way all the time. "I'm always picked on and ignored," he said. "I never get new things."

By then Courtney was creating quite a stir. Even more beautiful, she still excelled in sports and her studies, a tough act to follow in the best of times. Though Nicolas was natively brighter, he rarely worked in school. So he picked on Courtney, being the peacemaker who didn't fight back.

Then Courtney began having trouble again. Sandy called to warn me, "Allison, watch Courtney carefully. There's a suicide possibility here."

A week later Courtney was riding with an unlicensed friend in her parents' BMW on a rain-slick street when they were hit. Just as the passenger side was demolished, Courtney was thrown into the back seat unhurt. She hadn't fastened her seat belt.

Her concentration level at school had dropped to zero. If she studied an hour before an exam, she remembered nothing an hour afterward.

After a few weeks, I said, "I'm going to call the dean of students to tell him what's going on."

"Thank you," she answered quietly.

After describing her suicidal behavior to the dean, I said, "I'd like her teachers to know but not to talk to her about it or do her any favors."

"Fine. I'll tell them and call if there's a problem."

After seven months with Sandy, Courtney admitted that she was angry with Peter for deserting her. "I was so mad at him," she told me that night, "that I wouldn't let myself be satisfied with anything." After a pause, her brow furrowed, she said, "I can't believe I denied my anger all this time."

Courtney had another realization about her father her junior year. One Sunday she called me from Peter's house about some problem. That night at home she remarked, "I just noticed I didn't tell Dad my problem before calling you. Guess my best friend is my mother."

She also had a boyfriend, Robb, a tall, sensitive senior.

About this time, Nicolas started to give away favorite mementoes to his friends, one by one. Concerned, I suggested he might like to talk to Sandy.

"Absolutely not."

"It looks like you're finishing business with your friends and I want to know what's going on."

"Okay, I'll go."

The afternoon of his appointment I came home early to drive him in. He was doing homework at his desk. Courtney also happened to be home.

"Time to go," I said.

"I'm not going," Nicolas announced, clinging to his desk chair.

Courtney, hearing this, came to his door. Together we picked up the desk chair with Nicolas attached and carried it to the car. When he realized that we intended to put him in the car no matter what, he got in himself.

All the way over to Sandy's he was screaming, "Why are you making me do this when you know I don't want to talk to Sandy? I won't get out of the car. You're a horrible person! You've always hated me!" His face was scarlet and he began to lose his voice.

Trying not to react and focusing on the rush hour traffic, I kept saying, "Nickie, I love you. I'm afraid. I love you."

Just as we came upon the first vista of the city skyline against the fall sunset, Nicolas suddenly stopped screaming and said, "Isn't that gorgeous?"

"Yes," I said weakly.

We drove the rest of the way in silence and he went into Sandy's office quietly.

After the session Sandy took me aside. "You were right to bring him in. Now just keep an eye on him."

Later that winter Nicolas was talking with friends on the playground after school one day when an older boy, Hal, shouted, "Hey! Did you know Nickie's dad is gay?"

The children standing next to him said, "What a jerk! Who cares?" His best chum didn't even respond. But Nicolas was upset. When one of his friends got home and told his mother what had happened, they returned to the playground, found Nicolas hysterical and brought him home. They stayed until he calmed down. His friend was still there when I came home.

Nicolas didn't want to go to school the next day so I offered to drive him.

"Mom, I'm so afraid. I don't want my friends to hate me."

"See if you can go to school knowing it's Hal's problem," I said. "He seems to think so little of himself that he makes others look bad in order to look better. Ignore him. Your classmates will. If you don't let on that it upsets you, nothing will happen."

"I'll try."

As we drove to school I said, "If the worst should happen, I'll pick you up after school so you don't have to be alone."

No one said a word about it to him that day or since. Nor did he ever mention the subject to any of his friends.

Five months later Sandy called me. "Nickie's very angry with his father over the desertion, but for now I think he can work some of it out by himself."

During Courtney's senior year, Robb's family invited her to go with them to the Caribbean at Christmas. It sounded like a great idea and I decided to give her this trip as a combined Christmas and birthday present. Courtney asked Peter about it the next time he was at the house.

"I'd rather have you with me for Christmas," he said.

"Why do you say that?" I asked.

"Kids should be home at Christmas. My parents would like it."

"No, Peter, those kinds of arguments don't fly here."

He replied, "Kids have a duty to be home and we ought to insist."

"She lives here and I'm not insisting. So why should you?"

The following Friday night Courtney and I discussed the trip while Peter and Nicolas went out to dinner. When they returned Nicolas went off to study. Peter, pouring himself a drink, joined Courtney and me in the kitchen.

"Courtney can go," he announced, "the day after Christmas."

"It doesn't make sense," I said, "to fly alone a week later just so she can spend four hours of Christmas Eve with you. I've decided she's going when Robb's family goes and coming home when they come home. You're pressuring her unreasonably."

"I want her home because next year I might not be here."

"What did you say?"

"I may be dead."

"My goodness!" I cried. "What do you mean?"

"I was exposed two years ago to someone who has died of AIDS."

"Do you have it?"

"No," he answered, "I've tested negative and I'm well, but six or seven years after exposure it can appear."

Courtney ran out of the room.

I began screaming. "You don't have the disease! I could just as well say, 'Gee, I might get hit by a car crossing the street so I'm not going to work any more.' Peter, give me a break!"

He yelled back. "You're being flip about a serious thing."

"I'm sorry you've been exposed, but you will not use it to make your children's lives miserable. I won't stand for it. You're using what might happen as blackmail. How dare you!"

"But I haven't done anything!" he shouted.

"You've just said that you had sex with someone who had AIDS."

At that, Peter grabbed the garbage can and went out the door.

When he didn't return I went out to see what had happened. The front door was open, garbage strewn all over the walk and his car gone. Angrily picking up the garbage, I became frightened. "He's going to drive over a cliff or run into a tree on purpose."

Just then Courtney and Nicolas ran out, Nicolas crying, "He's probably going to kill himself. Let's follow him."

As we tore down the street in the car I thought, "This isn't rational." Aloud I was saying, "I'm so angry. I'm so angry."

The children were saying, "Relax, Mom. Calm down."

At the corner I turned back realizing it was a foolish exercise. Once home Nicolas and Courtney went to their rooms and I called Tom and asked him to let me know if Peter returned.

A half hour later Tom called. "Peter's coming up the steps and he's in one piece. So you can quit worrying about him."

As I hung up Robb appeared in the doorway. "Courtney called twenty minutes ago. She was upset and didn't make sense so I came over."

While Robb talked to Courtney I went into Nicolas' room and talked with him about AIDS until he fell asleep.

When I checked in on Courtney, Robb had calmed her down. Robb asked me to tell him about homosexuality. Sitting on Courtney's bed I explained it to him for about an hour—that it's something some people are born with and which cannot be changed and that it has nothing to do with being a good or bad person.

What I didn't talk about was my apprehension about the effects of Peter's gayness on Courtney's attitude toward men, or my own terror of being rejected by another man. Nor did I speak of my anger over Peter's alcoholism, his unwillingness to deal with it and his irrational stance on AIDS. Nor my fear that Courtney and Nicolas might follow in their mother's footsteps and enter into a dysfunctional relationship out of low self-esteem. After all, Peter's gayness itself has never been the central issue.

Your Mother Cared
Grant

Coming out of an eleven-year marriage in the early eighties, I transferred to Manhattan to a good position which paid well. Most of the people in the office were single, divorced or separated, and without children. After work a group of us would go out for a drink but there was no further involvement. It was a great life for a single, attractive man in his late thirties.

That's how I got to know Karen. Ten years younger, pretty with auburn hair, she'd left her husband two years earlier. Mentioning being battered, she sounded gutsy. I felt sorry for her because she'd had to leave her two-year-old son, Cal, behind because she couldn't support him.

That spring I applied to law school, deciding that I didn't want to move up the ladder at work. Karen and I started dating and soon we were in love.

Karen moved into my place just when her parents were in town and they stayed with us. I hit it off with them, especially her mother, Shirley.

I started law school that fall and Karen filed for divorce. When she phoned her father to tell him, I could hear him yelling, "How could you, and give up your son?"

Again I was struck at how gutsy she was, standing up to him. Yet she loved her father and all of her family. One of five children, she talked often about their dinner table conversations and holiday get-togethers.

The eldest of three, I wasn't close to my brother and sister. At seventeen I'd left school to join the army because my folks had trouble supporting all of us. My parents were not high school graduates, but they came to my graduation to accept my diploma for me.

That Christmas Karen invited me to join her family gathering in Syracuse and I found out for the first time what fun it was to be part of a close family.

In February Karen enrolled in a financial planning course, so we both had to go to school after work. By the end of the year we were grating on each other. She was always saying, "Oh, Grant, I'm sorry. I'm sorry"—not so gutsy, after all. She did everything alone, unlike me who liked to do things with others. Complaining that I didn't communicate, she suggested that we go to counseling.

"Sure," I said, thinking, "Let's help Karen."

I stopped after a few sessions. Karen continued and began talking more about how much she valued family. By December when her mother was planning a family reunion for Christmas, she brought up the topic of marriage, something we hadn't wanted.

"Well," I said, "what about it? Will you marry me?"

"Oh, yes, Grant," she answered, hugging me.

At the Christmas reunion everyone toasted us around the tree. Back home we had a small wedding in Karen's community church.

For the next two years we both worked and went to school. Karen brought in less than I paid in taxes. When my courses ended I took leave to study for the bar which I passed just as Karen finished her course work. To celebrate we took off in a recreational vehicle to tour the States for several months.

While on our trip we decided to quit our jobs and fulfill our dreams, hers to be a caterer and mine to be a trust lawyer. "It won't be the same money," we agreed, "but we'll enjoy what we have more." There was also my savings, stocks and pension.

We rented a cottage in White Plains and Karen began work in a delicatessen Tuesday through Saturday at below minimum wage. That Thanksgiving two of her co-workers, Rose and Joline, joined us. Neither woman appealed to me, especially Rose, who dressed like a ragamuffin, smoked, used drugs and swore a lot. But I thought, "They're Karen's friends. It's up to her."

For a year we talked about having a baby. The next spring Karen said, "Grant, I've been reading the statistics on birth defects and the mother's age. It's now or never."

She was pregnant by summer. We each dreamed that it would be a girl and after much deliberation decided to call her "Heather." We both went to birthing classes and doctor visits where, thrilled, I heard the baby's heartbeat. Then Karen decided to use midwife assistants with a backup doctor if needed.

Three months into her pregnancy, Karen, along with Rose and Joline, filed an equal rights discrimination grievance with the deli and left. She found another job closer to the city working late hours to make breakfast and brunch specialties. As time went on her work hours were scheduled later and later at night.

"Well," I thought, wearily, "if she likes it, I'll put up with it." At this time my savings and stock sales paid the rent since free-lance legal work didn't bring in much more than Karen's salary, now barely above the minimum wage.

In late March after a false alarm, Karen went into labor and we went to the hospital's alternative birthing room with its two beds, cradle, couch, wallpaper and stereo. I had my camera ready.

Suddenly Karen cried, "It's coming!" Since it was earlier than predicted, the assistants called in the emergency room doctor. Karen pushed once, twice, and out popped the baby into the doctor's arms. Snapping a picture, I yelled, "It's Heather!"

When Karen and Heather came home, aunts and Grandmother Shirley flew in to see the baby, who slept in a cradle beside our bed. Cal, Karen's son, came too, as a surprise. When Karen saw him peek in the door she started crying. Then they hugged and cried some more. Shirley stayed for the christening, performed by a woman minister in the church where we'd married four-and-a-half years before.

When Heather was three months old Karen went back to her late night shift. Weekdays she went to bed at eight and I about eleven. She left at two in the morning for work and I arose at six to take the baby to the sitter's. Karen picked her up at two.

"With my weird hours," Karen said one Sunday while we were out driving with the baby, "I can't see any of my friends except Rose, since she has the same crazy schedule."

Rose worked and lived in the Bronx, not too far away. She and Karen jogged afternoons and talked on the phone after supper, while Heather nursed and I watched TV or worked at my desk. Soon, Karen was taking the phone into the bedroom to talk with Rose, who sometimes called after eight causing Karen to lose an hour's sleep and be irritable the next day.

When the phone bill arrived I confronted Karen. "Every day you call the Bronx for almost an hour. You've racked up twenty-five dollars worth! You see Rose every afternoon, so what's left to say? What are you whispering when I go by the door?"

Karen looked startled.

"I'm telling any caller after eight that you're in bed," I yelled. "I'm tired of taking the brunt of it the next day."

The calling slacked off a bit. Instead whenever Karen had to work late, she asked if she could spend the night at Rose's.

"Sure," I said. "This way I'll know you're getting an hour's extra sleep. You aren't getting enough."

Because of Karen's hours we didn't make love often. One night that fall when we did, I was surprised by how smooth it was. Always before after a lapse of several months, it was a bit awkward. This time it was as if we'd been having sex every two days. "Has she been with somebody else?" I wondered. Then I laughed, "How could she, with work and seeing Rose all the time?" But something in the back of my mind said, "Make note of this, Grant." I feared pursuing it further.

A week later we were invited to a Halloween party. Karen asked to go separately. "Rose will take me and Heather."

"Sure! What time?"

"About seven. Would it be okay if I stayed the night with her since I have an early order?"

"No problem, if she'll let you."

By the time I arrived at the party Karen was there with Rose and Joline. Since I was driving I didn't drink. About 9:30 P.M., well past Heather's bedtime, I gathered up her and the diaper bag and left. At home an hour later, opening the bag, I found Karen's keys. "Damn. Now she can't get home or go to work."

I called Rose's. No answer. "Strange," I thought. "She said they'd leave the party by ten o'clock."

Once Heather was in bed I called again. Still no answer. Then I called the deli where Karen worked. No answer. In case I'd missed them at Rose's, I called there once more. As the phone rang and rang, I recalled another time when Rose hadn't answered because she was mad at Joline. "Oh-h-h," I groaned. "I'll have to drive there."

It was midnight when Heather and I arrived. Karen's car was parked where she'd left it after work. I rang the doorbell with Heather in my arms. When no one came after a couple of minutes, I peered in the front window to see if Karen was asleep on the couch. She wasn't. "Odd," I thought. "Well, she's probably in the back room." Starting around the house, I noticed a couple of cops on the corner. "Oh, oh!" I whispered to Heather and hurried to the car.

I drove out to the deli. Since it was still locked up I used the pay phone to try Rose's once again. Still no answer. "She's got to be there!" I muttered and drove back over to Rose's.

Lugging the sleeping kid in my arms up to the door, I rang the bell over and over, getting more and more ticked.

Then that little voice in the back of my mind said, "Go look in the window." Fearing what might be there, I didn't. But the voice said, "Make note of it anyway," as I unlocked Karen's car, put the ignition key in the glove compartment, placed the door key in Rose's mailbox and drove home. It was now 1:30 A.M.

The next morning when I called Karen at work, she said that they thought it was Joline ringing the bell.

"What would have happened if I'd needed to get ahold of you because something had happened to Heather?"

"God! I didn't think of that."

"Well, look in Rose's mailbox. Next time come get the keys yourself." I was beginning to resent Karen's inconvenient schedule.

That Christmas Karen's church held its annual potluck and dance. Though I didn't want to go, we went anyway and brought Heather too. I didn't like to dance so Karen danced with Rose since there weren't enough men to go around. Then it was time to take Heather home.

Outside Karen said, "Oh, I've got to tell Rose something."

"You just saw her two seconds ago."

"Yes, but I forgot something."

As she went back to the church hall I strapped Heather in the car seat, hearing that funny voice inside say, "Go look." But I didn't want to leave Heather alone or carry her with me.

Over the next few weeks Rose drove out from the Bronx occasionally to go to a movie with Karen or a spa Karen had discovered with a group from church or a local tavern.

Then one night Karen said, "I'm thinking of going on the church retreat this weekend to think about things."

"Oh?" I said, scared. "She's thinking divorce," I thought, "I won't let it happen. I've seen too many broken families."

The next day I sent Karen a bouquet of roses with a note: "I know things haven't been going well. I'll do anything to change but don't know how to start. I need your help. Let's talk. I know we can work this out." Since we were both coming down with a flu bug, I figured this might tip the scales to make her stay home.

She called when she arrived home from work. "Thanks for the beautiful flowers! I'm leaving now for the retreat. See you."

As the weekend went on I decided between nausea bouts that we had to get counseling. "We have to hold the family together."

Since Karen didn't say much when she returned Sunday night I thought, "O.K., I'll bring it up next weekend."

The next Saturday Karen had dinner at Rose's to talk about what to do. At midnight Rose drove up with Karen in the front seat.

"I drank too much and fell asleep so Rose had to drive," Karen said, stumbling in the door. Her eyes were red and puffy.

"Well, have you decided what you're going to do?"

"Let's talk tomorrow," she said and shuffled to the bedroom.

On Sunday as we drove to the city to visit friends with Heather in the back seat, I asked, "Well, what have you decided?"

"I'm going to leave."

"Leave? Why?"

"We aren't getting along. You don't communicate." She rattled on about things that didn't warrant that drastic a move.

In between her reasons I kept saying, "Give me a chance."

"You've had a chance," she said finally.

"How could I have had a chance if I didn't know I was being given one? I'll make any deal if only you'll stay."

"No, I've decided."

"Where will you go?"

"I could go to Rose's."

When Rose came to help Karen move on Friday I said, "Gee, thanks for letting Karen stay with you while she's going through this."

Sunday, I asked Karen to dinner on Monday. Taking off from work early, I bought Cornish game hens to stuff, vegetables for the kind of salad she liked, wine and candles. While Heather slept we had a nice dinner with lots of talk.

Then as Karen put on her coat to leave, I said, "Let's try to work things out. Come back. Give me another chance."

"No, Grant, I'm still leaving."

Once the door closed behind her I began to cry.

Every day that week when Karen came to take Heather to the sitter's and then to bring her back, I asked her to return.

When I asked on Friday she said, "No, I couldn't go to bed with you again."

"Who's talking about that? I'm talking about saving this family and making it work for Heather. I'll sleep on the couch."

That weekend I decided to write Heather a letter about her birth nine months earlier. It was important to put my positive feelings down right away as if Karen and I were still together so Heather would know her mother cared.

By then Karen had told her mother Shirley that she was leaving me. Shirley called Karen immediately. "I'll give you a year's salary to spend time with Grant and Heather so you can work things out."

Meanwhile one of Karen's church friends I'd asked for advice said, "She mentioned communication problems. Why not see a psychiatrist?"

Starting on Heather's first birthday in March, I saw a psychiatrist two or three times a week until October. "The faster you get to know me," I told her, "the faster you can help me get my wife back. Ask whatever you want. I'll hold nothing back."

I used up half her tissue box the first session. At the fourth session I said, "Maybe I drove her into being gay or something."

"Why do you say that?"

After describing our lovemaking incident the previous fall and the car keys incident after the Halloween party, I said, "I never followed up on these things until now."

In April Karen began to share Heather's care and Shirley came to visit. She stayed with me since my house had more room.

One night as we were having tea in the kitchen, Shirley said, "I told Karen that I'd watch Heather to give her more time with you. I also told her to get a decent day job to have a normal life with her family. But she said, 'No. No. No.' "

Shirley continued, "I told her there were only three reasons why she'd leave you: one, she has a terminal disease and wants to alienate everyone; two, she's had a nervous breakdown and doesn't know what's going on; or three, she's gay. She said, 'No,' to the first two and nothing to the third."

"Well, that's Karen!" I said, thinking she'd found the third reason too ridiculous to answer.

Over the next month my work went downhill but communication with Karen improved. "It took nine months for you to decide to leave," I told her one night. "I'm going to try at least that long to win you back."

Karen's son Cal came to visit that summer. I liked watching him and Heather play together with her toys.

Shirley visited again too, staying with me. One day Karen asked her to come to the Bronx to meet someone. Shirley took the train in and I agreed to pick her up. At dinner time she called to say that she'd take the train back and catch a taxi home.

When she arrived at midnight I'd just finished Heather's letter, describing her conception, the doctor, the delivery room, her birth and her baptism. My last words were, "We dearly love you and want only the best that we can provide for you."

"Shirley," I said. "I'll make you some tea and you can read Heather's letter to be sure there's nothing negative in it. I'm still hoping Karen will come back, you see."

Shirley read it in the kitchen with loud sobs as I watched TV in the living room. Then she came out, her eyes swollen.

"There's nothing negative, is there?" I asked.

"Oh no! It's very nice, Grant. Good night."

After Shirley left in tears the next day, I cried too. "Do I deserve this?" I asked myself. "I don't fight with Karen. I take care of her. I'm not a heavy drinker or drug addict or chauvinist pig. I was first to battle the company to get a woman in a top position. What's the real reason? If it's another man, I don't want to know it. But if I'm really nice to her, maybe he'll go away."

Six months after Karen left I told my psychiatrist, "Maybe she's homosexual. But it can't be. I know her."

Three months later Karen asked me to go see her counselor with her. "We'll drive separately," she added. "I don't want to be in the same car with you."

Once we were seated in front of the counselor Karen turned to me. "Grant, I've found myself. I'm gay."

"I thought so," I said, my eyes dry.

After we talked some, the counselor asked how I felt.

"Shitty. What do you think?"

For the next five days I sat in contemplation and cried. Unable to stop shaking, I didn't think I'd last the six days to my next counseling session. My dreams of a happy family were shattering and there wasn't anything I could do about it.

At some point Karen called to suggest that I do some reading about homosexuality. "I don't want to know any more than the little I know already," I thought.

Then I called Shirley, who said the evening she'd spent with Karen was a rap session with her gay group. Karen had told her that she thought she was gay and later told Cal. Shirley had urged her to tell me.

When I saw my psychiatrist, I told her with my eyes averted.

She drew in her breath. "I never suspected."

After the session I decided to read everything available on homosexuality. The only way to fight Karen on her level was to know as much as her.

I felt like I was entering a dirty bookstore when I went to the library. The whole world seemed to be looking over my shoulder, thinking, "Oh, oh! Look at that guy." I snuck around the stacks and used the microfiche reader when no one was around. After finding four books I thought, "Oh! I've got to check them out." Putting the one with "homosexual" in the title on the bottom, I opened it to the date page so the title was hidden. The librarian turned it over anyway, giving me a look as she stamped it. Then I grabbed the books, ran outside, threw them into the trunk and sped away.

The first book I read that night, *Whose Child Cries*, described five gay situations from the child's viewpoint. Turning each page, thinking of Heather, I cried and cried. At one point I even contemplated suicide but knew I could never do that to Heather, sleeping in the next room.

For eight weeks I read these and other books, writing down my thoughts and feelings in a notebook. It seemed like a lifetime. At the end any hope I'd had was gone.

In late September Karen and I met with her counselor to discuss Heather. "Joint custody is fine," I said. "But I won't agree to anything more. When Heather's ready for school, I want you and Rose to move out here so she can come to your place or mine and still go to the same school."

Over the next nine months we worked out a sharing schedule for Heather. Even on Father's Day I had Karen pick her up as usual in order not to change our routine. Karen arrived with a Father's Day card for Heather to give me. As she went out the door she suddenly turned back. "I want to hug you, Grant."

"O.K.," I said, keeping my arms at my sides.

"You know," she smiled, "You're a wonderful father."

"Yeah," I thought, "but a lousy husband." If there were a way to keep Heather and not have to deal with Karen, I'd choose it. But I tried to get along with her so our daughter wouldn't see us fighting.

Yet I feared that a custody fight was inevitable. "If there is," I told myself, "I'll ask for a home investigation to determine what's best for Heather and find a house that is better than hers."

Although I was broke, I started house hunting. Shirley offered to help finance it if necessary. I also advertised for a single mother with toddler to share a three-bedroom place with us, so Heather would grow up with another child and see a man and woman together at the dinner table as a role model.

A woman with three children answered the ad. "Great!" I thought. Then, I caught myself. "Wait a minute! You're helping out women again."

Within three months I had made a down payment on a New England style bungalow with three bedrooms and a front yard in a complex that had a playground and pool. It was a quiet place with plenty of kids in the neighborhood.

Five years earlier I'd have said, "Kids? No way." Now I was elated.

Two years later it is still top priority that Heather have playmates as well as a home with a father who cares.

I Love You, Jeff and Peggy
Frank

We made a perfect family: two rosebud children, Jeff and Peggy, not yet in school, Patty at home cooking up a storm and me at the university, supposedly making straight A's and preparing for my doctoral exams. We had a lot of friends and lived in a lovely apartment in Austin, after six years of temporary "homes" and separations while I was in the army. Making all this possible were the student loans we took out together so that Patty could stay home with the children.

Meanwhile I was being torn up inside, turning papers in late or not at all, running away from difficulty without telling anyone and inventing excuses to maintain my academic image.

Simultaneously, my homosexuality was growing more powerful. I felt confused, pressured and frightened. Any man or woman who's been there knows my pain—an incredible self-doubt, a contradictory yearning. I was too afraid to ask anyone what was going on and felt terribly isolated.

Our second year in Texas I met a man who pulled me across the line of my fear, from wondering to enjoying. Once across, I couldn't go back. Everything in my life became distorted, my judgment cloudy, my behavior erratic. I thought, "Here's this all-American, "Joe College" father having a secret romance with a young man and no one knows."

I learned how to lie, to cheat and be devious, not because I was a bad person but because I feared telling the truth and thereby suffering rejection and loss.

Patty and I could never deal with that truth. I recalled what Dad had said when we'd pushed up our wedding date. "Just as you're the product of your family and our values, Frank, and you can't change it, so Patty's the product of her parents' values and she can't change that. You two are so different in where you come from and how you see the world, marriage is premature."

Although I never opened up to Patty, she knew something was wrong. "I don't like you spending so much time with this friend of yours," she said one night. "It's quality time that you should be spending with us."

I stopped seeing him for the sake of our marriage. It took tremendous self-denial on my part to restore the sense of wholeness in my family life.

On that superficially happy note, our family set off for Germany for my doctoral research and dissertation. Kids in tow and spirits high, Patty and I thought only of my research and the experiences we'd share in Heidelberg.

Then one morning, in the university library, I made eye contact with Emil and life for everyone was never the same.

Young and beautiful, Emil was connected with the world of intellectuals. He was my intellectual equal. He was also gay. In a matter of weeks I was swept away. And Patty was swept under the rug. I'd discovered something greater than my education and family put together: the deep satisfaction of having something I'd always wanted and of moving into a world where everything was right.

Though Emil and I were together every moment I was supposed to be studying, I still gave a lot of time to Peggy, Jeff and Patty, convincing myself that I could live two lives. The children blossomed! Patty was speaking German marvelously. Then we had to move to a remote village for my field research.

By then I couldn't even move without involving Emil, who went with me to prepare the house that friends had lent us. The day Patty and the children arrived by train, he left to return to the city.

For the next four months the family grew closer and we explored a new part of the country. Jeff and Peggy were growing, learning German, attempting to swim and manifesting self-confidence. Patty was radiant, her skin glowing and her hair lustrous as she moved about in colorful Bavarian skirts. I missed Emil but knew I could manage for a while.

In September as my grant was running out, Patty returned to the States with the children so that they could start school. "I have to stay," I told her, "for additional research."

Back in the States Patty had to depend on parents and in-laws in New York and live in a state of waiting as she had during my army days. I returned to Heidelberg to live a gay lifestyle.

Even before Patty and the children left, I missed them deeply! Yet my heart pounded in anticipation of sharing every moment with Emil, of being free. Freedom didn't imply rejection. It meant the freedom to love someone.

My desire to love so overwhelmed me that I couldn't think through the consequences, not because I didn't care or wasn't frightened for Patty and the children and myself and Emil. I didn't know how to think and felt that no one could have helped me. If someone had said, "Get divorced," or, "Move home," I couldn't have done either. I couldn't see that my life needed simplification. Instead I wanted more and more of what I'd found, to wake up nestled against someone I loved without the fear of going home with a lie or an excuse.

Back in New York Patty and the children felt hurt. My mother knew something was terribly wrong with me because I wasn't with my children I loved so much. My brothers and sister, who had suspected my sexuality was confused, figured out why my life wasn't going normally. Out of caring for Patty and the children as well as for me, they talked with her one day about what I might be facing.

When they finished Patty became hysterical. "That's not true! You have no right to interfere in our lives!"

In late August Patty flew to Texas to find us a place to live near Austin and to start Jeff and Peggy in school. Without me, her main emotional support, she sought solace in a conservative church. The minister gave her the order in her life that she felt was missing, a structure that allowed her to make sense of things. Gradually she developed a reality system that included no ambiguity, no doubts, no unresolved matters. Things were to be the way she saw them because that way was right. Once the children were in school she organized a regular schedule for the three of them.

Meanwhile in Germany I was growing further away from who I had been before. I had a sense of wholeness as a man. I was gaining the confidence to express my true identity.

As summer ended my professor said my research time was up. In September I flew to Texas to resume teaching and begin the dissertation.

A very different family was waiting for me, just as a very different Frank was coming home. My hair was long and permed. I wore contact lenses. I was slender now, wearing tailored clothes and tighter pants, much different from the sloppy graduate students around me.

Peggy and Jeff were overjoyed to see me. Patty was shocked by my appearance and what she saw as effeminate behavior. She was angry that she'd carried all the burden of the children and that I'd been away so long.

The next four months were hell. I taught my classes but not well. I avoided responsibilities. I didn't know when I'd see Emil again and recapture the happiness we'd shared.

Because Patty insisted that we go to church I went, wanting to share something important to her on her terms. Her religious involvement over the years hadn't threatened my values in any serious way, although I felt more comfortable in churches in which instead of discussing Christian theology about sin and salvation, the congregation instead talked about the values of love and community with room for ambiguity.

Making a lot of moral compromises, I went to Sunday School and church and acted like a devout father and husband. It was the glue that held together the remaining framework of our crumbling family. In my dutiful role I was in fact, "crawling the walls." What was asked of me was too much for me to handle and I was ready to explode.

Being separated from Emil was part of the problem. Slowly several friends understood what had happened to me but they didn't offer support. Although I needed someone I could turn to, I was terrified to bring up the homosexuality issue with Patty. I feared losing the children because I thought she would be unable to deal with the situation. Then in my confusion, no longer able to deny my sexuality, I began to have casual sex.

In March, through my arrangements, Emil came to Austin for a symposium. Patty acted happy for me because she knew that he was the friend I'd lived with while finishing my research. Although Emil stayed with friends, I went out every night to see him. Every day while I was presumably at the university, I was with him. One by one, everybody close to us saw the reality except Patty.

Emil's part of the symposium was applauded by faculty members, students and intellectuals from the community. Patty, beautiful as always, helped me host the reception afterwards. It was an awkward occasion as I only paid attention to Emil.

The following day when Emil asked me for a commitment, I was like a jellyfish.

"O.K.," he said. "I'll return to Germany next month as planned and wait. If you choose to contact me, I'll come."

The next day I found out that I'd contracted a sexual disease from some casual sex experience during the preceding months.

All along Patty and I had continued to have sex. She was the only woman I'd ever had sex with. Now I'd exposed her to disease! I couldn't hide any longer. There was no escape, no denial left.

That Sunday afternoon I took her for a drive to an outlying part. As we walked along the path that circled the gardens I began. "Patty,

I'm finally going to tell you why everything's been going wrong, why I couldn't answer your questions and why our relationship is so messed up." Then, I looked at her, and for the first time in my life said, "I am gay."

Everything Patty had feared exploded in her face. She fainted right there on the pathway.

As I held her I knew that our confusion and love were over. Years of anguish were lifted from my shoulders. "My door's open now," I thought, "but it's opened a terrible trap for her."

When Patty came to, she asked, "Emil...is he gay, too?"

"Yes."

"Could I have been exposed to a sexual disease?"

"Yes, Patty," I said, "there's a serious possibility."

We went home in shock. Patty was dazed. I was too except I knew that despite the pain I'd caused I could now live my life openly.

Once the children were in bed Patty went to see her dearest friends and I left to be with Emil. Everything then fell apart for the all-American family. Fortunately Patty wasn't infected by my disease, but we didn't know where to turn to get help in saving our marriage and the family.

Our friends became angry at me for my treatment of Patty and told her to get rid of me. Our pediatrician encouraged us to think of the children's best interests. "Lots of people work out arrangements to maintain family appearances, letting each partner dally on the side. You can be discreet in our town." But even if we had decided to do this, we would still have had to face our communication problems. This was something our pediatrician couldn't help us work out.

Next we went to Patty's minister. This time I needed his help to gain stability.

Once he heard our story he said, "Frank, homosexuality is a sinful abomination and a medical pathology. If you want to save your marriage, be forgiven by Christ and not go to hell, you'll have to renounce your homosexuality and cure this sickness. The only way to overcome something this powerful is by electroshock therapy."

I was horrified! The idea of someone burning my body to force me to give up everything that I wanted, that I was! "How terrifying,"

I thought, "to condemn someone in Jesus' name for wanting to be honest with himself and his family!"

That night Patty and I stopped sleeping together. The next morning Jeff and Peggy asked why I was asleep on the couch. We didn't know what to tell them since we hadn't made any decisions about the future. Patty wasn't interested in counseling and I clung to the fantasy that something might work out peacefully. Emil hadn't left yet and hovered on the side.

Patty gave me an ultimatum within the month. "Frank," she said, "totally renounce your homosexuality or move out."

The next day I went to see the university psychiatrist. He listened and finally said, "Do you want to be gay?"

"Yes, I do. I want to be gay."

And that was that. I'd acknowledged who I was and accepted the fact of beginning a new life. All the years of hiding from myself and Patty, all my fear, denial and suffering came to an end. Yet with the joy of liberation came pain and a sense of loss.

Within the week Patty said, "The only thing for you to do now is to move out as soon as possible."

So we had to tell Jeff and Peggy. Sitting at the table after dinner that night we said, "Mommy and Daddy are going to get divorced. We don't love each other the way we did, but we'll always love you."

The two ran from the table to their rooms and then back to us, saying, "No! No! No!" and holding onto us tightly. Then we were all crying.

It was the end of Patty's and my journey together over fifteen years. Yet I knew that as parents we shared a bond too deep to be broken by any legal institution.

Patty felt like a spurned woman who had been betrayed. She'd been doing right and I'd been doing wrong. That was her view and it was shared by many of our friends, some members of her family and the church. All of the insecurities, intolerance and fear that I'd noticed in her over the years surfaced to protect herself and the children. This isn't said to condemn Patty because I accept her for who she is.

When we separated Emil went back to Germany. He was to return once my life stabilized or I'd go there so that we could finally live together. Soon my going abroad as an unemployed graduate student was out of the question in the face of Patty's monetary needs for her and the children.

Trying to work out an amicable divorce settlement was difficult since there was a climate of intolerance toward homosexuality due to Anita Bryant's anti-gay crusade. The local court staff also included a known homophobic. I finally hired a young attorney and desperate to end the fighting signed away my life and chances for a reasonable scale of living.

Besides receiving a cash settlement Patty kept all of the valuables, furniture and car. In addition to her attorney fees, I was to pay hundreds of dollars a month in child support, the children's health and life insurance and payments toward the student loans that we had co-signed. Finally Patty received custody of the children, although I was awarded unrestricted visitation rights with certain holidays that we would share on an alternating basis.

Through the end of the academic year I saw Peggy and Jeff daily, driving them on errands, baby-sitting, taking them out, sharing dinners with Patty—anything to stay as close to them as possible and show how much I loved them.

Meanwhile Patty was impatient for me to get a job so that she'd have the support to finish college and gain more security than she had with my graduate school stipend. This meant finding a job in a city that offered higher salaries in my field than Austin. In August I moved to Chicago to work on a federally funded project, thereby relinquishing the hope of ever finishing my dissertation.

When I left Jeff was seven, an energetic, happy and loving child. Peggy was almost five, a red-headed jewel with a sweet temper. I felt they were forever my children and that I'd been with them long enough to instill the values of love and kindness, playfulness and sharing.

Although I only had three hundred dollars a month left after paying child support and loans, I scraped together enough cash to visit Texas and see the children, my friends and Patty that fall. Patty was dating a fellow named George, a pleasant, proper person who was defensive of her, fine with the children and noncommittal toward me.

Later that winter Emil joined me and we have been together the ten years since, outlasting my marriage to Patty.

A year after my move Jeff and Peggy began to say, "We don't want to come to Chicago." Sometimes they had legitimate reasons, like missing camp. Other times their excuses were flimsy, like fearing flying even though they'd taken long flights before.

When they came they always had a delightful time. We visited the Museum of Science and the Art Institute in the spring, walked along the lake in the winter cold and the balmy summer and saw the expanse of the city from the Sears Tower. When they got home, even as they were writing me effusive letters about the visits, Patty said that they spoke only of the plane trip.

When Jeff and Peggy were with me, Patty wrote them and they found gifts or notes or prayers hidden in their suitcases. She was there all the time, never completely releasing them to me.

The next thing I knew they started calling George "Daddy" and me "Frank." They stopped sending me Easter and Halloween cards or even birthday and Father's Day cards.

When I asked why they said, "We don't have money for a stamp."

I was sending several hundred dollars a month in child support and there wasn't enough money for a stamp! Gradually they stopped writing altogether.

Soon each time visitations came up, Peggy and Jeff said, "We don't want to go."

Patty said, "If you don't want to see your father, tell him."

When they expressed reluctance to come for their next Christmas visit Patty told me, "You can't make us do it, Frank. They don't want to and I'm not going to force them against their will."

Several things were contributing to their resistance. But primarily it was because Patty saw me as a threat to her fragile security. She'd pieced together what was left of her life to have the kind of lifestyle I'd never been able to give them. She and George bought new cars and a new house. He was devoted to going to church with her and the children.

I was no longer welcome in my children's lives. I was barred from seeing Peggy's and Jeff's counselors or teachers to find out how they were doing. My mother and Patty's mother were prevented from meeting. I wasn't allowed to contact any of her relatives. The children never saw the Baker side of the family. The lines were drawn tighter and tighter until I was effectively cut off from my children.

I was too far away and too poor to take legal action against Patty. Instead thousands of dollars went out for plane tickets whenever there was an opportunity for the kids to visit our meager but happy Chicago apartment. Then I was transferred to Philadelphia.

The move compounded all the problems of visitation. The first time I invited Jeff and Peggy they said that they didn't want to come. When I insisted, Patty told them to fight. They didn't come.

The next year the children's stepfather signed on with a company in Detroit much closer to me. This promised easier access, cheaper flights, more visits. I was exhilarated.

They were not. The message was, "We want less. Just bug off."

Since my business took me to Detroit regularly I saw them anyway. While Patty and the children fussed and fidgeted, I visited with the kids out of rental cars and ran them around like a baby-sitter. When I called their new school to see how they were doing, I was told that their records were in their stepfather's name as their legal father. This was against the court decree.

Visits became more regular the next year although each was like pulling teeth. When Jeff and Peggy went with me to my mom's in New York, they were well-behaved but wouldn't let me touch them. They never said, "I love you." They never called me "Daddy."

Several months later they came to Philadelphia, saw the Liberty Bell, ate our food, stuck their noses in the air and then flew home. Seeing my little babies act so rude and unappreciative hurt and confused me.

Emil criticized me for acting like the rich uncle who entertained them twice a year for a couple of days. Other friends said, "It isn't Patty's responsibility to remind the children that you exist. You've got a role in their lives to influence who they are." But I didn't know how to father except to send money every month.

Feeling discouraged and abused after two years of this, I began to go to a gay married men's support group. The group became close friends. They held me together, held me up and simply held me. They gave me belief in myself, helped me affirm the contributions I was making to my children and encouraged me to fight for my rights as their father.

Throwing down the gauntlet, I reduced my next child support check by twenty percent. By then I was working two jobs, but Emil and sometimes my mother often had to help me cover child support, loan repayments, insurance and plane tickets.

The following week the sheriff walked into my project office and came straight to my desk with a summons that stated I was in contempt of court for violating the divorce decree. I found an attorney in Detroit who set up an initial meeting with the judge. The judge said that Patty and I were to find a mutually acceptable psychologist for family counseling in which all of us would participate.

The selected psychologist held sessions with various combinations of us five. We all hadn't met together yet when he terminated the process. "The mother has resisted discussing her feelings," he told the judge, "particularly in sessions with her husband. Her disbelief in counseling and her manipulation of the process has undermined my role in this case."

The trial took place in the spring. George's testimony was key. Speaking of "Mr. Baker's lifestyle," he said, "I just wish he didn't exist. Life would be easier for us if he weren't alive."

When the psychologist came to the stand, the judge reminded him, "You're responsible to the court to share whatever you in your professional judgment believe is relevant to the case."

"I found a few answers," the psychologist said, "It was hard to get cooperation." After reporting on the children, George and me, he continued, "The mother seems to be deeply conflicted, over-protective of her children, quick to judge, slow to forgive and still at an unresolved stage, experiencing strong emotions toward her former husband. Because these emotions aren't resolved," he concluded, "no other family issue can be effectively resolved."

At those words Patty shrieked, "That's not true!"

The courtroom came apart. The trial was adjourned until the next day.

The rest of the trial went as expected. Patty's lawyer tried to discredit my lifestyle, while I described the rather mundane goings on around my house: "I go to my job, do the dishes, clean house, go shopping, do the laundry."

Several months later the court made its ruling. Monthly payments were reduced to the amount I wanted. Then the judge stated, "The father's rights have been violated. He is entitled to unrestricted visitation, provided he discusses visits in advance with the children and lets them participate in decisions about when and where visitations take place. They will alternate Christmas, Thanksgiving and Easter holidays between the mother and father and spend a substantial amount of time with the father in the summer."

The following summer I invited Peggy and Jeff to Philadelphia. Lo and behold, they didn't want to come. Patty said she wouldn't make them and would stand up against the courts to protect their right not to come if they didn't want to.

Once more I went to the Detroit courthouse, this time to take Patty to court for contempt. When the judge sat Patty, the children and me down in chambers with George sitting in the back, he first addressed Jeff and Peggy. "I do not accept your disregard for the laws and constitution of this state and the legal processes of the courts."

Turning to Patty he said, "It's your responsibility to ensure that the children comply fully to Frank's right to visitation."

Then he looked the children in the eye and said, "I never want to see you in this room again. You have responsibilities and rights and a father who loves you. The court has spoken."

Then, from the back of the room, came the stepfather's voice.

"Hey! What about AIDS?"

"Silence!" the judge roared. "You are totally out of order."

For the next year I didn't return to Detroit and rarely communicated with Patty. She never sent me copies of the children's school progress reports or samples of their work.

Jeff and Peggy came to visit me. It was the best period we ever had. They came for Easter, two weeks that summer, Christmas week, the following summer, and Thanksgiving. When it was my turn for Easter again they said, "No."

I let it go. Instead Emil and I decided to go to the Upper Peninsula of Michigan and stop in Detroit for a day on the way home. When I wrote Peggy and Jeff about the plan, they said they couldn't see me because they were leaving to see their aunts that day and couldn't delay their departure. That hurt. Yet it had been only four months since I'd seen them and Detroit was their turf so I didn't pursue it.

Emil and I camped and hiked for two weeks in March, full of vitality. It was the honeymoon we'd never had. We came back on March 25. On April 3 I was diagnosed with AIDS.

By mid-April I had regained my composure enough to tell my parents. By May I felt strong enough to tell my children. Through the principal of Peggy's middle school, I found out when her graduation was scheduled. Well in advance I wrote her to say that since I had business in Detroit then, I wanted to attend the graduation and visit with her and Jeff.

I wrote to Patty simultaneously about the children's expenses.

I'm as concerned about finances as you. Since I have to be in Michigan anyway, it would be a good chance for us to talk privately about money questions related to the children, such as paying for college.

Both letters were unthreatening. Peggy's reply was not. "I don't want you within the state of Michigan during graduation week. I'll be ashamed if you come to my school."

I wrote back calmly stating that I would attend the graduation and wanted to spend time with her and Jeff the following evening. I wrote Patty again also, reiterating the importance of meeting. "If we don't talk," I thought, "it will be her last opportunity."

Next I called Patty's former minister to come to Detroit that weekend to support her after I told her about having AIDS. A month later I was on the plane.

Graduation night I drove to the school and followed the pack of parents to the auditorium. Peggy was standing by the door talking with friends. When she saw me she turned away. I kept walking.

Then the ceremony began. Soon I was the proudest father there. Peggy had tied down every award there was—just like her father— and graduated at the top of her class. Her name was sprinkled all over the program though not once as "Peggy Baker."

The next evening I took her and Jeff to dinner. Jeff was nearly eighteen and so poised that he waved to a friend coming into the restaurant, unconcerned about how to introduce me if his friend came over to the table.

After dinner we drove to Grosse Pointe and walked along the lake. Jeff talked about his college plans. All Peggy wanted to do was skip. So we skipped together.

Then we sat down under a tree in the cool, quiet evening and I began. "I have the most important thing to say that I'm ever going to as your father. First, I want you to know that I've always loved you. Do you understand that I've always loved you?"

"Yes, we understand."

And then I told them. "I have AIDS."

Jeff, his eyes full of tears, put his arms around me. Peggy sat paralyzed, not sure what to do, but understanding now why I had to come to her graduation. After a few minutes she held me too. We stayed a long time in the darkness holding onto each other.

Then we talked about AIDS. Both children seemed calm even when I told Jeff it would be harder financially now for his mom and him to cover college expenses.

"I've been reading a lot," he said, "knowing you're gay. I thought maybe you might get it."

I'd brought along a handbook from the AIDS Foundation, which explained ways families can help each other as well as the patient. Handing it to Jeff but speaking to both of them I said, "Don't be afraid of what it says or what you don't understand. I'll help you find answers if you're willing to ask the questions."

Then I asked, "Do you want to tell your mom or have me do it?"

"We'll tell her."

Then it was time to go. "I might not be here physically much longer," I said, holding them close, "but I'll always be here for you in my love and spirit. As long as my health lasts I'll do everything possible to see you. My home will be open to you as yours."

I drove them back to their house, told them I loved them one more time and watched them go inside. That was the last time I saw them.

Later that night Patty called and in a quiet, meek and secretive voice said, "I don't want anyone else to hear what I'm saying. I wish I could be there to hold you."

By noon the next day her minister described a different Patty. When he'd called to offer support she'd screamed, "How dare you get involved in my family affairs! I don't need or want anybody's support with this!"

"I guess she'd have preferred a letter, saying, 'I'm dying,'" I said. "She doesn't want to be exposed to pain so close at hand."

After that I wrote Patty three times trying to make her see that our reality as parents was changing. "I won't be here forever," I wrote. "My money will run out soon. We must discuss the children's education and insurance."

By the end of June my medical bills totaled several thousand dollars. I wrote Patty again. "To take care of my health, I've got to hoard every penny for when I can't work. So I can't realistically continue child support. Please understand."

She responded by phone. "Frank," she began, "you've gotten what you deserve. This is the consequence of the lifestyle you chose. It's God's punishment."

"This is the mother of my children?" I thought.

Patty was still talking. "This is just one more way to avoid taking care of the children."

I hung up on her. Then when I called back to apologize, she hung up on me. I called again and quickly said, "Before doing anything, take time to cool off, Patty. We share concerns about the children's future and have to plan for it. I've been thinking about a trust fund that could earn enough interest to replenish itself and pay for their college and beyond."

"That's not a good idea. I'll call when I'm ready to discuss it."

Instead of calling she went to court to garnishee my wages.

This time I knew how to find legal support. An attorney referred by the AIDS Foundation wrote me an ironclad will. My former lawyer in Detroit took my case at no cost. The Legal Aid office accepted my case in the "public interest." Many documents were prepared, specifying how many hours I'd been ill and what my medical bills were, doctor by doctor, month by month. Then I became too weak to work and it was a moot point.

"Let it go, Frank," my lawyer said. "There's nothing more she can do. You'll never owe her another penny."

"But what if AZT works for me?"

He smiled. "Frank, she tried to get you when you were dying. She'll probably sue you for surviving. We'll fight that battle when it comes. I'll be here for you."

It's been eight months now since I let the children off at their front door. Since then I've received one note from Peggy saying, "Thank you for my graduation present" and a Christmas card with no return address signed, "Sincerely, Peggy and Jeff." Not a call, not a card, not a message, not a peep.

Afraid to be hurt I've written them only twice. No more fights for me. I've run out of time and energy and purpose. There's no room left for any more tears. May my children realize some day that they are truly richer because I was their father, because I am their father, because I will always be their father!

I love you, Jeff and Peggy. My blessings on you always.

❦   ❦   ❦   ❦   ❦

Three months later Frank's parents, brothers, sister, lover and friends gathered on Chesapeake Bay to celebrate Frank's life, which ended peacefully in a small AIDS hospice. A picture of Peggy, sent a month earlier, stood on his bedside table next to a letter he had just received from Jeff. It read, "I love you. You're always in my prayers."

Balancing Children's and Parents' Issues

Little information is available on how parents can help children understand homosexuality and cope with homophobia. The hope is that the children will continue to think of their gay, lesbian or bisexual parent as the same person who loves and cares for them. With this basic understanding, it will be easier for them to learn how to handle homophobic encounters constructively. The challenge is how to guide them so that gay-related stress becomes grist for growth rather than trauma. In bridging the gay and straight worlds for the children, the straight parent often assumes the major burden, particularly if the gay parent has left the family circle.

Recent media accounts like the documentary, *Not All Parents Are Straight*,[1] suggest that most children of gay and lesbian parents don't feel that having a homosexual parent is a negative factor in their lives. Yet the children and parents interviewed in such presentations are not representative of the whole spectrum. In many cases children experience serious problems ranging from negative psychological and physical reactions to a parent's coming out or separation from the family to the other extreme of resentment towards the straight parent for pressuring them to take sides against the gay parent.

The following concerns appear to be common among children whose parents come out: insecurity because of the parent's "difference" and resultant disruption of the family; confusion about their own sexuality because of the parent's sexual orientation; discomfort with stereotypical mannerisms or the non-conventional lifestyle of the parent; lowered self-esteem from the prejudiced reactions or ridicule of peers; and conflicting loyalty to the parents because of polarized gay-or-straight attitudes in the community or family.

While there is significant literature about children of gay, lesbian and bisexual parents such as the 1986 study of post-adolescent children's recollections of coming to terms with their parents' homosexuality or bisexuality by psychotherapist Jay P. Paul, Ph.D.,[2] as well as *Homosexuality and the Family* by Professor Frederick W. Bozett, R.N., D.N.S.,[3] scant reference is made to the pivotal role of the straight parent in helping the children cope with the crisis.

Without clear guidelines, helping the children deal with gay-related problems may seem daunting, especially to the parent already emotionally overwhelmed. In the coming-out crisis, gay rights are no longer theoretical issues but tangible problems that real families face in an intolerant society.

Parental anxiety can be eased by remembering three axioms: a person's sexual orientation has no bearing on his or her capability as a parent; children's issues are separate from spousal issues and development of a child's healthy self-concept depends upon the love and support of both parents. Keeping these principles in mind can help the straight parent to act in the best interest of the children and to resist the temptation to sever the children's ties to the other parent should the couple relationship become strained or break up.

Five strategies help the straight spouse to be an effective parent and the family to survive the crisis:

- Maintaining the bond to the homosexual or bisexual parent
- Educating the children about homosexuality
- Helping the children cope with homophobia
- Practicing open parent-child communication
- Resolving fears about the effects of the coming out on children.

Maintaining the Bond to the Homosexual or Bisexual Parent

The straight parent's attitude toward the partner is a key factor in how the children will accept the gay parent's orientation and in many cases, departure. Keeping the child-parent bond alive is essential for the children's development of self-concept and confidence. This first strategy calls for reaffirming the role of the gay or lesbian parent and the two-parent family unit.

Whether or not the partner is physically present, he or she needs to be seen as a continuing part of the family. Without the support of both parents children often don't feel valued, as illustrated in "Dad's Girl and Mom's Boy." Peter's departure made Courtney, who felt close only to her father, feel as though she had neither parent left. She then became a "model child," believing that perfect behavior was the only way to keep both parents from abandoning her. Finally she collapsed.

Separation or divorce usually compounds the sense of uncertainty from the non-straight parent. Courtney's brother Nicolas was never close to Peter and developed more severe psychological problems when Peter moved out. It therefore becomes even more crucial for gay parents to take an active role in their children's lives to compensate for their absence.

To minimize the separation crisis, communication lines between the gay or lesbian parent and the children need to be kept open. If a healthy parent-child rapport is not already established, the parents may consider family counseling to develop it.

It is crucial that the spouse avoid the temptation of using the children as pawns in conflicts with the partner. Hearing harmful comments about the other parent however factual they may be weakens the children's confidence in and link to the gay parent. To avoid such possibilities and to reassure Heather of her mother's love, Grant wrote her a "Birth Day" letter. Sorrow and pain can be expressed without faulting the gay parent in statements like, "I feel sad about what's happening."

This doesn't mean that the gay parent should be idealized or excused for wrongdoings by virtue of being a member of an oppressed group. It is helpful to remember that the coming out doesn't change his or her moral character.

Nor does the coming out change the gay parent's family responsibilities, often neglected in the stress of the transition. If any neglect, undue criticism, overindulgence or denial of children's rights is noted, the spouse may need to point out the harmful effects on the children. Of course this applies to the straight parent's behavior as well.

If there is evidence of harm done by either parent, action has to be taken immediately even at the risk of severing child-parent ties. In such cases, it should be made clear that the purpose is solely to protect the child from the dangerous behavior and has nothing to do with the sexual orientation of the abusive parent.

Some spouses, believing that the partner's homosexuality is immoral, exclude the partner from the children's lives. While spouses have a right to their own moral and religious beliefs, keeping the children away from the other parent deprives them of the two-parent support needed to cope with the separation as well as the coming out. For example, when Patty used Frank's AIDS diagnosis as confirmation of his supposed immoral behavior, the children's communication with him stopped. Consequently their separation trauma was never completely healed.

Despite such obstacles children can maintain a connection to an outcast parent in memory and love. In the end Peggy and Jeff did contact Frank. How much richer their lives could have been if they had been allowed to enjoy continual face-to-face contact with their father. In contrast a nine year old in Atlanta was with his father as he died of AIDS, designed a square for the AIDS names quilt and organized a memorial dinner for his father's closest friends, all because the mother, although angry about the coming out, kept the father-son contact alive.

Interaction with the partner's relatives helps validate the parent-child bond. It is crucial that children know their roots on both sides of the family. However awkward it may feel, the straight parent should try to stay in touch with in-laws for the children's sake. In turn relatives need to continue calling and visiting as always just as Karen's mother did.

Children may experience a division of loyalties between the parents as a result of outside social attitudes. Children in conservative communities, out of a need to conform, may view the homosexual or bisexual parent as the bad guy and the straight parent as the good guy. In progressive communities, on the other hand, the non-straight parent might be seen as the underdog deserving sympathy and the straight parent be viewed as a close-minded homophobe.

Facing such conflicts, children may feel pressure to choose one parent over the other. Most youngsters do not want to take sides and many become so determined to stay neutral that they repress tension building up inside. Their conflict is heightened if the parents separate, especially if one begins to lead a gay lifestyle. Both parents can help alleviate their children's turmoil by reassuring them of their love and by explaining that the child's doing something special for one parent won't put down the other. No sides have to be drawn.

The task of preserving the parent-child bond and reassuring the children of joint-parent love is ongoing. Teaching them about homosexuality and helping them resolve concerns related to it is an essential part of this process.

Educating the Children about Homosexuality

Most professionals advise that children be told about the parent's coming out, especially if he or she leaves the family or begins an active gay lifestyle. However, if the gay parent lives at home, his or her gayness is well hidden from public view and it doesn't significantly alter the family relationship, the decision may be not to tell the children. This is risky since the children may be told by someone else in negative, stereotypical terms and suffer hurt from the parents' deception.

Children who aren't told may suspect but feel uncomfortable about bringing it up. "Adults can seek answers when they wonder about such things. Children need help," a mother in Denver commented. Many are afraid to seek the truth and remain in ignorance, feeling increasing stress. Some take desperate steps to end their pain. A nine-year-old in

Ohio, for example, confused over why his bisexual father lived else-where, asked for a gun at a family gathering to kill himself. Such pain can be avoided through open family communication.

It is crucial that three messages are communicated when telling children. First, homosexuality is a normal, though not common, sexual variation. It is neither a disorder, a sickness nor a perversion, as they may hear from others out of ignorance. Second, the partner's sexual orientation in no way affects his or her ties to the children. Mom or Dad is still the same parent. Third, the children aren't to blame for their parents' marital problems.

How the parents tell the children affects how well they accept the news. The most effective way is for parents to tell them jointly to demonstrate a shared concern for the children's well-being. For example, Allison sat by Peter when he told the children. This showed their united concern and reinforced the sense of family stability. The underlying message needs to be, "Our love for you hasn't changed. We're still your parents."

If the partner wants to tell the children alone, it is critical that the spouse know when and how it is done. If the children still have questions afterwards, the partner needs to be urged to talk again with them. If he or she doesn't cooperate, the task falls to the straight parent, a less desirable option because the information is secondhand.

If the partner tells only some of the children, arrangements need to be made to tell the others to avoid hurt feelings. It is critical that they be included in this pivotal event of their parents' lives so that they know they are a valued family member.

Once they are told, the partner may want the secret kept in the family. If the children ask, "If Daddy (or Mommy) is okay, why can't I tell anyone?" an effective reply is, "Yes, it isn't bad to be gay, but everyone doesn't understand that."

What the parents tell the children needs to be appropriate to their age-related stage of emotional, intellectual and social development. Since infants, for example, primarily understand loving attention and its opposite, anger, parents need to bury animosity when the baby is present. This is what Grant did.

Many parents with preschool children are ambivalent about telling them. On the one hand, they fear that the children might babble the secret to neighbors and playmates. On the other hand, they want to prepare the youngsters for possible taunting should the word get out. Fortunately, at that age, children tend to repeat what parents tell them and will discredit anything friends or neighbors say that differs from what they've been told by their parents.

The most effective and reassuring explanation for preschoolers is a simple, brief statement that they can understand and remember. A young couple in New York, for instance, told their little girls, "Daddy likes men, but he and Mommy still love each other." Although preschoolers engage in genital exploration, they have no conception of sexuality, much less homosexuality. The implications of having a homosexual parent are beyond them. They can understand love however.

For children from five to twelve years old, more facts and explicit reassurance are needed. As Patty and Frank put it, "We don't love each other the way we did, but we'll always love you." If the partner has a lover, parents may want to add that he or she now loves someone else. Most important the children need to know that their daily lives will remain the same, especially if the parents are separating. Peter reassured the children after saying that he was leaving to be with Tom, "You'll remain in our house and go to your school." Preserving some semblance of structure helps compensate for the disruption of the family.

Innocent of prejudices, the five-to-eight year olds in this age group typically accept the gayness as a matter of fact. To them love between two people is normal regardless of age or sex. Yet their acceptance may be deceptive. Many later act out feelings not understood at the time, especially in the case of divorce.

A parent's departure is especially disruptive for the nine-to-ten year olds, especially sons of gay fathers. This age group may experience reactions to divorce as intense as that of teenagers, according to the landmark study of children of divorce by Judith Wallerstein, Ph.D., director of the Center for the Family in Transition.[4]

Adolescents need special consideration in the coming out since they have the most complex needs. They require both information about the parent's homosexuality or bisexuality and guidance to assimilate it into their own growing awareness of sexuality. At the same time they sorely need reassurance of family security to cushion the insecurities of their growing independence.

Adolescents are the most likely of all age groups to have negative reactions about a parent's homosexuality even if it was revealed years earlier. In part, discomfort comes from regarding either parent as a sexual being. As Jay Paul notes in his study, "It's less that they are bi/homosexual than that they are capable of having sex at all."[5] However, the teenager's adjustment to divorced parents' dating or remarrying is intensified by the gay parent's unconventional sexual behavior. This helps explain why Frank's daughter objected so strongly to his attending her graduation.

The negative reactions of peers, along with prevalent social stereotypes about homosexuals, compound teenagers' turmoil. When film maker Kevin White was in his teens, he felt isolated when his father came out, followed seven years later by his mother. Now married, he can't forget "the pressure of having other people question my sexuality."[6]

"How can my parent fit such a derogatory image? Could I be gay too?" are typical questions that plague many adolescents in the coming-out crisis. By learning about the variations of sexual orientation and behavior, some of their anguish and worry will be relieved. Parents can provide them with factual information about homosexuality and offer frequent opportunities for discussion. Paul's respondents whose parents discussed sexuality with them, compared to those whose parents didn't, seemed to be better able to "recognize cultural myths and prejudices about sexuality...and to be better equipped to handle them...with peers and others."[7]

Adult children, who have established their independence and identity, do not feel as threatened by the parent's disclosure. Their reactions, however, discussed in detail in Part Six, vary according to the moral code they have developed and their relationship to both parents.

They too need information and support in order to understand their parents' sexual orientation and to continue to accept them as significant adults in their lives. Those not married, in particular, need to understand how important it is to clarify their own sexual orientation before contemplating marriage. They also should be prepared to explain their parents' homosexuality to prospective marriage partners who might be uneasy about joining a family with a gay, lesbian or bisexual member. It should be pointed out that children of gay parents have no more chance of being gay than children of straight parents.

As children grow older their needs become more complex. It is advised therefore that parents keep abreast of current facts about homosexuality and AIDS. It is useful to have factual literature available like the AIDS handbook Frank brought along in anticipation of Jeff's and Peggy's questions. Materials can be attained from bookstores, libraries, public health departments, universities and gay and lesbian organizations.

Unlearning homosexual prejudice, a paramount factor in educating the children about homosexuality, isn't difficult if the family already values individual differences. If they do not, it is important that the family learn together to accept homosexuals and bisexuals as ordinary human beings with the same feelings and concerns as heterosexuals. Children are educated in this direction through factual information, the example of the straight parent and continued association with the gay parent. Eventually the children will know to ignore misleading labels and judge others by their individual character. It may help for parents to reinforce the message that it's okay to be gay, though it's difficult to lead a gay life because of discriminatory attitudes in society.

Helping the Children Cope with Homophobia

No one can predict if, how or when a child will encounter homophobic reactions in the community. He or she may blurt out a problem during dinner or come home in tears because of a classmate's teasing. Often it's hard to determine whether the children's emotional problems are caused by the parent's sexual orientation or just ordinary growing pains. Since children will very likely experience traumatic incidents due to pervasive anti-gay attitudes in society, it is important for parents to be prepared to help them cope. This is a third strategy for handling children's issues.

Children's problems related to homophobia arise from three major sources: the homosexual parent's stereotypical mannerisms or non-conventional lifestyle; ridicule or rejection from peers; anti-gay attitudes in the community.

Some children are embarrassed by their parents' "gay" mannerisms or intimate behavior toward someone of the same sex. This is more likely for children whose parent lives a gay or lesbian lifestyle elsewhere. Courtney, for instance, was bothered by Peter's flamboyant gestures when he drank during her visits. Another young girl in New York recalled being upset when she glimpsed her mother and female lover nude together in the bedroom.

While it's important to maintain the children's contact with the homosexual parent, many straight parents feel that exposure to an unconventional lifestyle may be stressful for young persons, especially adolescents who are sexually sensitive and confused. Although adult fears are often worse than children's actual reactions, it may be best to minimize the possibility of children's discomfort until they become accustomed to the idea that the gay parent no longer fits the conventional image of a father, mother or adult in general. The parents can negotiate appropriate limits of exposure for the children and the gay parent may want to exercise discretion when interacting with the lover in front of them.

This doesn't mean forbidding the children from seeing spontaneous affection between the gay parent and lover. Difficult as it may be for the straight spouse to contemplate the partner and his or her lover acting warmly in front of the children, it is healthier for children to witness a loving, supportive relationship between a same-sex couple than hostility between a heterosexual couple. Over time many spouses become more comfortable with the children's contact with the gay couple.

Ridicule for having a bi, gay or lesbian parent, a second source of children's discomfort, usually occurs at school age when children are prey to classmates' name-calling. Taunting, however brief, is traumatic. When one boy blurted out that Nicolas' father was gay it caused him to fear abandonment by all of his friends.

Since children are vulnerable to assaults on their own and their parents' identities, they need reassurance about themselves and the gay parent. Parents can teach them not to take other people's teasing personally. It should be pointed out that others often don't understand what gay means and that the gay parent is still the same person as before. This knowledge will help them to not be ashamed of the gay parent's orientation and to not feel a conflict of loyalty between their peers and family.

Peer rejection can be used to the children's advantage as an opportunity for them to learn about the cowardice behind name-calling and to find out who their true friends are. Nicolas learned this when he returned to school and heard no more about the traumatic incident. It was the name-caller's problem as his mother had said. Dealing with teasing also helps many children learn to recognize valuable traits in friends such as trustworthiness and acceptance. [8]

A third source of discomfort for children comes from intolerance in the community. Children of gay parents who maintain a high public visibility are more likely to encounter anti-gay reactions from peers and others. It's one thing to attend a baseball game with a gay parent but quite another to have a mother appear in the newspaper as openly lesbian. This concern applies equally to straight parents who are openly involved in gay-related events, such as working a booth at a Gay Freedom Day event.

When contemplating "going public," parents need to decide if they are willing to allow their children to be stigmatized for something that isn't their issue. Many conclude that it isn't worth the risk of causing their children suffering, such as taunting from their friends. One such mother remarked, "A child's self-concept isn't an appropriate battleground for a parent's fight with society, however legitimate it is."

Children are more likely to be hurt by involvement in gay or lesbian events in conservative or rural areas where homosexuality and bisexuality are not widely accepted. In such communities gay parents often risk loss of their jobs or arrest if homosexual activities are discovered. If such a threat becomes a reality, the children's welfare needs to be considered first when determining what to do. For instance, when a married peace officer in a farming town was accused of sodomy, the family moved quickly to a progressive city in the East to protect their children from the traumatic publicity that had already sent their reputation plummeting.

Decisions about children's involvement in gay events need to be based on the individual child as well as other factors such as community attitudes. Being seen as part of a minority group in a controversial social, moral or political realm can strengthen some children and unsettle more sensitive youngsters. Under some circumstances possible loss of self-esteem may be too high a risk for some children. In other instances reinforcing the child's acceptance and understanding of minority groups may be an overriding benefit.

Parents often disagree about their children's involvement in public gay events. On the one hand participation in such celebrations enables children to see people outside of their families accepting and respecting gays and lesbians. This is a very effective way for them to discover the range of homosexual persons and to break down their prejudices so that feelings about their own parents can be resolved. It is also a safe way for children to learn how to deal with homophobic reactions with parents and other children at their side.

On the other hand the straight parent may not want the children to march in a gay pride parade in the city, fearing possible harm if they are seen on the evening news by schoolmates or neighbors.

The gay parent may object, saying that the spouse is using the children as an excuse not to stand up for gay rights.

An effective reply is, "I support you in this but feel that it's more important right now that our children endorse you as a parent than the gay cause that might hurt them." Parents can compromise by finding low-risk ways to involve the children in the gay parent's life, such as Gay Fathers picnics.

The task of helping children cope with homophobia may seem overwhelming initially, but can be managed if one incident is handled at a time with trust in the children's resilience and creativity—as well as in the parents' instincts and common sense. Assistance is readily available from friends, family and, in metropolitan areas, community resources, such as the children's teachers, counselors, clergymen, parenting workshops and parent support groups.

Practicing Open Parent-Child Communication

How well the children cope with the coming out depends largely on the parents' receptivity to their feelings and concerns. Children who feel that they are listened to have higher self-worth. Those who aren't heard, feel inadequate and guilty and have trouble expressing their feelings. Communication with parents is especially important for sons who, compared to daughters, tend to have more difficulty accepting a parent's bi or gay identity.[9]

Parents need to make sure that they listen carefully not only to what their children say, but to what they don't say. This kind of listening requires what M. Scott Peck defines as "the work of attention."[10] This involves "bracketing" concerns about oneself in order to concentrate totally on what the child is saying and the feelings being communicated. Parents who don't feel open by nature can practice listening with a friend or family member. One helpful technique in effective listening is to rephrase what the other person has said to clarify meaning and to show understanding. Parents can also practice being open with each other to model the kind of openness they desire for the children.

It is critical that both parents set aside a "children's hour," time available for talking and listening. Even ten minutes a day will do. Since most children tend to confide more in their mothers than fathers, gay and straight fathers alike may need to make a greater effort to develop a rapport with them. This is particularly important for separated or divorced fathers of sons, who desperately need the reassurance of a father figure.

If children resist discussing feelings, it's helpful to talk about nonthreatening topics such as their everyday activities and interests. They may need confirmation that their feelings and thoughts are valued before they dare to express sensitive concerns. Observing their parents discuss feelings openly may motivate them to do the same.

Signs of trouble like Nicolas giving away his mementoes need to be explored. If the child doesn't open up the parent can ask, "Is there something you want to talk about?" If done in a caring spirit, such questioning won't be construed as pressure or interference.

Parents may want to alert teachers to the changes taking place at home, even if the specific circumstances are withheld. Teachers can note behavior changes that may require professional counseling.

Expressing gentle concerns doesn't always guarantee that a child's pain won't remain repressed and become self-destructive. Each child has unique feelings and a different level of tolerance. Seven years after his father came out, an eleven year old in Texas tried to commit suicide. His psychiatrist explained that this happened partly because the family never expressed their hurt and confusion over the coming-out crisis. The most sensitive member, through his actions, did it for them. Children often take on the role of drawing attention to unresolved family conflicts.

Children may be more willing to talk with brothers and sisters than parents, especially when coping with peer prejudices. Other sources of support include a trusted relative, a knowledgeable therapist or other children of gay parents, singly or in support groups. Gay Fathers or similar groups of the Gay and Lesbian Parents Coalition often have children's groups. See Appendix B for contact number.

If a child needs counseling it's important to screen therapists or support group leaders for sensitivity to both sides of the closet. Some mothers report that because of a leader's exclusive experience with the gay side of the issue, their children have blamed them for being homophobic or causing their father's stress.

Keeping the two-way communication going can help prevent children's problems from reaching a crisis point as well as encourage the development of their coping skills.

Resolving Fears about the Effects of the Coming Out on Children

As immediate children's problems are resolved, the spouse's fears about long-term implications of the coming out on the children can be resolved. This is the last strategy of this stage of recovery.

Many parents worry about how the coming out will affect the children, especially in the initial months. Factual information and counseling can disperse what otherwise might become a debilitating obsession. For example, mothers who become paranoid about their children kissing an HIV-positive father or using his water glass need only to review the facts on how the virus is transmitted to realize that their fears are unfounded.

Another common fear, even among spouses who appreciate the importance of coming out and know that sexual orientation isn't hereditary, is that one of the children will turn out to be gay. Sociologist Terry Arendell, Ph.D., points out a related misconception that children of single mothers may develop homosexuality.[11] There is of course no factual basis for these myths. Having a gay parent only widens children's awareness of the range of sexual orientations possible, according to Paul's study.[12]

When parents realize that the chances a child might turn out to be gay are probably no greater than they are for children of heterosexual parents, they become less fearful. In the few cases it happens, there is a repeated sequence of shattered expectations, guilt and grief that the child is "lost" to a separate world. In time, the fact that the child can be his or her true self becomes for many spouses a source of pleasure. Furthermore, unlike coming out in marriage, the disclosure injures no one else.

Yet the stigma of being homosexual is bound to hurt the child. The straight parent may feel resentment toward the gay parent for modeling the behavior. Or others may blame themselves for having accepted the partner's homosexuality so openly.

This crisis too can be overcome with the support of friends, appropriate counseling and the inner work suggested in subsequent parts of this book. A professional woman in Chicago whose son died of AIDS two years after the death of her husband from AIDS, eventually resumed a productive life and remarried.

Another concern is that the children may repeat the parent's pattern and gravitate toward a mixed-orientation marriage. As a bisexual man's daughter divorced from a bisexual man said, "Like children of alcoholics who marry alcoholics, a bisexual man was what I knew and understood best."[13]

While it can't be determined in advance how the children's lives will be affected by the coming out, parents can help them avoid much hurt by explaining the importance of being clear about their own sexual orientation in creating a healthy marital relationship. Adult children whose marriages are based on honesty will have greater promise of success than their parents. If a homosexual orientation is discovered in a child's marriage, parents can point out that the couple will have a better chance of working it out if the gay partner comes out immediately.

The effect that separation or divorce will have on the children is perhaps the biggest source of worry for parents. One of the strongest motives for keeping the family together is the children's need for security. This concern is valid since children in any divorce situation suffer insecurity and pain, according to Judith Wallerstein's ten-year follow-up study of divorced couples and their children, *Second Chances*.[14] Several children of spouses studied for this book still have physical ailments such as ulcers, resulting from their parents' departures more than ten years earlier.

Negative effects of divorce are compounded by a parent's disclosure. A sizeable minority in Paul's study felt that the parent's gayness was more stressful than the divorce.[15]

Although parents can't insulate the children from the painful effects of divorce, they can give them the gift of how to cope constructively with such upsets of life. They can also minimize their children's distress by maintaining two-parent support.

Coping with parental concerns on top of spousal problems eventually takes its toll on the straight spouse. "Parenthood isn't easy under any circumstances," a mother in Phoenix remarked, "but with the gay issue, it's twice as hard."

At this stage, children's real feelings about the parent's being gay and the divorce often go unheard. "Even if I heard them," a divorced mother said, "I wouldn't have the strength to do anything about it." To reflect how long it takes for spouses to be able to tune into their children's long-term concerns, those issues are not explored until Part Six.

Within the first year or two of the coming out, the triple burden of damaged sexuality, shattered marriage and parent-spouse conflicts becomes unbearable for most spouses. Exhausted from helping everyone else, many wonder, "What about me?" How two wives and a husband answered this question is portrayed in Part Four, which explores the crisis of lost identity and ways to regain a strong, authentic sense of self.

four

WHAT ABOUT ME?

IDENTITY CRISIS OF THE STRAIGHT SPOUSE

Many spouses are startled to discover that in the process of accommodating to their partner's coming out they have lost their sense of identity. Most have had little time or energy to notice how they have been personally affected because of the demands to adjust to their partner's new identity and changed behavior, make the marriage work or cope with separation and divorce and care for the children's needs. Typically by the second year after the coming out, exhaustion forces spouses to attend to what little is left of themselves. The identity crisis that they then experience is the fourth hurdle of their recovery process.

When spouses finally take a realistic look at themselves, they may not recognize what they see. Often body, mind and emotions are depleted or numbed with addictions to alcohol, caffeine, cigarettes or food. Many experience an overwhelming feeling of helplessness and feel abandoned by their partners. They feel devalued as people.

When the pain can no longer be tolerated, many spouses begin to ask, "Who am I?" The resulting quest for identity is the major turning point of the straight spouse's struggle. The journey is arduous but offers the promise of lasting renewal. Though support from others is needed, the spouse ultimately has to rely on her or himself alone. Even support groups for straight spouses which are invaluable at first may begin to seem counterproductive as the spouse's individual problems diverge from those common to spousal issues.

As the spouse searches for traces of her or his former self, buried passions and interests may be uncovered. Eventually, through self-exploration, the authentic "I" can be recaptured—an individual in her or his own right, no longer defined in relation to the partner.

The stories that follow portray different ways of coping with the identity crisis as experienced by two wives and a husband during or after their marriages. The concluding section examines the issue of shattered identity and outlines effective strategies that help spouses to reconstruct independent selfhood.

Personal Stories

On Trial
Catherine

The first sacrifice was to forego a marriage license. Larry, a radical liberal, opposed all institutions, particularly Christianity. A tall, gangly man, he was brilliant. I was tiny but full of energy.

We became friends in high school. He dropped out of college junior year to become a potter. While I majored in history and earned a teaching credential at the university, he made beautiful things out of clay. Although he'd said he was gay when we met, he took me out whenever I was home in Bloomington, Indiana. After graduation I taught school there. Eventually I left the job to live with him in the rustic bungalow his mother had bought for us near West Baden Springs to the south. The first year Emily was born and then William two years later.

Larry was so antisocial, he never had affairs with men. Yet his gayness colored how I approached our living together. "I'll work it out," I decided, "with whatever sacrifice is necessary."

Before long Larry's antisocial stance extended to his mother, who then terminated financial support. I was painting and making jewelry by then. Together we built up a solid reputation in the arts and crafts fair circuit.

Under Larry's strict direction, I did most of the leg work for these productions. He handled the creative aspects. With our proceeds we collected Oriental rugs and Indian crafts to add to the artifacts from my history studies. While I kept our accounts, Larry kept the house swept and tidy and cooked exotic meals. Sharing so many interests with him made me feel valued.

It was a busy, satisfying life most of the time except for Larry's streaks of violence. On one occasion he tied up our cat in a bag and threw it out of the house. The kids and I took it to the vet without letting on what had happened.

When William was five and Emily was seven, Larry told them he was gay and began to show them his pornographic gay literature. Sometimes when William was watching TV, he would run into Larry's workshop to say, "Come see the good parts of the movie." When I peeked in to see what was so good, it was men's bodies.

Then one day while Larry and I were working in the studio-living room, he suddenly said, "If only you were a man, Catherine, you'd be perfect." This was the first of many such remarks, each one further shattering my sense of self-worth.

Larry was unhappy about himself too because he hadn't had many gay relationships. Since he avoided social occasions, there were few chances to meet men at all. Whenever he did meet one he'd say, "Not for me. Nobody's good enough. I want someone who doesn't look gay and likes Indian culture like me."

His hopes went up when he met Stu, a handsome, intelligent, radical "straight," who agreed to sleep with him. Stu enjoyed sex with Larry—and with me. We three had a grand time together until one day Stu told Larry, "I'm not going to sleep with you any longer. What do I get out of it?"

Stu's departure put Larry over the edge. After that everyone was either pro-Larry or "the enemy." If you were Stu's friend, you were automatically in the latter group. Larry began creating straw men of all kinds.

Stu remained a close friend of mine. So did our neighbor, Louise, a practicing Christian. I therefore became the enemy and Larry moved out, suing for divorce.

Our common law marriage complicated the divorce process. I couldn't afford a lawyer since I was teaching without pay at a private school, so that the kids could attend tuition-free. So my mother, though preparing to go to Europe with my aunt, dipped into her reserve to lend me money.

At the first deposition for the divorce, the judge said we could sell the house even though it was in Larry's mother's name.

We decided to put it on the market once Larry's things were out. I suggested that he take the furniture, his rugs and the exotic spices he used for cooking. He took his clays, glazes and kiln equipment but left the other things behind.

"He must have forgotten," I thought, putting them in his workshop to pick up later.

He came by the following week while I was at work and put everything in the workshop back onto the porch. Discovering the pile there that night, I put it all back in his workshop. The next week he returned the stuff to the porch. This happened over and over until I finally gave up.

Louise said, "Stop taking care of Larry and take care of yourself."

I wondered how that was possible now that the house was on the market. The morning of my mother's departure for Europe, she called all atwitter. "Auntie's ill and can't go. Pack your things and meet met at the airport at two-thirty."

A vacation sounded wonderful though I feared Larry would break in and take things in my absence. Louise, elated for me, offered to keep an eye on the house and take care of the kids.

When I called Larry about the trip, he said, "Give the keys to the realtor to show the house while you're gone."

"No. Not with my jewels here for my current project."

"Oh, I'll tell her to watch the people she shows it to."

"O.K.," I said and hung up, having to pack in a hurry. There were less than four hours to get to the airport, a two-hour drive away. In my rush I left the breakfast dishes in the sink.

Three weeks later when I returned, regenerated by my experiences in Paris, Florence and Madrid, I went straight to Louise's. "How did things go?"

"Not good. Not good. Have some coffee while I tell you."

In my absence Larry had borrowed the key from the realtor, telling her it was for a termite inspection. Instead he photographed the dirty dishes in the sink, the newspapers piled up for building fires, a dead mouse in the yard, cat excrement from somewhere and the piles of bric-a-brac in the living room that allowed us space for our craft work. No pictures were taken of eight-year-old Emily's room which was spotless.

Larry then took the photos to the divorce judge to ask for custody of the children because of the filthy house. Showing him the picture of cat excrement, Larry said, "This was in my daughter's room, but there's lots all over the house."

"If it's that bad," said the judge, "I give you temporary custody." The decision stated, "Catherine is an unfit mother."

The night of my return, Louise and I cleaned up the house in two hours. I photographed it the next day, then took the pictures to court and asked for another hearing.

At the preliminary hearing, two teachers, both gay men who had visited our house, spoke as witnesses. "The previous report is not true," each of them confirmed.

The following day a court-appointed probation officer inspected the house. At the hearing four days later, he stated, "The house was fine."

Larry spoke up. "Did you look into the cereal box? Emily discovered worms in it."

The judge ruled in my favor.

A week later we met with our divorce lawyers, who told us to divide our assets including the fifteen-year-old Indian collection worth about $30,000 and $35,000 earned from fairs.

"Well, the collection's mine," Larry said on the way home. "You can have an Oriental rug, a Hopi carving and some jewelry."

"And you'll have twenty-five rugs and thirteen carvings? What about my Indian things?"

Larry agreed to have a mediator help us divide our collection. When we entered the house with the man, Larry cried, "Open the window. I can't stand the stench."

Neither the mediator nor I smelled a thing.

The divorce trial took place several weeks later. Larry's theme was, "Catherine's a liar. She steps in and out of reality." As proof, he and his lawyer recounted false stories about what I'd done.

The judge believed both men. He was a narcoleptic with a heart problem. For most of the trial his eyes were closed.

When it was over, the judge delayed deciding the custody issue, while my lawyer tried to have him removed from the case. In July he made his decision. Larry was to have all of the money from the fairs, the craft tools, the Indian collection and all but two of the Oriental rugs.

By then I was seeing a psychologist. My mother and aunt lent me money to continue seeing him and to hire my lawyer to fight for joint custody.

When the psychologist heard that I wanted joint custody, he asked, "Are you willing to sacrifice your own happiness to keep the family together?"

"Oh, yes."

In August Larry called to say that he'd rented a house in South Carolina and wanted full custody. That required a court order, for which the four of us had to see a psychiatrist in separate interviews.

After the psychiatrist had met with all of us, he reported, "Emily talks as if she's thirty-five. Larry is manipulative and proscribes others' lives." Nothing negative was said about me or William.

At the custody hearing the testimony sounded like a classic case from *Mothers on Trial*. When the psychiatrist took the stand, I held my breath. He repeated his judgments about Larry but made no recommendations.

After the trial Emily asked, "Who won?"

"It was fifty-fifty."

"Oh. I wanted Daddy because of the mean things you do."

I gasped, not having suspected brainwashing.

That night she wet her bed and came into my bedroom. "It's too cold in my room. Can I sleep with you?"

"Of course."

She crawled in, hugged me and fell asleep, her arms around me all night long. Over the following weeks this happened repeatedly, especially when she had nightmares.

A few months later after a weekend with Larry, Emily complained of bleeding in her crotch. I called Larry to find out what had happened.

"Oh," he said, "she fell on the jungle gym."

When our doctor examined her, Emily said she didn't remember what had happened. While she dressed, the doctor whispered to me, "I can't say anything about sexual abuse without her testimony."

Emily didn't remember the way it was before Larry left either. William recalled the violence. "Remember when Daddy threw out the cat?" he said one afternoon as we sat on the porch. He also reminded me of the time Larry wanted the dog killed. William seemed neutral about his father's behavior. He wasn't brainwashed one way or the other.

Emily saw it differently. To accept her father, she had to agree with his entire world view. An unspoken theme lay under every reference she made to him: "Daddy needs William and me to make it all right. If I don't do what he wants, he'll die."

One afternoon that spring, I came home from marketing to find the house empty. The kids weren't at Louise's or with friends. They didn't come home that night or the next day. The third day, having traced down Larry's post office box number in South Carolina, I drove there without stopping, straight to the post office parking lot and waited for him to come pick up his mail. In two hours, up came his van with Emily and William in the front seat.

I reported this to the police and the next day they cornered Larry when he arrived for the mail, charged him with kidnapping and brought the children back to me temporarily while the court decided what to do.

Again the narcoleptic judge delayed a decision. Larry's lawyer, his personal psychologist who was gay and the court psychologist, a lesbian, kept stating that I didn't want Larry to have the kids because of his homosexuality. The psychologist recommended that Larry have either shared or full custody.

As legal proceedings dragged on, all but seven friends backed away from supporting me. Stu and Larry's brother stayed close by me; his brother at the risk of losing his inheritance since his mother was again supporting Larry. The five other close friends were women: Louise, Larry's brother's wife and three lesbian women from a women's rape organization who helped me work through the legal maze to prove my fitness as a mother.

Each time a crisis arose, I telephoned one or more of these friends to help me think it through and decide what forces to marshal. A minor problem meant one call. When the count went up to seven, I knew the problem was critical.

For months I had no energy even for housework. Toward the end of the year, Louise told me about a teacher's aide job in town paying $6.00 an hour.

"Well," I said, "that's better than lying in bed till noon."

At the interview it came out that I was qualified to teach adult education. On the spot they hired me to teach adults who had never finished high school. The job was low pressure but creative—perfect for my life at that time.

For the next two years, court negotiations over permanent custody continued. Twenty-three people wrote letters on my behalf. At home I learned little by little how to do the household tasks Larry had done, except for his magnificent cooking. One night when Louise was over, I reflected, "You know, I'm happier living alone than the times I was happy with Larry! Now I'm an independent person and finally know what I like and who I am."

The third year I made my first foray into a singles bar and discovered that men found me attractive. Then several asked me out.

The first invitation startled me. "What? Someone cares what I think, where I want to go?" By the end of the year, I was dating one man exclusively. I wasn't the frigid woman Larry had made me out to be.

At work there were ever-changing problems that challenged my resourcefulness. "This adult can't read," I'd think with each illiterate student. "How can he or she get the information? What do I do?" Then I'd improvise and the student would always learn to read, no matter what the difficulty.

One day a filing cabinet had to be moved in the office. "You're strong," I told myself. "You can do it." So ninety-eight pound Catherine carried the heavy cabinet while the men watched. What they thought didn't bother me because the strength I expected of myself was really there.

After three years of fighting for custody, I was afraid of what would happen to William and Emily if they had to live with Larry.

The more I read about brainwashing children through physical and psychological control, the more I feared. I knew from Larry's past behavior that he would control the children if he had custody.

Slowly it became clear to me what the trial was really about. Had I known in the beginning that joint custody keeps women who are in an abusive situation trapped in it forever, I would never have agreed.

೮   ೮   ೮   ೮   ೮

A year later, against the recommendations of the two gay psychologists, Catherine was awarded full physical and legal custody of the children with visitation rights for Larry. Recommendations from the court-appointed psychiatrist and the children's therapist, testimony from therapists who saw the family over the years and interviews with Catherine and Larry verified the truth of her story.

That summer Catherine married the man she'd dated for two years. The following year Emily announced that she didn't want to visit her father anymore because he had told her and William to hurt Catherine and her new husband and had given them knives and other implements to do so. When the sheriff came to hear Emily's testimony and collect the weapons, William claimed the tools were for gardening, fearing Larry's punishment if the court were to force visitations. The court ruled that there could be no further contact with the father.

Two Minor Miracles
Wes

With our two children, Alex, twelve and Kate, nine, we were the golden family in church, in school and in Scouts, but something was missing from our marriage. I never got a loving touch or embrace when I got home from my long photographer's hours. For two years I'd begged Milly that we buy sex aids, but she refused. So I made deeper commitments to church and increased my prayer life to where I was open to any message God had as to what was wrong with my marriage.

Then the doctor discovered my cancer and I underwent radiation. As I recovered, Milly agreed to join me in a couples healing retreat.

Husbands went away for one week and the wives a second. Family members and friends were to send agape love in the form of messages. On my week, while the other men received cards and letters, bags of them, not a single card came to me from Milly.

Then it was her week. The day after she returned, I found the pack of letters she'd received—love letters from Helen, my daughter's soccer coach and our close friend, involved in our children's activities and all our family and church events. One by one, the letters revealed Helen and Milly had an ongoing affair, by then a year old, which included a week in our house when I was on a trip the year before.

I was doubly traumatized by the deceit and the warnings people had given me. I'd ignored them, saying, "As Christians, you're out of line. Mill and Helen have the right to explore their relationship. They're happier than they've ever been. What's wrong with that?"

Now I thought, "How could I have missed the signals?"

When Milly got home that night, I was overwhelmed with shame. "I'm so stupid not to have known."

"Not 'stupid,' Wes," she said, "Just unaware. It was something so new to you that you couldn't have conceived it was possible."

"Well, this relationship with Helen should stop immediately. And...," I added, stricken, "I'm moving to the basement. Since you two made love in our marriage bed, I cannot sleep there again." I also didn't want Helen calling while we were making love or trying to sleep or share a book and have Milly run out or ask me to leave.

The next day it was clear they weren't going to stop seeing each other. I kept asking Milly, "How could you love me and hurt me too? You're just punishing me."

"No," she protested. "That's not it at all."

"How can you prove it," I asked, "if we don't sleep together one more time so I know you haven't been fooling me?"

That's when I heard about faked orgasms with clenched fists. "For christsake!" I erupted. "For twenty years my whole sex life has been one big night in a bawdy house. How could you make real love with Helen and not with me?" I screamed.

We'd both had affairs before; those women thought my body was desirable. Milly's words crippled my sexuality. "Even if she says she's capable of making love to me," I thought, "I don't think I can."

What hurt also was Milly's intimacy with somebody besides me, which the letters made all too clear.

One night I realized that Helen had everything I'd been working so hard to buy for Milly, like the trailer and mountain cabin. "You're not deserting me for a lesbian lover, Mill," I lashed out, feeling even less of a person, "but one with three times more resources than I."

I assumed Helen had told close friends among the coaches or our kids' teachers. But neither Milly nor Helen would tell me who knew. "Not knowing is killing me!" I finally said. "Every time I go to sports and school functions, her friends see me as some big fool!"

Soon, the lies Milly had couched as accusations in the past came marching back like soldiers. There was the Boston trip when the kids and I went to my sister's wedding. Milly wouldn't go. "We can't afford it," she'd said. "We'll never get out of the hole. I don't deserve this."

"I must really be bad," I'd thought, "but I'm going anyway."

Then to find out from the letters that she and Helen had made love in our bed that entire week, doing things with oils and bath toys—the things I'd begged her to do with me—was too much. I snapped.

I became a walking time bomb. There was no one to talk to. I couldn't talk to my pastor because he was Milly's, too, and she didn't want anybody to know.

Milly and I fought constantly as I became obsessed by the fact I couldn't have her and Helen could. Then, as it became obvious we couldn't mend things, Alex and Kate realized their dreams were shattered. You don't go overnight from being the model family to having a raging set of parents, unable to function or sometimes get out of bed, without the kids being involved. So they went into their shells.

One night Alex heard us fighting about Helen's being lesbian. The next day he talked to Milly. She explained how she loved Helen and he seemed to understand, but the fire and brimstone talk about homosexuals heard at church still disturbed him.

A month later, Alex went to a church youth retreat. At one of the sessions, the youth minister said, "Homosexuals will burn in hell."

When Alex came home crying and confronted his mother, she explained some more. He still wasn't convinced she'd be saved.

All this time, I was a crazy man. Many nights, I slept in my darkroom at work. If, on the way home, I saw Helen's car in front of the house, it made me physically ill. I'd turn right around and go see another movie or do anything but face the disappointment of going home.

Sometimes I went without sleep for two or three days. As I walked the streets, disoriented, it felt important that people get out of my way. I joined civilian walk patrols in Denver's rough neighborhoods and walked the meanest streets to pick fights with drunks.

Since I was noncompetitive by nature, this antisocial behavior was out of character. My rage was fueled by homophobic myths and my upbringing in a conservative Catholic parish. Then I'd gone straight into a protestant church that did much gay bashing from the pulpit.

Mostly, I believed I had done something unworthy and my wife and everybody else was part of a worldwide conspiracy against just me. The long term deceit and paranoia built up such anxieties that I found no peace in Milly's presence. So my body and my emotions rebelled.

I started seeing a counselor but didn't trust what he said. Then, Milly gave me a clipping she and Helen had on a straight spouse support group. Resentful they'd talked about me, I took it reluctantly.

The group saved my life. When I went to the first meeting, the biggest shock was seeing the room full of ten women and one man, going through the same thing I was. As the women told their stories, their feelings sounded exactly like mine. "Wow," I thought, "this isn't yet another thing about how disappointing it is to be a man. It's about how painful it is to be a person." For the next four weekly meetings, my anger persisted. With constricted face, wrinkled forehead and dark-circled eyes, I couldn't even finish words or sentences.

After a month Milly tearfully said, "Wes, you're not getting better. You're just getting more and more angry."

That wasn't it. I was bringing out things not thought about in twenty years and rehearsing what to say about them. "If Mill says this, I'll say that," I practiced. "Goddammit, I'm going to tell Helen, 'You hurt me and my family and here's how you humiliated me.' "

The counselor warned of damage to the kids if I continued to beset Milly. So I walked the streets to rehearse, angrily going over the stuff. The minute I'd see people, words spilled out in a sort of muttering.

Meanwhile, my counselor was trying to build me up. "Wes, how many women wouldn't desire a man who was sensitive?"

"Oh," I thought, "just one more lie."

Six months after I found the letters, Milly asked, "Do you feel you'll never attract someone else, since you really don't have a marriage?"

"Exactly! I don't see how anybody will ever want me with the baggage you're forcing me to carry around."

"So I'll move out."

After the tears, I began to wonder what would happen if she took the kids. "Will it turn Kate into a lesbian?" I wondered.

The thought propelled me into the kitchen where Milly was cooking. "You cannot take my daughter," I announced. "I'll move to Boston and you'll never see her again."

For a week Milly went a little crazy over that possibility. Finally, she suggested, "I'll move just a few blocks away so Kate can come and go when she wants. We'll say to the kids, 'we have to live in separate houses and you can live anywhere you want and just come and go. You'll have equal bedrooms and amounts of clothes in each house and feel comfortable in either place any time.' "

Over the next month, we divided the furniture and consolidated all the bills into one big bill for car payments which I got stuck with. Then Milly moved out with Kate and all her books and with some furniture. Alex stayed with his things. Each went back and forth, as planned.

Mid-July, I appeared, disguised, on a local TV show on straight partners of lesbians and gay men. I wanted to speak out as "everyman" so the public would know what husbands go through. The day it aired, my boss called me in. "I have a right to know what's going on in your life and when you make public statements about it."

The next week, I was fired.

Come August, I was leaving the mall one Saturday, when somebody yelled, "There's the guy who threw his wife out because she's a lesbian." Turning around, I saw two people from our sister church in Denver.

So after putting ten years into the church to become a respected officer, I fell in status so fast I was ashamed to attend services. "How could best friends," I wondered bitterly, "not support me in my crisis because it's controversial?" I soon shopped only at night.

That was the summer of the Colorado Amendment 2 campaign to remove gays from civil protection laws. As Alex became more upset about his mother's being gay, he talked to no one after school and stopped participating in any kids activities.

"Whoa," I said, "we've become second class citizens, too."

It was so hard not to cry about it, but my counselor warned me not to cry in front of the children. "They've never seen you cry, so it will be a shock and therefore upsetting."

If a favorite Carpenters song came on while I was cooking, I could hide the tears that flowed from its gut-level sentiment. But for big cries, I ran to the shower, hoping the kids would mistake my wailing for singing. As the hot water poured over my shoulders and my muscles relaxed, the sobs came until my shoulders ached.

The alienation got so bad I wanted permission to die. "It's impossible to find a partner who'll love me with my cancer and my emotional baggage, my wife and being out of work," I thought. "It's too hard to hope. Better to end my pain and let the kids have the life insurance."

No longer able to pray, I cursed at God.

One chilly night, when the furnace was out of oil we couldn't afford, I was too tired to fetch wood for the fireplace and knew I couldn't turn to prayer. I then recalled a Robert Schuller broadcast about a blind man who couldn't pray—only moan about losing his eyesight. So he began kicking his slippers under his bed, making him get down on his knees to get them out. At that level, he felt humble enough to pray. "I'll try it," I decided, "tonight."

After a few weeks, I was praying again by my bed in the basement.

One night a month later, after the kids returned from visiting their grandparents, Alex came down to the basement, looking strangely at me. "Why are you still sleeping here? Mom's been gone for three months. There's no reason to be cooped up here."

"My son has no motive to manipulate me!" I thought with surprise. "Maybe people really do want to help me."

By saying prayers and hanging up favorite paintings and new window coverings in the bedroom, buying new sheets and moving the bed, I transformed the room. Once the toxic influence of what had gone on there lost its power, I reclaimed my power and moved in.

Every room was as methodically detoxed, one by one. Then I decided to plan family events that I could control and avoid that made me a victim of my battered emotions. From then on, whenever Milly and Helen picked up the kids for something, I made a point of being elsewhere. Birthdays and holidays were carefully planned.

For Thanksgiving, the kids and I ate turkey dinner with another spouse and her kids at the home of her gay ex-husband and his partner. Kate and Alex got to see two gay men enjoying each other's company and working together in the kitchen. It was nothing like any family time we'd ever had, but we didn't sit around and sulk at home.

That spring, I met a woman whose ex-husband was gay. Over the next months, we went to dinner, the movies and to her church which was Catholic and liberal. Then, we began to pray together. To get a prayer life with a partner when you never had one—how sweet it is.

By summer, she and I began to share our sexual healing. We pretended we were sixteen again, an age when we'd been comfortable with our sexuality as something innocent—and open to delight in any new development that came along.

As for Milly and me, we no longer fought. We even hugged once in a while. But we were separate individuals with separate lives.

Kate still hadn't been told her mother was lesbian, though she probably knew. Alex didn't care a fig who his mother was with as long as she was happy.

For me, the two minor miracles were that I could find out homosexuals were everyday people and not only lovable but loving, and, second, that I could actually love my wife again. Things I'd always liked about her as a friend and parent of my kids were still there.

What's left is a need to wipe out bitterness from wounds that go back twenty years. Only I can say how long it will take to attain true peace and balance.

What the Buddha Said
Ling

Sometimes I look at Jack and think, "Why am I still here?" It's been eight years since he said he was gay. There's a lot of love between us—not passion but friendship from living together for twenty years."

It wasn't surprising that Jack married me, a Chinese student in graduate school at a midwestern university where he was a graduate student in religion. The Orient had fascinated him since he was a boy. College was his first chance to meet an Asian person. Most of his friends there were Asians.

He'd had two girlfriends at his rural high school and became engaged in college to a very American girl—blonde, blue-eyed and beautiful. They didn't have premarital sex because it was sinful and they broke up before graduation. Then he met me.

When we met I thought, "Oh, he's American. That's a barrier between us." As I became acquainted with this tall, blond midwesterner, his interest in Asia and fondness for Asian people impressed me. I felt so comfortable with him that sometimes I completely forgot he was American and chatted away in Chinese.

He'd smile and say, "Ling-Ling, please speak in English."

After a year I felt so close to him on all levels that I said, "Yes," when he proposed.

His folks wanted him to marry the "girl next door." They still lived in the isolated area where he had grown up with only his brother for a playmate. He was the "perfect" son, raised without exposure to outside influences.

My parents, too, were against us. "You cannot marry an American," they wrote. Then because Jack's letter asking for approval, which I translated, was so sensitive, Father agreed.

Jack didn't want us to have premarital sex. "If you get pregnant and I'm killed in Vietnam," he said, "You'll have a hard time raising a child by yourself."

"This is true love," I thought. "He's the most perfect man I've ever met."

When we married, Jack decided to work for a design firm in Seattle. I couldn't work, lacking training or license for anything in this country.

Our first years I felt happy "until death us do part." We had sex. We went everywhere together. The only problem was Jack's strict morals because of his religious background. We couldn't dance since he felt it was a primitive pattern of intercourse.

"Oh my goodness!" I thought. "He's square!" Though my family had strict morals too, I went to dances as I was growing up. Dancing was considered a beautiful art form in China.

His family also objected to alcohol. Once, when his parents were visiting, his mother saw my rice wine with a Chinese label in the refrigerator. Sniffing it, she asked, "What's this! Alcohol?"

Finally I told Jack, "I'm going to use wine in cooking whether or not your parents are opposed."

After that he gave up.

Four years after we married, Lionel was born and we moved to the suburbs. Janice arrived four years later. That same year Jack met a Japanese man and began inviting him to dinner and picnics. Fond of me, Michio became a member of the family over the next few years. One weekend he and Jack went hiking in the mountains while I stayed with the children. All this time Jack was very loving to me.

Then there was a local fuss about homosexual teachers. Reading the news stories about it, I came across the word, "gay," for the first time although I'd heard of homosexual bars in Taiwan where I grew up. One morning, reading about a petition to dismiss gay teachers on moral charges, I said to Jack, "That's terrible!"

"Society is terrible for persecuting gay people," he replied. Over the next few weeks he talked increasingly about the issue. The more he talked, the more I detected a change in him.

One day a friend was discussing another friend of ours, Walton, with me. "His friendship with Jack seems strange. Maybe they have something going on."

Other things began to come together. One night I asked Jack, "Are you gay?" Though I understood by then why people are gay, I didn't want my husband to be.

His face turned pale and he got tense.

"I'm not against gay people, Jack," I went on. "I'm a very liberal, calm person."

"Then why did you ask?"

"I've got a feeling something is going on."

"Well, if you say so. I think I'm a bisexual."

"Have you had an experience?"

"Yes," he said.

"Then you had homosexual feelings before we married?"

"No, honestly not."

"Well, is it Walton?"

When he said, "No," relief flooded my being. Then after I guessed other men we knew, he said it was Michio.

"You've had a relationship with both him and me for the past four years?"

He nodded, tears rolling down his cheeks. "I couldn't satisfy my sexual needs with you, so I began to explore. It would've threatened you if I'd found a woman lover, so I turned to men. When I discovered my homosexual feelings, I was upset and couldn't believe it. But the more involved I became, the more wonderful it was."

As he told me about dating Michio and going to discos with him, I thought, "Jack—dancing?"

By then Jack was in shock. "Now I've broken up our relationship, Ling, and Michio said he'd stop seeing me if you found out, not wanting to hurt you. That's why I covered up."

The next day when Jack told him, Michio kept his word. "I must stop seeing you."

Then Michio called me. "This is the Asian way. You know that, Ling. Both of us are very Asian and our thinking is the same."

Jack said nothing more about it except that he was unhappy. "If only my gay feelings could be turned off with a switch, I'd go back to being straight."

I was devastated too, but my one thought was, "Poor Jack. I have to help him." I was nonexistent. So I did a funny thing. I went to Michio's apartment and begged him not to break up with Jack.

"No, Ling-Ling! I must stick to what I said."

In August Michio found another partner, but Jack hung onto Michio. When we went to concerts that fall, he hardly paid attention to me or the music. Watching him, I felt pain and anger. "I'm your wife. We came to see the symphony and you're thinking about Michio."

Our relationship deteriorated. Not knowing why, I didn't want sex with him any more. By November Jack became so depressed that he couldn't perform at work, which brought pressure from his boss.

Just after Thanksgiving we gave a party. After the guests left about eleven, Jack called Michio. It was the first time in four years he hadn't been invited to one of our parties. After the call, Jack joined me and my sister, visiting from the city for the weekend, for another glass of wine before going to bed. Twenty minutes after he left us, we heard a loud noise from the bedroom and rushed in there. Jack was on the floor. We shook him but he didn't wake up.

"It's probably the wine," I said.

Since he was too heavy to move, we put a blanket on him where he lay. Then he half rose and we half dragged him to bed.

The next morning, a Saturday, the kids came into the bedroom at five as they always did weekend mornings.

I shook Jack gently. "Let's get up."

"Go ahead without me," he mumbled.

As we started into the kitchen, there was another loud noise. I ran back to the bedroom. Jack was on the floor again, his head bleeding. My sister, now awake, called 911. When the paramedics came, Jack was still drowsy. Once they took his pulse, they called an ambulance.

I stayed next to him all the way to the emergency room. At the hospital the doctors washed out his stomach, assuming he'd overdosed. By then he was unconscious.

I called Michio immediately. "Maybe he won't wake up. But, if he does, he'll want to see you."

Michio came at once and each of the next three days as Jack lay in a coma. Going home to check on the kids, who were being watched by my sister, I found an empty jar of sleeping pills in the bathroom.

The fourth day Jack came to. Over the next few days, he wrote a poem about wanting "to die for love, not for the family."

Reading it when he finished, I thought, "His love for Michio is so strong that he wants to die because he lost him. I'm the wife, but he loves somebody else deeply! It's terrible knowing that it's a man he loves. If Jack wasn't gay and had a woman lover, maybe I'd have the energy and purpose to challenge her."

Once recovered, Jack didn't want to break up the marriage or family, but wanted a private life. "If you really love me, Ling," he said, "you'll forgive me and accept the situation without questions."

That meant changing myself to accept his other lifestyle. At home he was still the same person who liked to be with family and close friends. But he never did things for the children's soccer and volleyball teams, never volunteered to help out at school.

In his other gay life, he acted macho. When he went out with a man, I got mad. When I objected, he got bitter.

For a year I talked to other women and counseling groups about how bad I felt about his other life, but it didn't help. After that, Jack and I discussed separating, but that ended in a fight. Then I just tolerated his double life.

For several years Jack hung onto Michio, even going to New York with him for two weeks. That didn't make me jealous because Michio was like a brother.

When Michio was with us, Jack was extremely good to me. He often said, "The threesome is nice."

The funny thing is that Michio never said he was gay. One day he told me, "I'm interested in a woman and want to get married."

"Please don't, Michio," I said, "for the woman's sake. Don't do that to her. She'd go through what I'm experiencing. Women are human beings, too."

"But that's our tradition. I have to have children."

When Michio found another lover, Jack wanted another gay relationship too, but was afraid of being hurt again. So he went out only on one-night stands.

Some months later with someone from his gay men's organization, Jack joined a support group for men who only wanted tricks. After two meetings they learned that it was a sex addiction not something related to being gay.

"O. K.," I said to Jack, "you're addicted to sex. So find one person. Reduce the chance of AIDS."

He responded with the same argument he always gave me. "You pushed me in this direction, Ling. You weren't interested in being a passionate lover. I wanted a two-way relationship. If you'd been..."

Finally I dropped the subject. After that I never knew where, how, or why he did anything and didn't ask. I survived by praying, "If this is your will, God, give me your strength to get through it. If not, show me a sign and then give me the strength to develop a new life."

My religious beliefs were based on both Christianity and Buddhism from my childhood. Buddhist nirvana is similar to the after-death of Christianity, but in nirvana you don't exist anymore, you just melt into nature. Not wanting to lose my soul to nothingness, I turned to Christianity when I became a teenager.

Though I was frightened by the Buddhist idea of seven bad natures of man which cause misery, it still made sense. Why struggle against suffering that is human nature when eventually there will be nothing anyway?

After four years of struggling with Jack's other life, I felt I couldn't handle the pain any longer. For three days I sat in the corner of the living room under my scrolls and next to a jade plant. I couldn't do housework or eat or take care of the children.

According to Asian tradition, when you're in turmoil, you have to take care of yourself and be strong. You may be mentally disturbed and need professional help, but you don't dare seek it because it's shameful. It shows you're weak. You must resolve your problems alone and not blame anyone else.

As I sat in the corner, I thought, "Why am I struggling like this? Eventually, I will be nothing." Then I meditated, repeating, "I'm struggling, struggling every day, staying in deep depression."

After three days when I couldn't stand the depression any more, I switched my feelings off, saying, "The hardship of the struggle gives me strength to accomplish whatever I need to do."

A month or so later I took a part-time job in a community center. Some time after that I began to think, "O.K., Jack has two lives. Why shouldn't I find a lover?"

When I told Jack this, he said, "I don't like the idea, but I can't tell you not to. I don't have that right." Looking hurt, he probably thought, "Ling's not going to take a chance on that." He was right. It was only a thought. I couldn't look for somebody else since I was married. From my mother, a school teacher, and my grandfather, a Buddhist priest, I had learned that women shouldn't be promiscuous but devoted to their husbands.

My grandfather had deep thoughts. "Have virtue, self-control and compassion," he often told me. "Don't stain morality." I respected his word, particularly after my grandmother showed me his beautiful will which was written by him in brush, the rice paper full of holes that moths had made.

Self-respect was important to me, too. I had to be a good woman since Jack and I were married and living in the same house with children. I didn't want to look like a cheap woman in front of my children, going out with other men. It's hard to change an old-fashioned attitude instilled over many years.

Because we argued each time I said anything against Jack's gay activities, I thought about divorcing as many of our friends had done. One afternoon ten-year-old Janice and I were talking about a boy in her class whose parents had divorced.

All of a sudden she said, "Mom, if you and Dad divorce, I'm going to kill myself."

That scared me. I stopped thinking about divorce.

About the sixth year after Jack had told me about Michio, he no longer let me know when he'd be getting home from a night out. Once he returned at 3:00 A.M.

Hearing his steps in the hall, I came out of the bedroom, "I was so worried, Jack. I couldn't sleep."

"You pushed me to do this, Ling."

A few weeks later a friend told me about a woman who was dating a man who had married and divorced three times. He had told her, "Women are passionate only until they win the man. Then they become cold."

I told Jack the story that night. "See, I'm not the only one. I loved you sexually in my own way."

The following spring the center held an evening meeting and party to which I had to go. I didn't tell Jack how long it would last.

When I came in at 11:30 that night, he came out of the bedroom. "Are you alive or dead? Why didn't you call?"

"There was no telephone close by," I said, exactly the words he used whenever he didn't call to say he'd be late.

Nothing more was said.

Jack's nights continued in the same pattern, with different people every time. That made me think again about dating and perhaps separating from Jack, but I was too scared to act.

Then one of Jack's best friends, Greg, got AIDS. "All my life," I told myself, "I have controlled my own and my family's life very well. Now I have to face things I can't control. Today or tomorrow Jack may say, 'Ling-Ling, I'm sorry, I have AIDS.'"

I didn't know what to do. Insurance would cover medical treatment, but was my faith strong enough to watch Jack die?

Again I sunk into a deep depression.

When it was over, I brought up his promiscuity one more time. "You have a family and a social obligation not to spread AIDS. If you can't control yourself, you better talk to a counselor."

"You're overreacting, Ling. AIDS is mostly hysteria. It's very rare to catch it."

He saw a psychiatrist anyway. One night while the kids were doing homework, he reported, "Dr. Robinson says that as long as you're wrapped up in anger, Ling, our problems won't be solved."

"He blames everything on me because he hears only your side. I thought you went for help to stop one-night stands."

"You don't have any right to control what I do. Why don't you just accept me?" There was bitterness in his voice.

"What you're doing worries me, Jack."

A week later, noting he was nervous, I asked, "What's wrong?"

"Well, Greg's lover wants me to stay there tonight so he can get out of the house. He's exhausted and needs space."

"I don't mind since you're not planning to spend the night with a lover. It's wonderful that you're offering to help a friend."

"Well," Jack said, "I've got to change and start doing things for people. I've been selfish. After Greg goes, I want to work with the hospice."

After we talked a while about Greg's condition, I asked, "What causes the pain?"

"I don't know. He is dying so slowly."

When Jack left I thought, "Maybe this will make him realize how much burden he would be to me and the children if he got AIDS."

All this time I was thinking more and more, "If Jack stops acting gay, I can live with him. But, when we're in restaurants or on the street, he looks at men. When the waiter comes, he stares at him. I want my husband to look at me and be attracted to me. Jack says he cares about me, but without chemistry it's as if he were a friend or brother."

I saw the need to start taking care of myself so as not to get hurt anymore. Separation seemed to be the only answer, but when I told Jack, it led to a clash. So I avoided the subject.

That summer we went to Taiwan to visit my family. Jack and the kids returned in August. I stayed on for a course on Chinese, thinking, "If I can live without Jack for two weeks, I really can separate."

On my return separation didn't seem so scary, but I still worried that Jack would get AIDS. For the third time I plunged into a depression.

Frightened, Jack called one of my friends to talk to me and to make sure that I wasn't about to commit suicide.

When I came out of it three days later, I took off my wedding ring. "Now I will be free of Jack," I told myself, "and available to meet someone else."

When he saw my bare finger, Jack said, "You're trying to punish me."

"No. I did it for myself. I love you, but I don't want my husband to be gay."

Jack, I'm sure, was thinking, "Dear Ling, she has said that for eight years. Eventually she'll accept my double life."

A month later I said, "You go your way and I'll go mine in the house. We'll eat with the children but have separate rooms."

That was a month ago. When I think of moving out altogether, the loneliness frightens me. When you're young, it's easy. In your forties and after twenty years of marriage, it's scary. Yet nothing stays the same. If eventually we are going to separate, why struggle to escape that suffering now? God will give me the strength to act.

☙   ☙   ☙   ☙   ☙

Two years after this story was told, Jack was diagnosed HIV-positive. Though Ling was angry about his promiscuity, she didn't want to abandon the father of her children.

She began taking classes toward an advanced degree and continued her part-time job.

The following year, Jack became infected with AIDS. Ling stopped her coursework to take a full-time job and to care for him. He prayed that they each would attain inner peace.

Two years later, Jack and Ling had reached a spiritual reunion as he died at home, the family around him.

Discovering the Authentic Self

The spouse's identity crisis starts long before he or she is capable of doing anything about it. Most spouses are too disoriented or emotionally paralyzed right after the coming out to examine their pain. "I'd go to bed naked and hug myself to sleep," recalls a wife from Detroit. "Who else could I share that hurt with?"

Whether spouses divorce at once or try to make the marriage work, it may take months to realize the profound impact that the partner's coming out has had on them. Those who divorce are preoccupied with separation problems and those who stay married are adapting to their partner's bi- or homosexuality and gay activities. In either case, their own identities are slowly buried in the process of accommodating to the coming-out crisis.

For many spouses, keeping the marriage intact and meeting the needs of the children seem worth their self-sacrifice.

One such wife, Erin, married after high school, chose to help her husband accept his bisexuality as "good" rather than "evil," as a Pentecostal group had labeled him while attempting to pray the devil out of him. Later in their rural town where they were respected citizens raising four foster children, she stood by him when someone threatened to expose his gay activities.

Through each crisis her personal interests such as metaphysical reading, as well as her own private love affairs, eased both her emotional pain and her physical symptoms including gastroenteritis and skin problems that had plagued her the last half of their fifteen-year marriage.

For most spouses the first clues of lost identity come sooner, some time in the second year after the coming out. Married spouses, in particular, often find themselves drained of strength from the cumulative effect of the day-to-day struggles. Many have developed severe symptoms from physical ailments to depression. The desolation that all feel can be overwhelming.

Such despair overcame one young mother, Pamela, in Los Angeles. Empathizing with her husband's remorse over his gay affairs while taking care of three children under the age of eight, she could find no one who believed or understood her story. She finally cried "I can't take it any more" and swallowed a bottle of sleeping pills.

Pamela survived and learned how to create her own happiness. So do most spouses, rising out of their nadir through self-nurturing, introspection, support from friends and family, therapy, peer support, outside activities and spiritual nourishment. Straight husbands, possibly because of their wives' abrupt departure, seem to plunge into the depths more quickly but they tend to recover faster than straight wives. Wes, despite his acute anger, found a partner within two years. Wives take much longer.

Discovering one's true identity involves exploring inner emotional, mental and spiritual resources. Applying the coping skills used throughout the coming-out crisis, such as asserting needs and setting priorities, can help the spouse to succeed in this long and challenging process. The ultimate goal is to gain the inner strength to handle blows in life without losing self-worth and confidence.

Four steps lead to rebuilding a strong self-concept:

- Healing body, emotions and spirit
- Learning from the past
- Discovering an authentic identity
- Changing self-identity from "spouse" to "I"

Healing Body, Emotions and Spirit

The exhaustion and depression that signal the onset of the identity crisis can be used for healing inner wounds, the first strategy of this stage of recovery. Many spouses feel that their sense of identity has been damaged by day-to-day compromises, criticism by the partner or their own self-blame. As a working wife in Tucson said, "In the process, I lost self-esteem. The scars will never go away."

Fatigue often makes it impossible for spouses to continue all of their activities. In many cases they find that they need to stop being "the good girl" or "good citizen" and cancel or limit community, school, career or gay-related commitments beyond the regular work schedule. Separated spouses often decide not to see their partners as much for awhile.

Domestic chores may also need to be decreased to derive the most benefit from this healing period. No longer can spouses drive themselves to be superwoman or superman. Rather, now is the time to seek help from others, a new experience for some spouses. This is when friends, family, and partner need to be ready to assist.

Self-nurturing is one of the best antidotes for the overpowering desolation that many spouses feel. Rest, balanced diet, physical activity, relaxation and recreation with children and friends are simple but powerful ways to restore physical and emotional strength.

It is best to minimize artificial supports such as alcohol, cigarettes and drugs in favor of psychological, physical or spiritual activities that help to relieve stress, release feelings and help each person discover his or her own inner resources. Letting the mind wander while allowing the emotions to have full play greatly enhance the spouse's recovery. It is a time just to let feelings previously held in check, such as sorrow or anguish, surface naturally.

Non-thinking experiences like listening to music can also enhance the healing process. Music often releases significant sorrowful emotions that the spouse has previously ignored out of concern for the pain of others. It is a time when tears, anger, despair and even daydreaming are to be welcomed, not resisted. Tears themselves contain chemical cleansing qualities that heal.

Over a fourth of the spouses studied in depth for this book turned to some kind of spiritual realm to help them come to terms with their own disorientation. Meditation, for example, helped some spouses to get in touch with their own inner strength.

Theologian and author Dody Donnelly points out that "Meditating for fifteen minutes per day can let God into our lives, nourish us with Her love and heal us."[1]

Ling removed herself from the eye of the storm to recoup her emotional strength. Through meditation in the Buddhist way, she concentrated on her suffering until she could let go of it as an unnecessary burden.[2] Reaching inner peace, Ling was then able to switch back to her daily life and withstand the tension of living with a husband who was leading two lives.

Other spouses gained enlightenment from spiritual readings found in every religion, from Sufi texts, to the Hindu *Bhagavad Gita*, to Navajo stories, to Old Testament psalms.[3] For example, the repetitive verse form of the psalms of lament, biblical scholar Walter Brueggemann explains, leads the reader "into the darkness to face it, then through and out of it."[4] Equally important, notes psychologist Jeanne Paradise, Ed.D, "Hope is interwoven with these laments."[5]

As their physical, emotional and spiritual stamina is revived, spouses gradually feel that day-to-day survival is no longer impossible. They realize that they can continue to cope with their problems and take care of themselves at the same time. Now a single manageable goal to benefit themselves alone can be met such as taking a walk or reading poetry or calling a friend. It is a time simply to be.

Learning from the Past

Even with physical and emotional strength recovered, the spouse's sense of self may remain fragmented. An effective way to discover individual identity is to examine memories of the past, the second step of this stage of recovery. Looking back one can find what remains, what has changed and what has been squashed or forgotten. Questions such as, "What used to make me happy or sad?" or, "What meant something to me then?" can help arouse memories that illuminate the true self. Discovering such clues to identity reestablishes continuity with the present.

Reviewing the past can help uncover self-identity. Childhood, school life and marriage come into view, forming a collage of favorite places, games, books, friends, hobbies, all once treasured. Gradually these positive recollections form a person with a distinct personality who was once responsive to life. Negative recollections that engender pain or sorrow also help clarify the spouse's self-identity. Reflecting on the marriage or the partner's coming out may be especially illuminating. Rather than turning away from such unhappy memories, the spouse may find it instructive to examine them by asking such questions as, "Why did I feel that way? What does this say about me?"

Many spouses, while reviewing the post coming-out period, experience an outburst of angry feelings hitherto repressed. Auerback and Moser, in their study of seven support groups, report that it took five three-hour monthly sessions before wives expressed delayed anger at their husbands. Some never returned after their outbursts, unable to deal with their negative feelings.[6]

The tumultuous rage of this stage is normal and necessary. This feeling is different from fury over damaged sexuality. Instead, there is a deep resentment at being devalued by the partner. There may also be bitterness, a feeling that the partner's problem has killed the joy in the spouse's life.

Reflecting too long upon unpleasant parts of the past, especially those concerning the partner's coming out, has its pitfalls. Since the spouse is looking back from a weakened self-concept and feeling tremendous anger, the tendency is to magnify problems and to forget positive, happy times that also occurred. Such selective remembering can sabotage the process of learning from the past.

Sometimes spouses may need to realize that the goal of their retrospection is to learn more about themselves instead of punishing themselves or anyone else because of what happened in the past. The point is to put the good and the bad aspects of past experiences into perspective. Since recollections of marriage may be the most difficult to view objectively, it helps to compare memories with partner, friends and family members.

Good times in the marriage need to be recalled and savored. Positive emotions felt then were valid under those circumstances. Imagining oneself in such situations can reveal many forgotten clues to self.

Discovering an Authentic Identity

Building on clues from the past will help the spouse to revive a sense of her or himself as a unique and valued person. This is the third and perhaps most difficult task of the coming-out crisis. The goal is to reactivate desires and interests which provide significant insight into who the spouse really is. Concentration on the self is crucial. Concerns related to the partner or marriage need to be set aside. To keep focused on self-exploration, it helps to use language that emphasizes the "I" nature of what is being done. This can be accomplished in a journal or by talking to oneself using self-dialogue such as, "*I* am going to work. *I* am crying. This is *me*."

Self-dialogue is a powerful technique for self-discovery. As clinical psychologist Pamela Butler, Ph.D., explains, it "determines the direction and quality of our lives...(and) can make the difference between happiness and despair, between self-confidence and self-doubt."[7]

Some spouses may need the help of a friend, therapist, support group or clergy person to turn their attention on themselves. For example, Catherine needed Louise's gentle push to stop putting Larry's needs first. When Catherine did, she rediscovered her love of teaching which had been set aside to live with Larry.

A first step for spouses is to resurrect interests long forgotten. One effective strategy is to engage in solitary pursuits and follow the natural impulses that arise. Any activity, whether serious or mundane, can stimulate the buried self. This can entail writing in a journal, singing in the shower, swinging on a park swing, walking in the city or country, anything as long as the activity is enjoyable. With no one else distracting the spouse, all kinds of elements can come freely into play.

In the pursuit of interests, the spouse needs to keep alert to the least flicker of something loved or yearned for. Once detected, such insights can lead to self-recognition. One husband, Cliff, recalling how he used to look as a slim six-footer, methodically started a diet that succeeded in reinforcing his self-image.

Through reactivating dormant interests, the spouse will begin to gain a clearer sense of self. For example, Erin, the wife who stood by her bisexual husband in each of his crises, began making pillows after she recalled a forgotten yen to sew. Discovering the tactile pleasure of this hobby, she expanded to giving massages. Through these pursuits, Erin realized that the sensual side of her nature was a significant part of her identity.

Introspection and solitary pursuits need to be balanced by human contact to reinforce the development of a clear self-concept. Rather than participate in large social gatherings, it's usually better to be with close friends who can nurture the person hidden behind the "coping spouse" image. The spouse may need to seek out friends who have the patience to support the spouse in her or his inner work for as long as it takes.

Old friends are invaluable aids in ferreting out parts of the self that have been ignored or repressed to make the marriage work. Even brief contact, such as a telephone call, can bring powerful results. A professional in Los Angeles has lunch or an after-work drink with an old friend every week. Each encounter puts her back in touch with a meaningful part of herself.

New friends who share common interests with the spouse can be of tremendous help in reinforcing self-confidence. Though it requires self-motivation to meet new people, they can readily be found through a wide array of activities available in most communities such as those offered at the local gym, adult education school, community church, city museum, concert hall or sponsored outings to the mountains or seashore.

Individual therapy is extremely valuable at this stage since it focuses on personal development. With a knowledgeable therapist, the spouse can learn ways to correct her or his distorted self-concept created in the mixed-orientation marriage and to sustain the growing sense of self-worth. For example, a therapist showed a teacher in Ohio how to use creative visualization to affirm herself and not be torn apart by her husband's double life.

It is critical to find a therapist or counselor who understands the effects of the coming out on the straight spouse's identity. One young wife saw four different psychiatrists before finding one who, knowing that her gay husband couldn't change his behavior for her, helped her see that only she had control over her inner happiness.

Support groups for straight spouses may be less helpful at this stage than groups that focus on identity issues such as self-esteem and co-dependency. Many of these groups stress the Twelve-Step recovery process that affirms self-acceptance and self-love and is based on the premise that every person is responsible for his or her own life, not others.

A number of excellent books such as those listed in Appendix A provide information and techniques for self-discovery. Literature can be useful if based on acknowledged theories of cognitive, behavioral or emotional development, and backed by research, clinical practice or personal experience. Particularly helpful is *How to Survive the Loss of a Love*, by Melba Colgrove, Ph.D., Harold H. Bloomfield, M.D., and Peter McWilliams.[8]

Gradually spouses get in touch with who they are. In many cases, they find that they have become far different from the person they were before the coming out and even before the marriage. Ling's experience is typical of spouses who feel uncomfortable about the strangers they have become, acting in uncharacteristic ways. Deep in her psyche, Ling wanted to be a loving companion to Jack yet hated his gayness and yearned for her own sexual life. While respecting her Asian upbringing that emphasized self-respect and virtue, she wondered if she was courageous enough to date and if she could support herself without Jack.

Once spouses discover the hallmarks of their authentic selves, they can use these characteristics as a basis for reviving their identities. Ling returned to her homeland to try living separately from Jack. Wes, by reclaiming his prayer life, could reclaim his home and, gradually, self-worth.

It may take months or years to resolve contradictions between the valued self and the artificial person that the spouse has become. Recalling Reinhold Neibuhr's invaluable prayer adopted by AA may help spouses discover themselves: "Give me the serenity to accept what I cannot change, the courage to change what I can and the wisdom to know the difference." Through constant practice of valued behavior, undesirable characteristics will gradually disappear and be replaced by a stronger identity. After two years, Catherine, formerly under Larry's control, could decide for herself whether to move heavy furniture, if not mountains. With her revived self-esteem came the confidence to be herself, married or not.

Changing Identity from "Spouse" to "I"

Once the spouse feels that he or she is a valued individual, the final step is to shed the image of spouse (or former spouse) of a gay, lesbian or bisexual partner and become an independent individual. This means no longer being defined in terms of the partner or ex-partner.

To redefine themselves according to their individual identities, spouses often begin to describe themselves in a different way. Some stop using any terms that signify the married relationship. Wives may refer to their husbands and themselves by name rather than by role, "Jack," for example, instead of "my husband." When meeting new people, a spouse might say, "I'm Cliff," without adding, "Pris' husband." Former spouses speak of ex-partners as "the children's father (or mother)." One former spouse changed her entire name.

If still married, doing things independently of the partner helps reinforce the sense of separate identity. Timothy Wolf, Ph.D., in his 1982 study of twenty-six couples, suggests that having outside interests, friends, job and sex life helps wives compensate for the "sense of incompleteness in the less than exclusive relationship."[9]

Going out alone with friends, plunging into a new project at work or buying clothes without consulting the partner can also create an inner and outer picture of an independent "I." A wife in Richmond, who changed her hairdo and wardrobe, found a job and attended social events alone, was seen as an independent woman. Many acquaintances didn't realize she was married.

Often the partner's criticism or blame may threaten the spouse's fledgling identity. Self-confidence can be reaffirmed by seeing such attacks as symptoms of the attacker's own pain, a method described by psychiatrist Gerald G. Jampolsky, M.D., in *Love is Letting Go of Fear*.[10] Viewing the partner's actions from this perspective may help the spouse realize that such criticism is unwarranted.

The identity crisis recurs each time self-concept is threatened by criticism or adverse events. Each threat provokes more soul-searching and struggle to regain peace of mind. In order not to be drawn back into the morass of lost identity, it helps to focus on solving the problem that has prompted the attack by expressing personal feelings about it as well as affirming oneself with such nurturing thoughts as, "I am a worthwhile, lovable person."

Each time the spouse withstands a challenge to his or her identity, feelings of self-confidence increase. On the other hand, if interaction with the partner continues to weaken the spouse's sense of self, leaving the relationship may be the only way to preserve identity.

As spouses begin to think and act as autonomous individuals, either within the marriage or after leaving, a surprising shift takes place. Spouses no longer act only in response to their partners, for example, by being sympathetic, defensive or rebellious according to what their partners do. Instead, spouses now act according to their own needs and wants. Many begin to love and appreciate themselves for the first time.

As a stronger authentic self-concept is forged, many spouses gain a detached perspective on the coming-out crisis. Some even develop an ironic sense of humor about their situations. One such ex-wife calls her support group, "United Single Women in Search of Men Who Aren't Gay, Married, or Hung Up on Their Mothers."

Restoring self-confidence and autonomy are prerequisite for handling the most complex issue of the coming out, one that haunts many spouses for years. This is the partner's deception in hiding his or her sexual identity and, often, same-sex activities. Part Five examines how spouses work through the perception of being deceived to rebuild integrity and regain control over their lives.

five

POWER OF THE LIE

THE SHATTERING
OF INTEGRITY

Although not all mixed-orientation marriages involve deception, the vast majority entail deceit to some degree. Because of guilt, fear or repression, only a small number of bisexual or gay men come out before marriage or tell their wives once they acknowledge their same-sex attraction. Many stay closeted and often active for a period; others never disclose. On the other hand, many bisexual and lesbian women, among whom same-gender attractions tend to develop later than for men, tell their husbands soon after they acknowledge their sexual identity. Some form relationships with women before disclosing; others never tell. In the nineties, the number of lesbian wives coming out seems to be increasing.

When husbands or wives come out, the profound effect that the deception has on their straight spouses isn't readily understood by others, especially the partners. However understandable or valid the partners' reasons are for keeping their sexual identity a secret, the severe stress that spouses suffer as a result cannot be denied. Betrayal by the person loved the most, in the most intimate of human relationships, shatters their trust not only in the partner but in others and themselves.

More devasting to spouses is the realization that they have been living a lie without knowing it. There is no certainty left about the past, present or future. Without confidence in their ability to discern fact from falsehood or right from wrong, spouses find it difficult to be true to themselves or act with moral integrity. While the partner's integrity is affirmed in the coming out, the spouse's integrity is shattered.

It usually takes a year or more before the spouse is ready to face the deception issue and another year to restore integrity. Only after the spouse has resolved pragmatic issues and gained some emotional distance from the coming out can she or he handle the more complex problem of deception. Even then the process of regaining control of the moral quality of his or her life is often prolonged by empathy for the partner's plight, anger at being duped or continuing spousal love. "If only I had an off button to stop loving him!" said one woman, four years after separating from her husband of twenty-eight years.

Since deception more often affects straight wives, only women's stories have been included in this part to illuminate the issue. Wes' story, "Two Minor Miracles," however, could just as well appear here. The two narratives that follow portray the most severe type of deceit— the partner being actively gay before coming out. The final section examines problems that both husbands and wives encounter as a result of being kept in the dark and explores ways by which spouses can restore trust and integrity.

Personal Stories

I Hope You Never Find Out
Tracey

"Herb will be a better husband than Juan, mark my words," Mother said.

Juan was my boyfriend from high school until I was a twenty-one-year-old technical student in Pittsburgh. I was still cutting my blonde hair the way he liked and wearing the shade of green he liked. I broke up with Juan in March, met Herb in April, became engaged to him in May and married in October.

Heavily-built with brown hair, Herb joined the Army after high school to get away from his mother. On his return he worked at a machine plant in Scranton, where he became engaged to some girl. Two weeks before the wedding, he claimed that he'd called it off. Then he started working in Pittsburgh. We met at the church where he assisted the director of the Catholic Young Men's Group.

During our engagement, a friend told me to break it off. "Tracey, you'll never be happy with Herb," he said.

I couldn't break it off. I was pregnant.

After we married I kept working as a medical lab assistant, except for maternity leave with our first son. Two years later when I got pregnant again, Herb made me stop working. Two years after that son was born, I bore another making the total three sons, David, Edward and James, all under the age of six.

Those were the best times. Christmas shopping in toy stores, I'd grin watching Herb pick up the trucks and trains. "You're a bigger kid than they are!" I joked lovingly.

After James was born, it was a struggle to get Herb out to do anything. He'd come home from work, open a beer and then another until we ate. After dinner he slept on the couch until ten, when I went to bed tired from being with three babies all day. He stayed up with the television until two. The next morning twelve empty bottles awaited me on the kitchen table.

We had sex so often that I sometimes thought he was oversexed. That was all right. It was the weird things he wanted to do that made me uncomfortable. Whenever he suggested something like oral sex, I said, "That's stupid!" or "No! It's too perverse."

"You're just prudish," Herb said. "Your mother filled your head with garbage. Whatever a married couple does is fine."

"O.K.," I said, "as long as both parties agree to it."

Some things I did just to please him. Afterwards I hated myself, thinking, "Instead of enjoyment, I have turmoil."

When Herb got up to drinking five cases of beer a week and weighed 280 pounds, I sat him down in a sober moment and said, "You're passed out drunk all the time killing yourself. Worse than that, you're taking yourself away from your boys and missing so much important growth! It makes me angry."

"O.K.," he said. "What can I do to make you happy?"

"You know, what would be nice is if we went for a walk."

"That's crazy! Let's go out to dinner!"

So we went out to a nice restaurant, something grandiose that impresses people. We also went to Atlantic City three times with couples from the neighborhood though we couldn't afford it. "Everybody's going!" Herb reasoned. These times we spent with others were the happiest.

Home life was different. Each weeknight when Herb got home, I asked, "How was your day?" and listened to what he said about a job I didn't understand. Then I told him what happened at home including what went wrong with the kids and how I handled it.

Each time he jumped in, "That was the wrong thing to do!"

That hurt me and I eventually decided to see a marriage counselor. I told the counselor, "I expected someone who could give, like me. But his hugs have stopped—not even an encouraging word when I need it. I want to get out, but I don't want to leave my babies. What'll I do?"

"Go back to work."

All along I'd been working, though without pay. I organized food baskets and sold newspaper ads for the Lions Club, served on the PTA board and organized the Mothers' Sports Club for my older boys' teams. A paying job would be different.

Herb didn't like the idea. "If you go back to work," he said, "that's the end of the marriage."

"Listen," I said, "I need help. Go talk to this counselor. See if she can help you help me."

"No, it's your problem. I'm not going to sit in front of some woman. You women stick together."

So instead we agreed between us that I wouldn't work until James was in school all day.

The question then was which of us would take the responsibility of birth control. The pill was out because of my varicose veins. Dismissing vasectomy, we decided on rhythm.

During our ninth year of marriage, Herb went on afternoon shifts getting home after midnight and arising at noon. After an hour to shave and shower, he would eat and leave again at three.

At first I'd wait up for him to come home. While he watched television with his beer, I'd try to tell him what the kids had been doing that day.

"Can you wait for a commercial?"

"O.K.," I'd say and go upstairs. At commercial time he would come up, have quick sex with me and then go downstairs again. Once I called out as he left, "Just leave the money on the dresser!" Finally I didn't wait up and he didn't come up to wake me.

When James started kindergarten, I took some courses to get into social work. I also lost thirty-five pounds in three months for myself. The new life ahead excited me.

The next month I didn't get my period. I was pregnant again.

Eight months later, Paula was born. Still in postpartum depression, I telephoned a marriage counselor. "I can't take any more!" I cried. "I want to run away. Everything I do is wrong."

This man kept me talking for an hour and a half, getting me back on track. Then he had me make an appointment.

"It hurts so much," I said at my first visit, "that my husband puts himself first and can't give."

For five months the counselor gave me hints on how to get Herb to talk and how to show understanding rather than criticize him. "If you've got something serious to say," he said, "do it in public where he can't scream at you and you won't get off on a tangent."

These things helped for a time. Then the counselor said, "Without Herb working with you, you can't work on the marriage."

Herb refused. "You don't need your counselor. You need this," he said, handing me *The Total Woman*.

While continuing therapy for another month, I read the book from cover to cover, how the lady slipped suggestive notes in her husband's lunch box and how, wearing just a trench coat, she rang the doorbell and when he opened the door flashed him.

"O.K.," I thought, "We'll try it." I slipped notes into Herb's lunches. I called him at work to say I wanted his body, blushing later whenever I thought of it. I used perfumed oils, raspberries and cream, everything.

One night I lay on the living room couch in the buff while he watched television. "Hey, Herb!" I called, every few minutes. "Yoo hoo!"

"In a minute. In a minute!"

After half an hour I got up and threw the book into the fireplace. "This is it," I said, lighting a match to it. "I'm done trying, Herb. It's your turn."

Four years later the recession of the early eighties hit. Working only eight days a month, Herb drank more, smoked more and slept more. Worrying about unpaid bills made him irritable. I couldn't talk to him. The kids couldn't talk to him. We had no sexual contact for four months.

Come spring I said, "Herb, we're getting deeper and deeper into debt. I'm going to get a job."

"Where the hell do you think you'll get one?"

"I'll get one."

That afternoon the coordinator of social services at the local hospital hired me on the spot. Nervous about going back to work, I chose the midnight shift to be at home mornings to get the kids off to school and evenings to help with homework.

My high school had a reunion that September. Afterwards thirty classmates came back to my house, including my old boyfriend, Juan.

His wife had gone home ill. Long after Herb went to bed, the group left, all except Juan, who suggested we take a walk to catch up on each other. Five months later he called.

"How about lunch sometime?"

"I'd love it."

We arranged to meet on the first day of May. In late April my mother was hospitalized with cancer that had spread to most of her organs. I was the one who had to tell Dad that she was dying.

Because of my part-time schedule, I was able to stay with Mother on nights off so that Dad could go home to sleep. Then I went home, got the kids off to school, did my washing and cleaning, dozed, got dinner, did the dishes and got back to the hospital.

Herb visited her only once. "As always, I put others first and he doesn't," I thought angrily.

Several times a week my brothers, Web and Mel, came to the hospital. One night Mel sat with me, talking about his wife.

"You really love her, don't you?" I asked.

"Oh, yeah. She's everything. She keeps me going. She picks me up when I'm down."

"God, it must be nice."

"Tracey, what's the matter? Aren't you happy?"

"I haven't been happy for so long, Mel, I can't tell you when I was," I sighed. "What love we had has been slowly chipped away. One day I'm going to divorce Herb."

"Well," he said, "when and if you do, let me know. I have something to tell you."

"Tell me now."

"No. When the time comes, I will but only if necessary."

The day Juan and I were supposed to have lunch, I left a message for him to call. When he heard about Mother, he came to sit with me for four hours.

He came the next two nights too. The first was Mother's seventieth birthday. The second night I told Dad to let her go. "You're just prolonging her agony," I said.

Four hours after Dad left, Mother died. There was nobody there for me, except Juan.

He and I were beginning to feel an attraction between us though we didn't know whether it was just a midlife crisis or us trying to be fifteen again. When he hinted at an affair, I said, "No. I've got to give the marriage one more try."

In June Herb and I vacationed with some couples at a resort. The first night I came out of the shower wearing a lacy black thing bought for the occasion and stood between Herb and the basketball game on the television.

"Can't you wait?" he said. "It's a good game."

My heart sank. "That's it. I can't give any more."

Once the basketball game was over, we had sex. The nightgown wasn't mentioned.

We had sex in August too, the third and last time that year. After that when he went by me in the house, I flinched. In bed I prayed he wouldn't come up. If he did, I pretended to sleep or kept reading so he'd go to sleep first.

One night as he got into bed ready for sex, I said, "No, Herb, I don't want you near me. I don't know what's wrong."

"Get your hormones checked. Must be a change of life."

The next morning a doctor at the hospital took several hormone tests and reported, "Everything's fine."

When Herb heard that, he said, "Then see a psychiatrist."

"No," I thought, "all I can see is getting a divorce."

In September I found another counselor. "I don't have the guts to divorce," I said. "Teach me how to be strong enough."

But the counselor wanted me to work on the marriage so I stopped seeing him. I went back to my obstetrician who told me to see a psychiatrist. Instead I just tried to keep on with the kids' sports, school activities and daily needs. On vacations I took them along so that Paula and I could share a bed and Herb had to sleep with the boys.

Then I got depressed and began to lose weight. The kids often found me crying when they got home.

When I bought my oldest son, David, a four hundred and fifty dollar car for his job and school, Herb screamed, "What did you do that for, Tracey? It's just junk."

A few months later Herb's mother called me frantically to say his father was in the hospital. He'd been ill for years. "I need your help, Tracey," she implored.

For the next three weeks, I went every other day to see Herb's dad and check on his mother. Herb went three times. The twenty-first day as I sat with his dad, my son Edward called to say that my father was having a stroke and needed me to get him to the hospital.

I drove to my father's house, put him in the car, got him into the emergency room and went back up to Herb's father's room. He had died. So I had to tell Herb's mother, all the brothers and sisters and my husband as they came to the hospital one by one.

Herb didn't cry when he heard.

"It's okay to cry," I said. "It's your father."

"As far as I'm concerned, he died when he first got sick."

The viewing of the body in the funeral home took place a few days later on a hot and humid Saturday. The whole family met at Herb's mother's house so that we could car pool.

When we got into our car, I said, "Follow David. His car isn't running right." Then as we pulled away, I cried out, "Wait! We're missing a kid. I didn't see Paula come out."

Herb kept on driving. "You're crazy. They're all here."

"Let's check your mom's house to be sure."

"She's in someone's car, Tracey. Don't worry."

Just then David's car stalled. As Herb made a U-turn to get behind him again, he started shouting at me, "I had to watch the damn kids when your old lady croaked. I was stuck babysitting the damn kids when my old man croaked and now I'm stuck babysitting again. All I asked for was some support during this time. You haven't given me anything."

Stunned by the violence I heard in his voice, I thought, "This isn't grief. This man hates me." With growing anger I recalled what I'd done for him and his family and what he hadn't done for me.

By the time we were at the funeral parlor, I was in tears. As I opened the door, I asked, "Does anybody here have Paula?"

When no one spoke up, I turned to Herb, "Look, you're the oldest son. Take your mother in. I'll go back and get Paula."

"No," he said, turning toward the door. "You no-good mother. You can't even keep track of your children. I'll get her." As he passed me, he gave me a shove.

"Herb," I whispered, my voice shaking, "if you walk out the door, the marriage is over. I've had it."

He walked out. I took off my wedding and engagement rings and threw them on the floor.

"Tracey!" his brother-in-law said. "I'll get Paula."

Everyone stood paralyzed. "There, there, we understand," one sister-in-law said. "It's only a year since your mom died."

Another whispered, "We know. Herb told us that you're seeing a counselor."

After Paula arrived and we viewed the body, I left with the grandchildren and some girlfriends to prepare the post-viewing dinner at Herb's mother's house. It was ninety degrees, one hundred percent humidity by then. When the others arrived, David took me home. By the time Herb got home that night, I was on the couch with my pillow and blanket.

"What do you think you're doing?"

"Filing for divorce. I'll never get in the same bed with you again. It's over. I'm tired."

He stood at the end of the couch and laughed. "You know, you really are sick!" he said and walked upstairs.

I filed for divorce a week later and slept on the couch for a year until it was final.

Herb was served the papers on our eighteenth anniversary. "Why are you doing this?" he asked. "Letting you work was my mistake. Those divorced women you hang out with gave you this idea. I gave you everything a woman could want, a beautiful home, luxuries, travel. What more did you want me to give?"

"Yourself."

After this exchange I began wondering about the secret my brother Mel had mentioned. One day, talking with my other brother's wife, I couldn't contain my curiosity. "Mel has some secret he wants to tell me," I began. "Gosh, I wish he would. I should know."

She started crying. "Tracey, I hope you never find out."

"You know?"

"Yes," she said, "Web told me years ago."

"Years?"

She nodded. "I hope you never find out."

That night I thought, "This secret must be powerful." Then I remembered a scandal about the director of the Catholic Young Men's Group, something about pornographic photos and fondling some boys. "And Herb was his assistant," I thought. "It's the only thing explosive enough to be kept secret."

The next week I went to watch Edward play field hockey. As I sat on the bleachers with the other Sports Club mothers, one began telling me how she'd discovered that her "ex" had chased women during their marriage.

"Did you know about it, Tracey?"

"Uh huh. He chased me for a month until I stopped him."

"Why didn't you tell me? You were my friend," she said.

"Because you seemed happy." I squeezed her hand. "Don't worry. My brothers are keeping a secret about Herb from me."

"Do you have an idea of what it is?"

"Uh huh. I think it has to do with sexuality."

"You're right."

I sat up rigid. "What do you mean, 'I'm right.'"

"About his sexuality." She stopped for a minute and then took a deep breath. "Herb went around the Men's Sports Club asking friends and neighbors you know for sexual favors."

Shock, anger and hurt shot through me all at once. My husband, my partner, the father of my children, doing this?

Regaining control, I crawled off the bleachers and went to the school pay phone. The only number I remembered was Web's. "Web," I said, "I want to know the secret now."

"Mel will tell you. He brought it up."

"I know. But I want to know how you know that Herb is bisexual."

Web was quiet. Then he asked, "Are you okay?"

"It's the truth, isn't it?" I persisted.

"Yes. Remember when I was hospitalized and Mel spent the night? Herb came to visit once and pounced on Mel. When he resisted, Herb said, 'There's nothing wrong with it. I did it in the Army.'"

"'Well,' Mel said, 'not with me. I'm getting out of here. You do this again and I'm telling Tracey.' The next day Mel talked to a counselor who told him to inform you."

As Web talked, I wondered if Herb had been drinking or was joking. Maybe these guys had misinterpreted what he said. "How did Herb say it?" I asked.

"Well," Web said, choking a little, "I can't say exactly."

Driving to work in agony, I wondered, "Why didn't Mel tell me? Maybe he thought that what I didn't know wouldn't hurt me." By the time I arrived at work, I couldn't function. The next day I called Mel. "Did Herb approach you?"

"Yes, three times. The third time was when you all came for dinner at our house. I came home late and took a shower. When Herb came in to use the bathroom, he made a grab for me."

"Well, that's that!" I said, hanging up. "I can't protect Herb from this as I have with the drinking and his other faults."

That night I called New York to talk with a male neighbor Herb had supposedly approached years before. Only his wife was home.

"Yes, it's true, but I assumed that you knew about it," she said, "and that you and Herb had an arrangement."

Since the holidays were coming up, I kept the secret inside me until Paula's birthday in January when we all went to eat at a restaurant in the mall, somewhere public enough to discuss it.

When the kids were off playing video games, Herb asked, "Tracey, why don't you stop the divorce!"

"I can't now."

"Why not ?"

"I have to ask you a question, first. Are you bisexual?"

"Yeah. So what?"

As I told him what Mel, Web and the neighbor had said, he nodded, emotionless.

"Now what about the Young Men's Group? How could you work so closely with the director and not know?"

"I never was aware of it."

Then I asked, "Have you ever touched one of our sons?"

"No."

"That's all I want to know."

The subject came up once more one night when he was drinking. "You never pleased me as a woman, Tracey," he said. "That's why I had to get it from men. No woman would want me this fat."

Over the next few weeks, I called friends who might know something more. They told me that he was involved in the Young Men's Group scandal and that it was his first fiancee who had cancelled their wedding at the rehearsal dinner. Some people thought I knew. Most believed my happy face and didn't want to rock the boat.

The more I found out, the more I suffered abdominal pain, vomiting, diarrhea, headaches. My best friend didn't want to talk about it. The girls at work were no help since they had no experience with it. I couldn't find any books on being married to a gay person. In February I went to a psychiatrist.

Then one afternoon in March, the left side of my face and left arm became numb. "My God, it's a stroke!" I said and drove myself to the hospital. Going up the steps to the emergency room, my left leg gave out so that I had to drag myself to the door.

They were about to admit me to the cardiac unit when they called my doctor who said I had a chronic blockage in my nervous system. "Give her tranquilizers and send her home," he said.

When I called my doctor the next day, he said he didn't tell me before because it was something one can live with.

Three months later my co-workers noticed my left cheek drooping and my eyelid half closed. When they took my blood pressure, it was 150/110. Once chest pains started, they got me to the emergency room at which point my heart rate was jumping all over the place and my blood pressure was going up and down. This time I was admitted to cardiac care and a cardiologist was called to see me.

All I was aware of was the kindness and caring in his eyes as he asked calmly, "O.K., what's the problem?"

He heard me out. Then, after asking if I wanted an AIDS test, he told me about his own bitter divorce and the emotional and physical symptoms that many people experience in such trauma. "We'll do some testing, but I think it's apprehension and anxiety. We'll get you through it."

After thirty-two hours I was sent home with orders not to do anything but sleep until testing on Monday. Not wanting to call on Herb for anything, I had my neighbor drive me home.

On Saturday Herb came home with a swollen arm. Taking one look, I sent him to the hospital clinic. It was a blood clot. He was admitted for five days.

The first day I was able to rest. The second day Herb called wanting clean underwear. The next day it was something else. The fifth day he asked for a ride home. When I arrived, his mother was there with her car.

Over the next five months, we just existed waiting for the divorce to be final. I went to work, exercised on the treadmill in the cardiologist's office and helped the kids with school activities. Herb moved out when the divorce was final.

We put off telling his mother until the holidays were over. In February I took her to lunch to tell her gently.

"I knew something was wrong," she said, wiping her eyes. "Oh, Tracey, don't let me lose the grandchildren."

"You won't," I said, putting my hand over hers.

"I hope we can still be friends," she smiled. Then she asked, "Is there anything else I should know?"

Afraid that she'd find out from the other family members I'd told, I said, "Yes, one more thing. It's a big one."

When I told her, she said nothing for a moment. Then she asked, "Tell me, did a Francis Locke ever call Herb?"

"Yes."

She started crying again. Francis, I found out later, was a known homosexual Herb had hung around with after the Army. The family knew about him and didn't like the relationship.

Except for her, that was the last time I saw or heard from Herb's family, though they spoke of me to others saying that I'd had affairs with men at work through the last years of the marriage.

For weeks after the divorce, anger and guilt plagued me. As I folded laundry, I wanted to rip up the clothes. I kept saying to my psychiatrist, "I busted up a marriage and family."

"Listen to yourself," he finally said. "What other choice was there? Did you want to stay miserable all your life?"

"Well, maybe I'm the type who likes being a martyr."

"No, Tracey, you're not!" he said.

I went to my priest with my guilt. "I was taught by the nuns that marriage is forever and not to be selfish. This is the first selfish thing I've done. It benefited nobody but me."

"In order to take care of others," he said, without a pause, "we must take care of ourselves first."

Then my fortieth birthday came. As I woke up that morning, lying in bed, I vowed, "This is the day I'm taking a step forward. I am not ever going to take a step back again!"

Siempre Manana
Caitlin

I had a traditional image of what life would bring me. I'd go to college, become a teacher, marry, have kids and stay home, working for the PTA and volunteering. Life would be wonderful for me.

In high school, I didn't date much. In college, I saw my male classmates just as intellectuals I could have wonderful discussions with. That's how I controlled relationships.

My heart was first touched doing community work in Washington. Miguel was bright, attractive, popular and had a tremendous amount of energy and skills. When he said that he planned to get a doctorate from Harvard, I thought, "I can't believe my luck! It's everything I wanted and more."

Miguel grew up poor, the son of Puerto Rican immigrants. He was the first of his family to graduate from high school, not to mention college. His parents were so proud! When he wanted to get a master's degree, they were impressed but could no longer identify with his goals. When he joined the Peace Corps and then wanted to get a Ph.D., they sat back and smiled.

Education was the way Miguel could leave his background. He dreamed of financial security, professional acclaim and a close family that he hadn't had because of his father's absence from home working long hours to make ends meet. Like me, he'd been raised as a good Catholic and shared my values to be loving, kind, get married and have kids.

So we became engaged. We were a handsome couple, Miguel with his brown hair and flashing eyes and I with auburn hair and the translucent skin of the Irish. We were two liberal kids of the sixties.

One weekend after our engagement, we went to lunch on the coast. Watching the fog circle outside the window, we felt close. All of a sudden Miguel stopped talking and his brow furrowed. Frightened, I wondered what I'd said wrong. After two days he came out of it. All was well again.

After we married, we found an apartment in Boston where he got a job and started graduate school. Then he quit his job to study full time, day and night.

"That's O.K.," I said to myself. "We can put off quality time until he finishes school."

Our sex life wasn't terribly exciting but it was regular. When Miguel's course work was finished, we decided to have a baby. We moved to Hartford, within driving distance of Harvard and both found positions in the school system. Miguel planned to finish his dissertation later.

Gradually our sex life improved and I got pregnant. I stopped teaching just before our son, Felipe, was born. Fifteen months after his birth, we decided to have a second baby. Lo and behold, it was twins. Confined to bed toward the end, while Miguel travelled and started his dissertation, I kept thinking, "Of course, he has to do this for his career. So what if I have a toddler and a difficult pregnancy! I can handle it. My husband is going to have his Ph.D. A few years of struggle are necessary for life to get better afterwards."

Lucy and Maria were born in the fall. Once I regained my strength, I shared babysitting with friends so I could do consulting work in the schools again. My career took off.

When the twins were a year old, we decided to adopt. Good community-minded people of the sixties, we'd planned to adopt two underprivileged children after having two of our own. Since we now had three, we decided to adopt only one. A month after our decision, a friend of Miguel's family asked us to adopt her baby, due in a month. After therapy and much discussion, we said, "Yes, we should do this." Carlos arrived well and happy.

Miguel continued to work on his dissertation while I took care of the four babies, all under three, did some consulting work and kept things going financially. When my mother questioned my load, I answered cheerfully, "Once Miguel finishes his degree, we'll have the life we want."

Meanwhile the pressure of Miguel's research was turning him into a basket case. He began having horrible nightmares and losing momentum.

After each nightmare I said, "You have to finish or you'll always question yourself. I can sacrifice whatever's needed."

For months we went without sex. "I just don't have the desire because I'm so stressed," Miguel explained.

I wasn't concerned. "So what? Life isn't perfect and what a marvelous husband I have!"

When it was time for Miguel's oral examination, I went with him. "This is great," I thought, sitting in the Harvard Yard. "Finally, the eleventh hour! My husband is taking his orals and I'm here to cheer him on and to hold his hand when he gets anxious."

After graduation Miguel became severely ill. He was so sick physically and emotionally that work was impossible for months. Our sex life was still nonexistent. Since he had always been an overachiever, I figured he was just getting sick to extremes.

Yet his depression scared me to death. With my encouragement, he went into therapy, choosing a psychologist in Boston, an hour and a half away. "Why not?" I thought. "Maybe they have professionals of higher quality in Boston."

I also suggested that he think about making friends. "Why not join a men's group of some kind?" I said one day.

Miguel chose a group concerned with men's issues. It turned out that three-fourths of the men were gay, but I encouraged him out of my open-mindedness to continue going to meetings.

Soon Miguel began to stay out until two and three in the morning several evenings a week. When asked about it, he said, "I need some alone time to think."

"Yeah," I answered, "it's hard to think with four kids in the house." I thought, "He needs time to tend to his own needs after these years of struggle." But his absence began to annoy me.

When I brought it up, Miguel said, "Caitlin, I love you. You're wonderful. Just give me time to work things out about myself. Please be patient."

Before long I began to lose sleep, worrying that he would commit suicide from depression. Soon we began arguing about his late hours, we who had always been nice to each other. I finally made an appointment to see his therapist.

"Is Miguel going to get better or have a breakdown or what?"

"I don't think he'll have a breakdown," he said, "but if he does, you must think about your own needs. What if he never changes? Can you live with that? Does the marriage meet your needs?"

"Sure," I thought.

That Easter we were putting the kids to bed when Miguel said that he wanted to talk. Downstairs he handed me a six-page letter. I sat down on the sofa, turned on the light, and began to read.

> Please do not hate me, Caitlin. I really do love you. That's why I married you, but it has become obvious that I cannot love a woman the way I love a man and that I am gay.

I drew in a deep breath and kept on reading. As a child he'd felt attracted to other boys but fought the urge. A few homosexual experiences freshman year in college scared him into going to a psychologist who said, "Don't worry. You're eighteen and haven't had sexual experiences with women yet."

"I'm not 'strange' after all!" he told himself and repressed his homosexual feelings. Although he dated girls, he avoided sex by keeping busy with jobs and a full course load. He went with one girl for many years until she mentioned marriage. When the next girl he dated became intimate with him, he ended the relationship.

Then he met me, the epitome of the woman he wanted in his life. "You didn't press me for a physical relationship," Miguel's letter said. "You were nurturing and understanding." As he fell in love with me, he again questioned if he was gay.

The psychiatrist he went to for a year told him, "You're not gay. All you need is a good woman. But don't tell Caitlin."

Somewhat reassured, Miguel subdued his fears by keeping a frenetic schedule, always under pressure from work, school and community activities.

> "My breakdown started," Miguel's letter went on, "when I was staying several weeks at a time at Harvard a year and a half ago. I met a master's student who turned out to be gay and we started an affair. Because of his fast life of bars and parties, I

ended the relationship after a few months. Then I met another person at the university....

I became sick trying to avoid the issue. I knew it was wrong and I still loved you and the children. So I got help from the therapist in Boston (who is gay), the men's group, and a gay advocacy group until the pressure finally broke me."

As I finished reading the letter, not totally surprised yet still in shock, I said, "Well, let's not panic. I can deal with it. Let's figure out what to do. Poor Miguel! Look at all you've gone through. I'm so sorry. Don't worry. I'm not going to hate you."

Miguel came over and we sat together, holding each other and talking. Then he mentioned Ed, his friend who had visited us often. "He's more than just a friend, Caitlin."

Miguel had met Ed in the men's group. When Miguel brought him to our house, I liked him. A good-looking man, he seemed warm and friendly. He came for dinner several times and once we set him up on a blind date with a friend of mine. Recalling this, I couldn't believe what Miguel was telling me.

When he finished, I said, dry-eyed, "This doesn't mean our marriage is over, but I need you to be honest with me. If we're going to make this marriage work, it's got to be based on honesty. I don't want any surprises."

"Sure," he said. "No surprises."

Then I stood up, saying quickly, "I need to take a drive."

Calling my friend, Judy, I asked, "Can I come over now?"

Before leaving for Judy's, I telephoned a college friend in Washington. "Can I come for the weekend? I can't tell you why."

"Of course!"

When I arrived at Judy's, I said, "I've got to tell you something." Then I began to cry.

She held me as I talked and sobbed until I was calm enough to go home.

That weekend none of my Washington friends were surprised. "We figured it had to be that. Nothing else would upset you so."

On my return Miguel met me at the airport. As we drove home, he said, "I'm not sure you realize that Ed is still my lover." Then he explained that they had already been sleeping together when I invited

Ed for Thanksgiving and Christmas, thinking he'd like a family dinner since he lived away from home.

"Remember that weekend retreat my therapist recommended?" Miguel continued. "Ed had a job in the area that weekend and stayed with me in the cabin."

"My father's cabin? You two were having sex in my father's cabin?" I cried.

As I was digesting this news, I discovered that while I was in Washington Miguel had hired sitters and gone out after reading to the kids and putting them to bed. Hurt and annoyed, I said, "You can't even give up your social life for the family!"

Two nights later I had Miguel invite Ed over so that I could talk with him. While Miguel stayed upstairs, we talked for four hours. "I'm not going to be ugly about it," I told him. "I'm not against gay people. You're not going to ruin Miguel's life. If it had to happen, I'm glad it's you."

He replied, "I like you, too. I'm not going to be strange or try to take away the kids or ruin your marriage. I told Miguel not to tell you so it wouldn't be ruined."

For the next four months, I kept telling myself, "This is part of my life now. Miguel is gay and has to have time with his lover. I can deal with that. I'm going to be loving, supportive, rational and think about the needs of the family."

For a while our sex life improved. Miguel kept telling me how much he loved me. Soon we worked out a system for him to be with Ed two evenings a week, Friday and one other.

"I'm not ready for you to spend the night with him," I said. As it was I cried every evening he was with Ed.

Next I spent forty dollars on books to read all I could on homosexuality and on marriage. I located a support group of wives of gay men in Boston and met a woman who had been with her gay husband for thirty-five years after he'd come out. They had raised their kids together. She'd become his friend, confidante and mother protector. She'd made him get one man out of his life because she thought the man was "weird."

As I looked at this overweight chain smoker and apparent alcoholic, I thought, "Wait! I can't let this happen to me."

Going to the support group was like coming home. The other women understood where I was. As I listened to their experiences, some more ugly and painful than mine, it became clear that my increasingly negative feelings were normal.

In the group the image I projected was "We have a wonderful marriage. I'm going to make it work." Everyone was impressed with how positive, cheerful, strong and capable I appeared. Even I believed it. It was true because I'd worked hard at realizing this image I'd always had of myself.

Inside I was thinking, "Something's destroying my life, my marriage and my fantasy."

Finally I agreed to let Miguel spend Friday nights with Ed. Yet I cried when he was gone, despite his saying, "It's a wholesome experience, much like having sex with a woman."

Bit by bit I discovered underwear decorated with cupids in his dresser and cards from gay baths and bookstores in his wallet. Though I knew looking for them wasn't right, the discoveries forced me to finally see reality.

Four months later, after I could no longer stand my jealousy which was alien to my nature, I said, "Miguel, I can't think clearly about this. I need space. Please move out."

We told the children, "Daddy needs time out. He's really tired."

I helped Miguel move into an apartment ten minutes away. All six of us spent the first night there. The second night just the kids stayed with him.

Once he was in the apartment, jealousy overwhelmed me. "What's happening to you?" I asked myself between crying bouts. "You're usually such an accepting, supportive woman."

A few weeks later en route from visiting my parents, the children and I stopped by Miguel's apartment. "I need to see him," I thought as I rang the bell. "Ed may be there, but that's okay. The kids should see their father."

When Miguel answered the door, I saw the candlelight dinner the two men were having. They both looked embarrassed. "I don't care how they feel," I thought. "I'm the one who's hurt."

Because Miguel lived so close, we were still a couple, seeing each other every day. We still loved each other tremendously and felt like best friends. I wanted him to share everything he was doing in his life away from me, even intimate details about his sex life. Each time he finished telling me, I thanked him, welcoming the hurt.

Then Miguel received a job offer in Washington. He let me decide whether he should go, as he had with the Ph.D.

"Go," I said. "Take the job." I'd started consulting work again, juggling it with the care of the children and our large house. Having him out of town was what I needed emotionally.

Once he was gone traveling for his job, it was hard handling the kids by myself. With energy only to survive, I didn't realize the trauma his absence was causing me. The pressure of keeping his secret compounded my turmoil. One day, when picking up Felipe at a playmate's house, the mother, whom I didn't know well, asked how I was.

Without thinking I blurted out, "My husband's gay."

Though she was conservative, she held and comforted me. As I left I thought, "This secret isn't as awful as I'd imagined."

When our anniversary came around in May, we spent it together in New York. For my birthday a week later, we met in New York again.

The following weekend I called him. "Let's try again. Let's see if we can make it work."

"Fine."

"I want the next year to be just us," I continued. "I don't want Ed nearby."

"O.K."

Though I didn't like making all of our decisions, I sold the house, left my job, packed up our belongings and moved the four children and myself to Washington before school started. While house hunting, the children and I stayed in a motel and Miguel remained in the house he rented with several straight men.

Right away Ed moved to Miguel's house. When we found a four-bedroom house for our family, Ed took Miguel's place in his old house. Once again he and Miguel spent Friday nights together. Once again Miguel traveled. Once again I put up with it because we were trying to redefine our marriage.

Miguel's lifestyle made me tense especially when he and Ed went to the baths, even though he said, "We don't do anything with anyone else. It's the only place where we can be together publicly."

I didn't believe him. I couldn't trust him any more. There was no way to know if what he said was true or not.

By then our lovemaking was infrequent. When we made love, it wasn't very good. Miguel was also having work-related stress. To get the bills paid, I took a good-paying job unrelated to my field.

Then our anniversary came around again. I gave Miguel an azalea plant as a sign of growth. He gave me nothing, though we had dinner at a restaurant we found at the last minute. Although I understood that his money was tight, I was disappointed that he hadn't thought ahead. I can't recall whether or not we made love that night. By then I didn't want to anymore because of the possibility of getting a sexually transmitted disease.

The next week I vowed, "If this marriage is going to work—and, by God, I'm going to make it work—it will be sexless. I'm going to give up my sex life for this marriage. I'm going to find love in other ways, not necessarily sexual. Lots of friends will nurture me. This is not going to ruin me."

That weekend I told Miguel, "I've given up my fantasy of being Donna Reed in a blissful Hollywood marriage. It's hard to give up so much. I will need support." Tired and weak, feeling physically ill, I counted on his help.

My birthday was the following Saturday. Friday night I was alone since Miguel was with Ed. After I took the kids to stay with relatives, I rented movies and a video machine to binge on something other than alcohol or food. Stretched out on the couch in front of the TV, I watched movie after movie until well past midnight.

The next day Miguel and I went out to lunch and walked among the cherry trees. Before dinner I said, "Please don't drink too much. I'm too tired to drive having watched movies so late last night."

Miguel drank at dinner and then at a show bar we went to afterwards. He slept all the way home while I drove.

When we arrived home he asked, "Are you disappointed?"

"Well, yes. I know money's tight and I appreciate spending the day and evening out, but I didn't get a present or a card from you. Birthdays are important to me. You know that."

Suddenly he screamed, "What more do you want from me? I didn't have time to buy you a card. I didn't even have time to go to the bathroom all week!" Then he stormed out of the house.

I was furious. It was the first time I could remember being angry with him.

The next morning Miguel came home. "Sorry, Caitlin," was all he said.

A few nights later while I was resting on my bed listening to classical music, it suddenly became clear. "Why am I giving up my whole life for this marriage?" I thought. "What do I get out of it? Give me crumbs and I'll stick around? I can't even have sex with anyone else. I can't be an unfaithful wife."

Then my thought switched. "Wait! Miguel's the one who's unfaithful. You don't even have a marriage you morally agree with, Caitlin. It's not based on faith and trust. Your image of right and wrong is screwed up. What Miguel is doing is wrong. Therefore this marriage can't last."

There was nothing more to do. It had taken two and a half years of trying to make the marriage work for me to see that it was over. I'd wanted my fantasy to come true so much that I'd compromised who I was and what I believed to make it real.

Of course my fantasy couldn't come true! Until that was blatantly obvious, I couldn't let it go. Now I could finally let it go and deal with reality.

Reversing the Negative Effects of Deception

The deception revealed by the partner's coming out presents a painful enigma for the straight spouse to unravel. To some extent the partner's deceit may seem motivated by good intentions such as the belief that love for the spouse will override the partner's sexual orientation, the desire to keep the marriage going and the family together or to not hurt the spouse. Yet to the spouse it can appear as if the partner did it primarily to serve personal interests. While the partner's closet may have provided him or her protection from sexual or moral confusion or anti-gay discrimination, in the marriage it created a false world in which the spouse unwittingly helped carry off the masquerade. With the discovery of the partner's sexual orientation, the spousal role may seem like a charade and the marriage a sham. In the spouse's eyes, the real partner was hidden behind a misleading mask. As a professional woman, formerly married to a gay man, commented, "Our husbands were the best actors!"

For many spouses the deception implies that they have been living a lie without knowledge or consent, through the misleading behavior of the beloved partner they trusted. Discovery of the truth destroys their world as they thought it to be. As sex therapist Sharon Nathan comments, "(It) robs you of some sense of continuity with your own past."[1]

Some spouses, quickly deciding that the partner's betrayal nullifies the marriage contract, divorce at once. A more common reaction is to ignore the deception as too painful to address right away. Divorced or married, it takes months for spouses to sort through the moral issues surrounding the duplicity and to determine a moral compass to guide their lives.

Rebuilding moral integrity involves eight stages:

- Sorting out the truth from lies
- Assessing the power of the lie
- Using anger constructively
- Understanding both sides of the closet
- Rebuilding trust in others and self
- Sharing the secret
- Reconstructing moral values
- Acting with integrity

Sorting Out the Truth from Lies

When spouses finally realize the discrepancy between the truth and what they assumed it to be, their reactions can be explosive. When Herb yelled at Tracey that she was a bad mother, she, unable to reconcile such an unfounded accusation with reality any longer, cried, "It's over! I'm tired," and filed for divorce. When she realized the extent of Herb's duplicity later, severe psychosomatic symptoms erupted.

Until the marriage is recast in a framework of honesty, the first task in restoring integrity, the spouse rarely feels certain about anything in her or his life. As one twenty-year-old said, in trying to get her husband to tell her where he'd been overnight, "Everyone needs the truth."

In retrospect, layers of lies are usually found woven into the marriage, often from the beginning and almost always from the time the husband came out to himself. Most lies appear as omission of facts, projected blame, rationalizations or cover-ups—what some wives describe as "mind-bending" by their husbands. Explicit denial occurs rarely and usually in response to a confrontation.

The screen of rationalizations used to hide the secret may have seemed plausible at one time. Being late or absent because of gay encounters at teahouses, bars or designated places in the community can be camouflaged by believable explanations—extra work at the office, heavy traffic or overtime at a construction site—excuses that any errant partner might offer. Actual events like meetings or choir practice can provide gay contacts. On the other hand, an excuse like, "Let's not go out with the so-and-so's. He's too dull," may turn out to be a smoke screen for the husband's fear that he'll make a pass at the other man, as Tracey's husband did.

Once the truth comes out, it may seem incredible that it could have been hidden and that the spouse didn't suspect. Many spouses wonder if they were accomplices to the deceit through a naivete that made the charade possible or an unconscious wish to deny the truth out of loyalty or fear of being hurt. There may also be nagging guilt, feeling somehow responsible for their partner's life.

Often spouses continue to discount the truth by playing "What if" and "If only" games. For example, wives who have separated and divorced may tell themselves, "If I'd only known, I could have done something to make the marriage work before it was too late." Dwelling on hypotheses that can't be proved isn't constructive. It only perpetuates more self-blame and prolongs the denial of reality.

Some spouses, unable to accept the betrayal, may seek out further proof of the painful truth. The result can be upsetting as Caitlin found when she walked in on the candlelight dinner of Miguel and his lover. Such hurtful encounters help cure disbelief, somewhat like cauterizing a wound. Yet enough is enough on top of the guilt and growing anger of this stage.

Gradually as spouses sort out the truth, they begin to understand more clearly why their partners blamed them for sexual or other marital problems. Whether or not the blame is at all merited, placing all accountability onto the spouse is a way to deny the real cause and to substitute a false culprit. Such psychological projection erases the partner's culpability.

Assessing the Power of the Lie

Assessing the impact of the partner's lie on the spouse's life, the second task of recovery from deception, may be one of the most unsettling parts of the coming out for the spouse. Without knowledge of the sexual incompatibility in the marriage, it is impossible for the spouse, no matter how capable, to resolve sexual and marital problems. If Tracey had known Herb's sexual orientation, she wouldn't have tried to attract him nor suffered the subsequent humiliation. More devastating was the realization that Herb, knowing his sexual orientation, let Tracey continue her futile attempts to seduce him.

Wives whose husbands knew but didn't reveal they were gay or bisexual before marrying, feel doubly hurt because one of the primary factors for deciding to marry was deliberately hidden from them. Although some men marry believing it will help cure or overcome gay inclinations, their wives nevertheless have no say in the decision that affects them as well. One such woman, an intensely sexual "flower child" of the sixties, married a doctor who promptly stopped making love to her and groomed her into a doctor's wife. He made no effort to satisfy her frustrated sexual desire. Finally, thirteen years later, he revealed that he was gay.

When asked why he had married her, he responded, "I expected to have a sexless marriage."

"Who are you to tell me," she exploded, "how I'm supposed to live my life?"

Ultimately many wives feel stripped of power over the quality and direction of their lives. As Sissela Bok, Ph.D., explains in her classic study, *Lying*, applicable to straight spouses, "...to be given false information about important choices in their lives is to be rendered powerless. For them, their very autonomy may be at stake."[2]

The negative effects of a partner's deceit can have serious consequences for the spouse beyond psychological problems. Lisa, a twenty-three-year-old mother of a toddler, had her tubes tied because of her husband's anger over her second pregnancy. After the truth came out and they divorced, Lisa had to cope not only with his deceit but with the fact that she couldn't bear any more children should she remarry.

Even after the coming out, many spouses' lives are dominated by deceit as their partners ask them to keep their secret in strict confidence. Many spouses feel powerless and alone in their predicament with no one to turn to. As their partners suffer from the social stigma, so do they, as Wes felt in "Two Minor Miracles."

Some spouses find themselves caught in the cross fire between their partners and a homophobic society. In one extreme case reported in a metropolitan newspaper, a Catholic Archdiocesan Tribunal annulled the marriage of a straight wife on the basis that her ex-husband was actively gay before the marriage and did not tell her. Although he admitted the fact, he sued the ex-wife along with the archdiocese for several million dollars over terms used in the privileged document, such as "personality disorder." Nearly three years later, with the suit still pending and a non-refundable retainer fee spent, the wife feels like a pawn in the larger social-moral controversy.

Feeling victimized by the lie, many spouses struggle for a long time to shake off its negative effects. They feel robbed of their lives and experience intense rage at their partners, the gay world, homophobia and themselves for having been taken.

Using Anger Constructively

Anger at deception can predominate spouses' thinking for months and years, diverting them from regaining control of their lives. Such fury generally stems from expectations about what the partner "should have done," presumptions that Albert Ellis, M.D., founder of the International Institute for Rational-Emotive Therapy, calls "irrational beliefs."[3] Although anger is a normal reaction to feeling duped, it does not change what the partner did or might do in the future. Harboring resentment or hostility tends to color interactions with the partner, preventing constructive resolution of subsequent couple problems.

Spouses can learn how to use their anger as a tool for positive growth, the third step in restoring integrity. This is done, Ellis explains, by perceiving anger as resulting from a specific feeling such as frustration, disappointment, irritation or pain. Spouses can determine which feeling actually underlies their rage by asking, "What am I really angry about? Am I mad because things didn't turn out as I expected, I didn't get my way or my partner's behavior is bothering me?" By handling the specific feeling aroused by the circumstance, the spouse may be able to distance herself or himself from the debilitating anger and move towards resolution of the problem.

For example, the fury that a wife feels when her husband goes out with his lover can be recognized as disappointment at not having him at home. Rather than rant about his behavior which she cannot control, it's more productive to plan ways to avoid similar disappointment in the future. In this case, the wife may decide to go out or invite a friend over the next time the husband leaves her to be with his lover, thereby replacing the disappointing situation with one that she enjoys.

Constructive use of anger can be practiced on everyday problems such as waiting in line at the bank. Rather than fuming over what the teller should or shouldn't be doing, energy can be used to do something productive like thinking through a problem at work. That task will then get accomplished and the spouse won't be so upset over the inconvenience of waiting in line.

Understanding Both Sides of the Closet

As anger becomes more controllable, spouses can begin to unravel the perplexities of why their partners hid the truth. The dilemma can be resolved by understanding the partner's motivation and, conversely, by helping her or him comprehend the spouse's hurt. This twofold task is the fourth streategy in rebuilding integrity.

It is critical to understand what was at stake for the partner to have carried out the deception. The purpose isn't to excuse what was done, but to understand how guilt, fear and other motivating factors can cause bisexual and homosexual persons to deny the truth to themselves and to hide it even in marriage.

In seeking to understand the partner's behavior, it is important that a spouse hear the partner's side of the story without refuting what may sound like rationalizations. Typically gay husbands may say, "I didn't want to face the possibility myself and didn't want to upset you," or, " I'd rather have died than tell you I was gay. I didn't want to lose you and the kids." They may also say that they dated men because cheating with women would have threatened or hurt their wives more.

When listening to such statements, it is more effective to concentrate on the partner's underlying emotions and to resist the temptation to argue. It helps to remember that the aim of this dialogue isn't to "catch" the partner in more lies, but to comprehend his or her motive. Trying to understand feelings shifts the tone of an otherwise adversarial discussion to one that is mutually supportive.

As spouses begin to comprehend the powerful role that guilt and fear play in their partners' lives, incomprehensible actions like husbands leaving telltale clues around can be explained. Often the rationale in that instance is "I've put out the signs. It's up to her to act upon them." According to Diane Vaughan, Ph.D., this is a common ritual used to break up a relationship without hurting the other person.[4] The irony is that the spouse does get hurt anyway.

Living a false life may hurt the partner as well as the spouse. In prolonged deception, Bok explains, the pattern of covering up becomes hard to reverse. At the same time, living in constant fear of being found out slowly erodes integrity.[5] If the partner has a lover, the need for secrecy becomes even more complex, Vaughan points out, as both the sexual identity and the affair have to be hidden from the spouse.[6]

The partner's deceit—often to him- or herself as well as to the spouse—can also lead to severe physical problems or self-destructive behavior such as alcoholism or suicidal thoughts. One husband who married thinking his graduate school affairs were behind him suffered severe chest spasms eighteen years later. As he hovered near death, his wife took him to several doctors who were unable to determine the cause. Undergoing further treatment including massage, rolfing and Reikian therapy, he finally revealed what had been buried in his frail chest. After he disclosed his homosexuality, he left the doctor's office pain-free.

When partners finally tell their spouses the secret, they feel tremendous release from guilt and pain. Many are proud of their courage to be honest. Before the impact of the deception hits them, spouses often empathize with their partners. They may even encourage their mates, as one said, "to stop hiding behind this facade." Only later do they begin to see how the duplicity has hurt them.

As spouses realize the extensive role that deception has played in their married lives, it is important to express candidly to their partners how much pain the deceit has caused. The aim isn't to punish the partner or arouse more guilt, but to raise his or her awareness of the spouse's side of the crisis.

Spouses may find it hard to suppress their resentment or anger when explaining how the deceit has affected them. Yet the surest way to be heard is to communicate negative feelings calmly and directly. For instance, when a husband responds by saying that he didn't want to hurt the wife by telling her, she might reply quietly, "Well, it's really the other way around. Not telling me hurt far more."

In many cases the partner may counterattack, especially if the spouse is agitated. From her counseling of straight spouses, Aurele Samuels describes how a gay husband often reacts to an angry wife. "She is accused of homophobia, being crazy, overreactive, hysterical, and unreasonable. Her dilemma is discounted in preference to his."[7]

Such a response is counterproductive and inaccurate. The wife may be hysterical, but expressing her hurt is not a homophobic attack. The husband has no right to deny the wife her feelings. By listening to her underlying emotions, he may better understand her position and become more sensitive to her concerns. If the couple is unable to discuss their problems constructively, they may need the mediation of a counselor.

To hear each other out requires patience and objectivity on both sides. In particular, understanding the spouse's perspective can help the partner to become less defensive about his or her actions and to be better able to examine the consequences of his or her coming out.

Rebuilding Trust in Others and Self

Having been duped by the most important person in their lives, many spouses experience difficulty in trusting others and themselves after the coming out. The loss of trust is one of the more damaging aspects of the deceit, since trust is fundamental in any healthy relationship. Rebuilding trust in others and self is the fifth task of this stage.

After the disclosure, spouses often begin to distrust everything their partners say or don't say. "He must have other secrets," many think. For example, wives may wonder if their husbands have "quickies" in men's restrooms or how often they make "eye contact" with other men in public places. Worries arise, such as "Does he really practice safe sex elsewhere?" or "Will he tell me if he tests HIV-positive?" Repeated protestations of love, typical of this period, may also become suspect. Many spouses wonder, "How can he love me if he's gay?"

As wives realize the extent of betrayal, their distrust increases. After repeating, "Poor Miguel," with empathy for his pain, Caitlin was horrified to hear that he had used her father's cabin for secret trysts with his lover. Then when Miguel went back on the agreement not to see Ed for awhile, Caitlin's buried suspicions about his reliability surfaced and she stopped trusting him altogether. Honesty was to be the basis of their marriage after coming out.

Increasingly cynical, many spouses now lose confidence in everyone, including themselves. Straight husbands and wives alike often suffer from the distorted impression that anyone of the opposite sex may be secretly gay. Spouses may also doubt the reliability of their own judgment in having placed such unquestioning trust in their partners. Many wonder why they weren't able to perceive their partner's homosexuality when friends or family were able to.

Recently during a TV talk show on straight wives, an older woman in the audience asked one of the panelists, "Why couldn't you tell, being married for twenty years? I could three months after we married just by the way he talked and walked and dressed. Anyone who stayed in the rest room as long as him had to be gay."

"But my husband didn't look or dress differently from other men I knew," answered the panelist quickly. Afterwards, her confidence vanishing, she said to a friend, "Why didn't I see other clues!"

To lessen unnecessary mea culpas, it helps to remember that until recently there was little information on gay-straight marriages. Through the seventies, common belief held that married persons with children couldn't be gay. Although the spate of comings-out in the eighties proved otherwise, reinforced by a steady if not increasing number in the nineties, many people still assume that marriage and homosexuality are a contradiction of terms.

Moreover, the majority of gay men and lesbians don't display stereotypical behavior or dress. Many are indistinguishable from their straight counterparts and are found in all walks of life, just as some straight men who use effeminate mannerisms may appear "gay" and straight women may appear "butch."

As information about gay-straight marriages becomes more widespread, there will be more likelihood for such marriages to be based on honesty and trust with more chance for success. Yes, there are progressive centers across the country, but also are pockets of misinformation in some communities and subcultures since sexual attitudes are partly the product of cultural values. Hispanic groups, for example, who place high value on macho behavior, as well as African-American groups, who adhere to religious sanctions against homosexuality, tend not to recognize the existence of gay men. Recently the blind trust of a widow of a Latino in Dallas turned to agony when the cause of death was listed as "AIDS from multiple partners."

Most spouses eventually decide that in general it was far better for them to have trusted than doubted their partners. Their only regret is not having had the courage to explore issues when deceit was first suspected. The legacy is loss of trust in others.

Another troubling issue is the partner's distrust of the spouse. Many wives, wondering, "Why didn't he trust me enough to tell me?" begin to doubt their own trustworthiness. Dispelling such self-doubt can be a long and painful process.

Spouses can restore confidence in their own trustworthiness by performing a self-trusting activity each day such as fulfilling a promise to call a friend or to help a relative. To reinforce self-trust, it helps to record each accomplished task in a journal.

The process of rebuilding realistic trust can be reinforced through positive interactions with close friends. Friends can be especially helpful by acting as models of trustworthiness. Gradually the spouse will realize that trusting others doesn't always lead to hurt and that her or his own judgment of others is reliable.

Sharing the Secret

Learning to trust is particularly important for spouses who haven't yet shared their partner's secret. Until they tell a trusted friend or relative, many spouses are plagued by such questions as, "Aren't I guilty of deceit too? Whose secret is it? Whose responsibility is it to tell the children, friends and family? Do they have a right to know?" Spouses who have disclosed the secret to support groups and counselors but not to the key people in their lives often feel similar disquiet. Resolving the dilemma of secrecy is the fifth step toward the reestablishment of integrity.

Keeping the secret isolates spouses from the reality check that outsiders may provide. Consequently, their judgment may become distorted and they may sink into depression. Stuck in the closet, it's common to exaggerate the horror of their situation. For example, when Caitlin blurted out her tale to her conservative acquaintance, the woman expressed empathy instead of repulsion. Caitlin then realized that her secret wasn't as terrible as she'd thought.

"We're only as sick as our secrets," says a character in Libbe S. HaLevy's play, *Shattered Secrets*, about incest.[8] Such stigmatizing secrets have to be destroyed in order for moral healing to begin. Telling others does just that.

Revealing the truth isn't easy. Yet as moral conflict increases, it becomes crucial to tell someone—counselor, support group, trusted friend or family member.

Friends or family who suspect or know the secret can help by gently informing the spouse. However discreetly it is done, however much support is given, the truth will hurt but less so than perpetuating the silence as Tracey's friends and family did.

Each spouse's approach to handling the secret varies according to what is most appropriate for her or his particular circumstances. Some, valuing their privacy, never tell. But many eventually find that tension from leading a double life overcomes the compulsion to protect their partners and themselves from anticipated discrimination or rejection. When they finally share the secret and explore its moral implications, the downward spiral of their lives can be reversed.

For Wes, in "Two Minor Miracles," his support group provided the audience needed to arrest the pathological momentum of his anger. Sharing was a first step toward clarifying his moral stance toward Milly.

Reconstructing Moral Values

Once the secrecy issues has been resolved, spouses can rebuild their moral code, the seventh step toward regaining integrity. To reverse moral disintegration is a complex and demanding task that calls for reconstructing concepts of right and wrong. Eventually, most spouses regain the moral strength to be true to themselves.

First, moral sensibility needs to be nourished. This is achieved most effectively in solitude. Simply reflecting on their moral confusion allows spouses' repressed notions of moral values to emerge. Some spouses find that listening to music or engaging in creative activities allows buried sensibilities to flow freely again.

Reading biographies of admired persons can broaden a spouse's moral perspective. So can seeing movies and plays on ethical issues. Another helpful exercise is to imagine how the deception might be viewed by people whose values the spouse respects, such as a former teacher, deceased grandparent, ancient philosopher or spiritual leader.

Unexpectedly, the spouses may sense a flickering response to the morality of something in their lives. As Caitlin listened to classical music, for example, her true feelings about Miguel's double life became self-evident. This recognition is the first clue that the inner work is bearing fruit.

Most spouses find it hard to put such feelings into words because of the long period of confusion and compromise. Even a tentative expression, however, is a crucial step toward reformulating a moral code.

Talking with other spouses who face the same moral questions helps clarify the half-formed concepts that have arisen. Writing about them in a journal will trace their genesis. Eventually, the spouse can formulate a moral opinion about everyday events in thought, conversation or journal. A judgment call might be made on a children's prank, a friend's oversight, a stranger's generosity, a miscalculated grocery bill or a news story on crime. Statements may be simple, like "Good!" or "That's unfair" or "Here's a error." However short, each remark is a giant stride toward regaining control of the moral quality of the spouse's life.

The next step is to explore deeper ethical questions about events, such as, "Does this action harm anyone? Does it infringe on the rights of others? Is the action responsible?" Working out answers heightens moral perception. Discussing them with friends will sharpen the spouse's discernment.

Some spouses, feeling powerless from the deception, exaggerate the power of their own views and fear that taking a position contrary to a friend's may ruin the friendship. By trying their opinions out on a confidante, they may see that friendships aren't affected by expressing different points of view. Besides feeling more comfortable asserting their position, they also realize that their moral values have power to influence only their lives, no one else's. Reclaiming that power now seems possible.

Clarifying one's moral values takes a long time. For example, a Reno housewife, married to an HIV-positive man who has been arrested in public rest rooms twice, remains stuck in her caretaker role with him and their children while she awaits inner "voices" to reveal the meaning of her suffering. While spouses like her may not feel ready to make a moral judgment about their lives, waiting too long may lead to chronic depression, chemical dependency or other self-destructive behavior. This can be averted if they work on trusting their own moral sense.

Acting with Integrity

With moral values in place, spouses have a foundation from which to take control of their lives and to act with integrity. This final stage of moral recovery involves two steps: first, forming a judgment about the moral dilemmas raised by the coming out and second, guided by their moral compass, resolving how to live life with integrity. Spouses need to make major decisions about their positions on homosexuality, rights and responsibilities in the marriage and the ethics of deceit. A realistic resolution of these issues can be attained through decision making that balances moral concerns with compassionate understanding.

A spouse's personal views on homosexuality are fundamental in determining what role their partner will play in their lives. For many spouses, courage may be needed to explore the idea that homosexuality is a natural sexual variation, a position that runs counter to the prevalent view of society and their own moral standards, forged since childhood. A number of spouses are naturally accepting and not bound by tradition. Others, despite strong religious convictions, are curious to know why some religions accept homosexuality and others don't. They begin to wonder, "If gays are rejected only for being sinful, who then is acceptable?" Still others choose to work through stereotypical ideas and moral discomfort to look at bisexuality and homosexuality from a fresh perspective.

Challenging long-held moral views can be difficult and threatening to many spouses. However, many gradually transcend earlier ideas and develop a more positive view of homosexuality.

Acceptance of homosexuality is supported by a substantial body of Judeo-Christian biblical and theological research, as reported by evangelical authors Letha Scanzoni and Virginia Ramey Mollenkott. This view holds that accepting gay, bisexual and lesbian persons is as Christian an act as respect for any other human beings. Moreover, loving, caring, committed relationships between people of the same sex are consistent with values about love and relationships found in the Bible and early Christian history.[9]

"Ultimately," says Reverend James DeLange, "the issue is not how do we reconcile homosexuality and homosexual behavior with a few Bible passages that purportedly address the issue, but how do we reconcile the continued exclusion of gay and lesbian people from full participation in the life of the church and society with the gospel of Jesus Christ? I don't think it can be done."[10]

While some accepting spouses go on to take strong positions against anti-gay discrimination, others go the other way to reject the possibility that gay persons are normal or good. In a painful situation like a coming-out crisis, it is very hard to entertain a view that contradicts beliefs upheld by family and religion. Yet Scanzoni and Mollenkott caution, "The refusal even to consider the possibility of such transcendence may well lead to moral rigor mortis."[11]

In many cases the coming out and the partner's new lifestyle raise the moral concern, "What is a just balance of individual rights and joint responsibilities in a mixed-orientation marriage?" Many spouses conclude that the partner has a right to express gayness, but that it must be weighed against family responsibilities. In creating a new lifestyle, the partner is not entitled to deny the spouse and children the right to a stable family based on trust.

Many spouses conclude that sexual orientation isn't a matter of choice, but bisexual and homosexual persons can choose how to handle their lives responsibly.

"If they hurt others by their chosen behavior or lie about it," one straight wife stated, "that is wrong." This is not to say that the partner can't be forgiven for wrongdoings, only that hurtful behavior can't be condoned.

Spouses also need to examine how they are handling their own responsibilities and rights. For instance, spouses who seek an outside affair need to consider how it affects others in their lives.

The AIDS crisis heightens the morality question for mixed-orientation couples. Bonnie Kaye, founder of Spouses of Gays, a national network (no longer operating), reports that over seventy of the two thousand wives she counseled between 1983 and 1985 have contracted AIDS through their husbands. For some, that was how they discovered their husband's secret.[12]

To diminish the chance of infecting their wives, actively gay married men have a moral obligation to tell the truth to their wives. Yet denial and fear remain powerful deterrents even in such grave circumstances. No one knows how many AIDS-infected husbands haven't told their wives. However, a wife on the East Coast reports that four of the five husbands being nursed by their wives in the AIDS ward of a public hospital have not yet disclosed their homosexuality to their spouses.

The final moral question straight wives face is what to do in response to their partner's deceit. While spouses may feel they originally had little choice in marrying their partner, they now can choose how much support to give him or her, how much priority to give their own and their family's needs and which situation—marriage, separation or divorce—would best serve their own moral imperatives.

No single resolution of the issue is common to all. Most women who have already divorced find that the consequences of the deceit confirm their decision to end the marriage. For many women still married, the extent of the deception or betrayal of the marriage vows influences whether or not they leave the marriage. The longer the deception, the more likely it becomes the major reason to separate or divorce. Only a minority of wives decide that love and marital satisfaction supersede the hurt of deceit. If honesty has been reestablished in the relationship, they are more likely to choose to stay married.

Divorce itself may present a moral dilemma. Though Tracey's reluctance to break up the family vanished when she discovered Herb's deceit, guilt remained until her psychiatrist helped her realize that only divorce could end her misery. Her priest dispelled her lingering feelings of selfishness when he told her, "To take care of others, we must take care of ourselves first."

When spouses finally make a decision based on their own moral values, whether it is to stay married or to divorce, they experience liberation. For the first time in a long time, they are acting without fear or guilt. They are finally in control of their lives.

With moral compass in place, straight spouses who are also parents feel secure enough to move beyond survival concerns and to look more closely at family needs long neglected. Now, they have the strength to listen to the voices of their children and other family members without fear of painful reality or candid criticism. They can more objectively assess what has happened to the family so that decisions about the future may more likely be appropriate for everyone. Part Six examines long-term issues voiced by family members, in particular, the children.

<u>six</u>

FAMILY VOICES

AFTERSHOCKS IN THE CHILDREN'S WORLD

Trusting oneself to act with integrity remains an abstract exercise until real life challenges arise, especially if loved ones are involved. At this stage, when spouses are more confident and calm, those with children face the dilemma of how to balance family responsibilities and personal needs.

In many cases, family wounds from earlier decisions made out of frustration, anger or confusion in the chaos of the partner's disclosure remain untended. To begin the healing process, spouses need to widen their field of vision to encompass the entire family, in particular, the children.

Children's needs lie at the heart of the family. Deeper than the initial day-to-day problems discussed in Part Three, children's cumulative concerns related to having a gay or lesbian parent, call for their parents to "be there for them." Now that the spouses' shattered identity and moral compass are repaired, they can better hear the children's voices and determine ways to minimize further pain and to improve everyone's well being.

The new sexual identity and way of life of the bi, gay or lesbian parent prompt positive and negative reactions from children. At the same time, their feelings and coping strategies change as they experience each stage of cognitive, social, psychological and moral development. Adolescents and young adults struggle the most as they deal with their own sexuality, isolation, trust and identity issues.

The majority of youngsters are or will be in a divorce situation and therefore confront a double crisis. Issues surrounding the coming out are knitted into the divorce trauma that all children of divorce suffer. Of the two traumatic events, the breakup usually causes more stress than Mom's or Dad's homosexuality. Yet, the stress of each exacerbates the pain of the other.

Children invent a variety of coping strategies to maintain their equilibrium in the midst of the tumultuous changes brought on by the coming out and, in most cases, the divorce. Their private struggles are affected by how family members interact with one another. They are also influenced by attitudes about homosexuality and gay-related activities voiced in their neighborhood, school and community. In the end, most children resolve their issues alone, though not until reaching adulthood. By then, most develop inner strength and a coherent belief system.

The following stories illustrate how four daughters and a son, aged eleven to seventeen, coped after their parents came out. The discussion at the end explores typical concerns expressed by children of all ages, reactions of other family members and family strategies that children want and need to resolve their issues constructively as they grow toward adulthood.

Personal Stories

Tired of Keeping It a Secret
Lynn

Sunday morning after the Midwinter Ball, my parents called us into the den after breakfast: Andy, thirteen, Dirk, nine and me, fifteen.

We moseyed in, not thinking it was major. My parents were both crying. Dad, white as a ghost, was pacing and muttering. Mom was on the big chair, trying to keep herself together.

Dad had a speech written out. "This is about integrity and my love for all three of you," he began. "We're going to get a divorce."

Andy, Dirk and I looked at each other. It was the last thing I expected to hear, because my parents had the perfect marriage.

Then Dad said, "We're divorcing because your father's a homosexual."

My mouth fell open. Shaking, I asked to go upstairs.

Up in my room, I called all my friends until I found one home. "Hank, meet me at the park."

The minute I saw Hank, I said, "My parents are splitting." Then I wept, while he hugged me and said, "It's gonna be all right, Lynn."

It was the longest day of my life. "I don't want to go home!" I cried. "What'll it be like? Dad's going to stay for another week until he finds a place. It'll be awful."

When it started to get dark, I went home. It was too quiet and empty. The next day I went to school, without homework done and scared about what was going to happen. When I told my best friend, Liz, about the divorce, my eyes filled with tears for the millionth time in twenty-four hours. A jumble of questions raced through my head. "Who am I going to live with? What will our friends say?"

I'd just stopped therapy for anorexia and had felt so happy.

Now I began to see the therapist once more, as the first weeks became a blur of depression and crying all the time. It was hard to picture Dad wanting to be with another man. "He's been with Mom twenty years. How could he not know?" I kept asking myself. It made me angry that he didn't know when they got together and had a family and brought me into the world and then said, "Oops, that's not who I really am."

Mom and Dad made a deal he'd still be home every night and eat dinner with us. "We want to stay together as a family," Mom said.

The first few weeks Dad came home religiously every night. It was comfortable. Then, gradually, his visits tapered off.

Those three weeks, I didn't tell anyone about Dad. It felt like a long time. One noon, sitting in the cafeteria with Liz, I suddenly felt, "I can't keep this a secret any longer. If I can't tell my best friend, who can I talk about it to?" So I started, "The divorce isn't for the usual reasons..." I broke off, crying.

"What, is he gay?" she joked, trying to make me laugh.

I stopped crying and looked at her.

"No!" she said.

"Yes." In the next few seconds, I wondered if she might walk away. She stayed.

Over the next three months, I told all the friends who mattered. When they heard, jaws fell, mouths gaped open, eyes went wide. Most asked, "Didn't you know you could talk to me about something like that?"

Two friends faded out of my life once they heard. The last thing I needed was to lose a friend as my marks dropped significantly.

At home, changes in the family structure were frustrating. I wanted to scream because I couldn't deal with so much at the same time. It was as if twenty zillion people were talking to me at once. I felt like I was insane. There was so much anger, I couldn't do anything with it. So I took scissors or knives and carved up myself, sitting in my room. "I'm all alone. No one else in the world knows what I'm feeling," I said, stabbing at myself. Then I saw my arm bleeding. "Why did I do that?" I thought. "It's stupid." So I just sat and cried.

Since it was winter, no one saw my wounds, covered by my long-sleeved shirts. Even Mom never knew.

There was a lot I wasn't talking about, but, after a few months, I stopped stabbing myself, trying to commit suicide. Where I put the anger or where it went or whether or not I just ignored it, I didn't know. But it didn't go away. The anger was just there. It still is.

Andy, who's quiet and puts things inside, wasn't talking about anything related to Dad. One day, a kid in his eighth grade class called him a "faggot." Andy took it personally and got in a fight with him.

Mom forced him to go to therapy. He went twice, pouted about it and refused to go again.

"Andy," I said, "It's going to catch up with you soon. I'd like to be there for you when it does."

Shrugging me off, he went out to play basketball.

Dirk, ten, asked Dad lots of questions like "Do you and Buzz sleep in the same bed?" But he didn't talk much about it with us.

That spring, Mom started dating Ernest. I didn't like him. He smoked, too, which started Mom smoking again. Then, when Mom told me she'd slept with him the first date, I couldn't believe it. "That's stupid," I told her, "something a teenager would do."

Ernest made a real effort to be nice to me, but I ignored him and gave him nasty looks as I waltzed up to my room. Then I walked about upstairs, slamming doors, being really immature.

Because Ernest took up a lot of Mom's time, I felt he was taking her away from us. She'd also returned to college, so she was away half the day. When she got home, Ernest called and she was right over there. We became latchkey kids. This was last on my list of expectations.

I lost a lot of family, especially grandparents. When Mom told her parents about the divorce and why, they didn't like it. Each time we talked on the phone, they asked, "So, did your dad's friend sleep over last night?" or "How's the fag doing?"—rude, stupid questions. They also said, "I can't believe your dad would do that to you. How can you live like that?" I wanted to hang up. Love is love, no matter what sex you prefer.

Dad's father was dead but his mom, I'm glad to say, still loved him.

Junior year, my grades went back up and I made National Honor Society.

In class, kids sometimes said "fag" and "lezzy." It bothered me, but I kept my mouth shut. If I objected somebody would say, "What are you talking about?" or think, "Lynn must be one."

When I turned seventeen, I grew up a little and was nice to Ernest. It actually came from the heart, which was good because it took a lot of energy to hate him. In my first relationship, I also began trying to understand Mom. "She's in love, too."

Sometime in the spring, I began to wonder about my own identity and what kind of life I wanted to lead. Dad's coming out had changed my views. If I saw a guy walk down the street, it was "Ooo-ee." If I saw a girl, it was also "Ooo-ee." Some days I was so sure I was lesbian and some days, so sure I was straight. "If my boyfriend could hear my thoughts, he'd have a cow," I told myself.

By then, Dad came over only occasionally after work at dinnertime. When we finished eating, he'd say, "I hate to eat and run, but..." and rattle off a list of things he had to do.

I saw Dad about every ten days, mostly when he wanted something, just like he called Andy because he wanted his car washed or grass cut.

Andy and I could drive and take care of ourselves. But Dirk, eleven, lacked in the parental guidance department. I wasn't in charge like before. Dirk could make his own food, so he was pretty self-sufficient but totally neglected without a father and a mom never around.

One weekend, late that summer, Mom was out of town with Ernest so Dad stayed with us. Liz spent Saturday night. At two thirty a.m., Dad and Buzz walked in both drunk, which made them act feminine. They started prancing around while we sipped our sodas in the kitchen. Then they went out for a swim and frolicked around the pool.

"Oh, no," Liz burst out laughing. "This is hilarious."

To me it was yuck. I'd never seen Dad drunk with his lover and in the pool. It was embarrassing that Bonny saw him like that. "This is gross," I thought. "What will the neighbors think, three o'clock in the morning, and two guys screaming in the back yard?"

Two weeks later, school began, my senior year. In psychology class we got into a discussion about homosexuality. This ignorant jerk said, "You choose to be gay. You're not born that way."

"Bull," I said, standing up and seething. "Why would you want to choose that lifestyle when you see how homosexuals are treated around the world? Why would you want everyone to dislike you so much?"

After class, the guy looked at me funny, but no one said anything.

That was a month ago, when my anger began to resurface. The stuff I have to deal with gets to be too much sometimes. But I'm glad

I'm dealing with it myself instead of shoving it to the back of my mind or running to the shrink.

Nothing's been easy, but the one good thing is that Dad's coming out made me more open-minded. I feel worlds ahead of my peers. I take people for who they are. Their race or religion or sexual preference doesn't matter. It's what's inside that counts.

Dad's being gay doesn't bother me, except when he's drunk at three in the morning. It took courage to come out with three kids, a wife and a business. I admire him for that and hope I can be like him.

But I'm tired of keeping it a secret, very tired. Since this is my senior year and I no longer care what people think, I don't want to keep it any longer. But I also don't want to put it on my younger brothers, coming up through the lower grades.

I can't wait for college. I can keep my mouth shut for that freedom.

He Screwed Up Really Bad
Adrian

I'd seen little tiffs between Mom and Dad the year before Dad told us. He'd be gone for a weekend and come home late or not at all and Mom would be depressed. You could almost see fear in her eyes because she didn't want anything to happen.

The next year, when I was seventeen, Mom was out on her midnight shift and I saw my dad downstairs with some dude he had over. It made me want to kill him. But I told nobody.

A month later, after dinner when my sister was home from college, my dad said, "We need to talk." That's when he told us he was gay. "I had no choice," he said. "It's just the way I am. I've known since I was seven."

We sat a while, no one saying anything.

Then he asked me, "Adrian, do you have anything to say?"

"Well, no. I've got nothing to say to you."

Since I already knew, it wasn't as much of a shock as it might have been, but I didn't have nothing to say. I knew everything else from there. You can't go on being a Beaver Cleaver household after that.

Later, Mom and my sister and I talked. "Saying he's been gay all along?" I said, "that's bull shit."

I had to mature really quickly in the next weeks and pretty much became the man of the house. It really sucked.

No one outside of our family knew. Keeping quiet was the hardest thing for me, because I'm the Talk of the Town person for my friends. I'm "The Mouth." Friday nights, I get ninety calls about parties: "Where are they?"

When friends heard Mom and Dad had split, they asked, "Where's your dad?"

"Well, I have no idea."I didn't like other people knowing and felt I had to keep it quiet, because of how my friends worked, especially with the "guy thing" men have at that age. A lot of them weren't mature enough to handle it.

As far as my emotions and beliefs about Dad being gay, I dealt with them on my own. I'm strong enough inside to handle anything. While my family raised me really liberal in Los Angeles, a liberal community, I had my own set of morals as well. "There's no problem with people being gay," I decided, "as long as Dad stays out of my life." That he was gay and also in my life were two huge negatives against him, totally against my morals. They still are.

But no one needed to know my feelings. Your emotions are your emotions. You're going to feel how you feel. It doesn't matter if it's bigoted or racial or what other people think.

That was almost two years ago. Now I'm in junior college. How do I feel about my dad now? I hate him. I have pretty much nothing positive to say about him and nothing to say to him. If he had no choice being gay, he shouldn't have started a family. He started something he couldn't finish. Now he should stay out of our lives. He's trying to relate, but it just don't work anymore.

I don't foresee sharing it outside the family ever. Certain things are other people's business. This is family business. Especially if I move back south where my mother's thinking of moving, I'll never mention it. In the suburbs, you can't even say the word, "gay."

The only easy thing is Mom's seeing this Joe guy, which makes her happier. It's my job to make my mom happy—not to make my dad happy any longer. Mom was so depressed for so long that seeing her happy, because she is dating this guy, makes me happy.

It's done with. I can't do anything about it. It's time for me and my sister and my mom to go on with our lives.

There for Each Other
Anne and Joan

Anne: I was eleven when Mom, who was divorced, brought home a woman who didn't leave that evening. I figured it out because, about eleven o'clock, I snuck near the bedroom and heard voices. My sister, Joan, was sleeping over at a friend's so I couldn't run and tell her.

The next day, when Joan came home, I told her, "Mom's gay."

"I don't believe you."

"Yes, she is," I said.

"No, she's not."

Joan: We went back and forth until I became angry. Though not a physical kid, I jumped on my bike, which I never rode, and rode to my best friend's house. She wasn't there. I don't know what I'd have done if she had been, because I never did tell her for seven years.

So I rode back and waited with Anne at the top of the stairway for Mom to come home so we could ask her.

Anne: As soon as Mom opened the door, we asked, "Are you gay?"

"Girls, we need to talk," she said, going into the living room.

We followed, and she told us she was a lesbian.

"How could you do this to me?" we each screamed. "You've ruined my life! This is disgusting. We're the only people in the whole wide world who have this kind of family. How weird! How horrible!"

Joan: I was angry. Two years before, Mom did something I didn't like and I'd said, "That's 'gay,' " a term used to put people down.

"That's not nice, Joan," she'd said.

"Why not?"

"Because those are people."

"Well, are you gay?" I asked.

"No, but I have friends who are."

So it became something I could cross out forever.

Now, I yelled, "You told me you were never going to get a divorce and you did. You told me you weren't gay and now you're saying you are!" I was furious. "How can you do this to me?"

Anne: Fortunately, Mom suggested we see a therapist.

Thank God I loved him. Most eleven-year-olds don't like even the idea of therapy, but he was the only person aside from Joan who I could talk to about Mom. Joan didn't like him and never went back.

Joan: Mom had been planning a trip for us to take the following weekend with her and a friend. For weeks she'd said, "I want you to meet her. You'll really like her."

Wondering what the big deal was, I'd said, "We'll have dinner with her and if we like her, we like her. If we don't, we don't."

Usually I did what I was supposed to do, but when it became clear the trip would be with the woman who'd spent the night with Mom, I thought, "This is disgusting," and said, "I'm not going."

We went. As we drove up to Washington, Anne and I sat in the back seat with Mom and her friend, Lil, in the front, holding hands. We kept sticking our fingers down our throats, gagging.

My parents had never touched each other. So any touching between people in a loving way was strange. Actually, holding hands was all I ever saw between Mom and Lil, except quick kisses and hugs.

Anne: It turned out we had a great time. Lil was so damn funny, so brilliant. We became close to her and loved her.

Joan: We absolutely adored her. For months we kept asking Mom, "When is she moving in?"

Each time Lil left the house, I asked, "When are you coming back?"

Lil eventually moved in. She was very afraid of people finding out, though, so I couldn't tell my friends. "If it isn't O.K. with Lil and Mom," I thought, "it certainly is never going to be O.K. with me."

Anne: We had this wonderful family in this tiny house that we couldn't share with anybody outside.

It was a struggle not to tell. I had a big fear of people hating and harassing me and of not having any friends come to my house.

My next door neighbor, a close play friend, constantly asked, "Who's this woman living with you?"

But I couldn't say. I didn't even tell the guy I went out with from freshman to senior year.

Joan: I was terrified friends would find out. If friends were coming over, Anne and I took down photos of Mom and Lil and hid the love notes they left for each other on the kitchen table. I spent half my day wondering, "How can we get into the house without making it look obvious when we run to the table and grab something off it?" On the way home, we'd freak out, thinking, "Oh my God, the notes will be there even though we'd asked them not to leave any."

At my father's house, we couldn't mention Mom's name in front of him because it would set him off. If we'd done something with her, we said what we'd done but not that we did it with her. Though we still lived in the house he'd left, we couldn't call it "home." When we went home, we said, "Bye, Dad, we're going to Graham Street now."

Every time one of my friends met my father for the first time, I said, "He hates my mother. Don't mention her name in front of him or he'll blow up." I didn't say it would make him talk about her sexuality.

Mom's sexuality was at the root of Dad's horrendous outbursts. He'd say, "Your mother's a lesbian" with such disgust, I figured it must be the worst thing he could say. Then he'd add, "Wait till you're old enough to understand what your mother did."

I knew she was with a woman but, at thirteen, couldn't understand her sexuality. Yet, every time Dad said, "Your mother's a fucking lesbian," I felt such absolute rage, I swore back and left.

Anne: At eleven, I couldn't understand that this man was hurt by his ex-wife and unloading on an eleven-year-old wasn't appropriate.

Joan and I had no dialogue to deal with it. We didn't know how to say, "Dad, look what you're doing to us. How do you think that makes us feel?" So there was much blowing up and crying.

We were learning to communicate with Mom and Lil. To become a family that really cared, we had to talk about it. That was wonderful compared to the hell in our heterosexual family, which I'd avoided by creating paper villages in my room while Joan bore the brunt.

When I turned fifteen, Lil left. It was the most horrible loss because I absolutely loved her. On the other side was relief I could bring home my friends.

Joan: When they told me, I said to Lil, "Please don't leave. I'll never have anyone over again. I'll do anything you ask."

"Joan, that wouldn't be fair of me to ask you to do that. You can't not have your friends in your home for me."

So this woman I adored moved out. We lost another parent absolutely. It was a second divorce, and I couldn't tell anybody. She had lived with us for three years and been with Mom for four. She'd brought me up. I went to her for advice. I went to her for money and for rides.

Depressed, I went into therapy, as we lost complete contact with her. It was one of the hardest things I've ever gone through.

Anne: After Lil left, friends could come over, but we still kept secret the fact Mom was lesbian. The therapist was the only outside person I talked about it to until high school graduation.

My coming out as the daughter of a lesbian began when I went to college. Joan, who had met someone from the Gay and Lesbian Parents Coalition International, called me that fall. "This man wants us to go to this conference to take care of the little kids."

Joan: We'd never known anyone else who had gay parents, and suddenly there's a room with fifteen kids all going through the same things. Our stories were different—some people lived with violence and others knew only gay and lesbian parenting—but we had a common bond. It was powerful. So, at nineteen, I began my own coming out.

Anne: It was amazing. I cried the entire two days and started to be more open about who I was and who my mom was.

From then on, if people couldn't accept those two things, I didn't want them in my life. I was no longer afraid people would hate me.

Joan: Back home, I found out that friends had known all along. In the end, no one ever left me because my mother's a lesbian.

Mom, meanwhile, had become completely different from the woman we grew up with. She had been miserable then and not fun to be around. Now, she was warm, loving, funny, everything anybody would want in a friend or parent.

Every time I came home, her growth amazed me. "You're so able to listen, so willing to learn," I'd say or, "God, I can't believe it."

"What better gift," I told Anne, "than to be involved with somebody just sprouting and blossoming."

Because Mom was able to be open, I was too. Sometimes, it wasn't pleasant. Issues would all of a sudden come up when we were out for dinner and I just laid a childhood memory on the table and nailed her. "This is what you did. You really sucked and I'm going to tell you why." How many kids, I wondered, could say things like that?

Other times, I said, "Ma, you're not listening."

She always thought for a moment and then said either, "You're right," or came back with, "Joan, you're being this way... or that way."

Through it, I learned to listen, and we developed the close relationship we'd never had.

I continued going to the yearly gay and lesbian parents conferences and then started lecturing with my sister and mother on having a lesbian mother. Anne and I also began facilitating children's groups.

Anne: By then, we could say Mom's name in front of my dad. When Joan graduated from college two years later, we had a graduation dinner with Dad and his wife, Mom and Joan's friends. This year for mine, Dad's wife was sick, but they would have been there otherwise. That was wonderful in itself.

I feel lucky. Though it was a struggle to go through this experience, it opened up my mind. It made me stronger and more conscious of diversity. To get over what I went through at such a young age gave me good coping skills. Talking about it helped me deal with other things and communicate in my job and school.

Being involved in the gay community is part of my identity now. Some friends say, "Anne, there are so many other problems in the world. Life is not going to end because your mom's gay."

"This is like a revolution," I answer, "something I'm passionate about. Everybody struggles with knowing somebody in their family who's gay, a cousin or brother or cousin of an aunt."

I'll work with kids of gays and lesbians until I die. It's close to my heart. I'd love to get paid for it so it could be a full-time job.

Joan: It's been a twelve-year process. I wouldn't want my life to be any other way or my mother to be anybody else. I wouldn't want my experiences, except for some, to have been different, or I wouldn't be the same person.

My goal is to give the children the message, "There isn't anything wrong with being gay even though society teaches us there is!" I tell them, "Look at our families. We love each other, support and enjoy each other. Even when things are difficult to listen to, we listen."

If the little kids can see that I don't care who knows about my mom and live a happy and healthy life, then they can realize that they can have the same thing. Some of them fear real violence and it's terrifying. I want them to know, if I could get through that, they can too.

My Abba
Xan

An eleven-year-old never knows what the future holds. My mom was an artist, and my father—I called him Abba—was a salesman who was away a lot. I thought they were happy together, so when they told me about the divorce, I ran to my room in shock.

I always put this poster under my door so you could open it only three inches. My dad opened it that much, took the poster out, came in and comforted me.

"Oh," I thought, "Abba still feels the same way toward me, his daughter. The divorce doesn't change that."

Dad moved to a two-bedroom apartment in Manhattan. He came twice a week to see my younger sister, Tobie and I, and brought dinner to cook, usually chops. We spent every other weekend with him. Then, funnily enough, he grew a moustache.

Tobie turned ten two months after they told us, and I turned twelve a month later. Then Mom started acting as if she was the child and I, the thirty-eight-year-old. She didn't want to take care of us and wanted me to be her peer. Soon it felt like I was raising Tobie.

That summer, we went to the city for a bar mitzvah. Tobie and I stayed with Dad. After introducing us to his roommate, Rob, Dad showed us the sofa bed where we'd be sleeping.

"I don't want to sleep with my sister, Abba."

"O.K., Xan. You can have Rob's room."

"That's weird," I thought. "Rob's supposed to sleep there or it wouldn't be his room. Why does Abba want me to sleep in the same room with a guy I barely know?" That's when it occurred to me Dad and Rob might be sleeping together. I had no idea what "gay" was, but I'd read a book where the main character's boyfriend was bi. She was negative about it, so the relationship lasted only ten pages. "I can't think of my father as gay," I thought and pushed it out of my mind.

One night that June, when Mom and I were unloading the dishwasher after dinner, she said, "Xan, your dad is gay."

"Yeah, right," I said to myself. "You're being weird again. This is my dad who had me and Mia. How can he be gay?" I decided she was just being mean, trying to alienate me from him.

Two months later, my father sat me down in the living room. "I love Rob, yes, but there are different types of love. It's in a different way than I love you." Then he paused. "Do you have any questions?"

Stunned, I said, "No, Abba, not really."

That fall, I went to public school, the first time in four years. I knew no one. Since it was junior high, every other person was going through puberty too, and my father was gay. That was bothersome, one other thing that made me different.

About then, Mom asked that child support be raised, and Dad stopped bringing dinner. He also stopped buying us clothes.

This manipulation made life difficult. Mom's complaints about Dad escalated. At one point I hated him, not because he was gay but because of what she said. She never said anything positive about him. She became so blatant, I felt stuck in the middle. That's exactly why I felt depressed for seven years.

While Mom acted childish, I tried to be non-childish. "It'll take care of itself," I thought, as we lived on TV dinners. "Yes," I'd say, the third time we had chicken pies during a single week, "This is great."

Mom was also going out with men a lot and not spending time with us. She didn't care what we were doing and paid more attention to men than to her daughters. Once she dated a married man. "Oh, he's divorcing his wife," she told me when I asked about it. He never did.

I wasn't secure talking with Dad, either. He never said anything bad about Mom, but it was like, "We're not going to do anything nice for her." That was fair, but not when talking to young children. Worse was when he said, "I enjoyed sales trips so I didn't have to deal with your mom"—not the nicest thing for a twelve-year-old to hear.

At school, going through the trials of puberty, I felt alienated. I had few friends and was teased for being a hermit or dressing weird. Most of the time I was happy to go off in a corner and read. Books were the one thing I loved. They were beautiful things. Sometimes, I fought and was beat up on my thirteenth birthday.

I told nobody about my father. If I spoke of him at all, I cried. At one point, someone introduced me to two boys who had a gay father, but one was seventeen and couldn't be seen talking with a thirteen-year-old girl and the other was younger than Tobie. I wasn't going to play with some crummy little boy.

I wanted attention and wasn't getting it. I also needed to talk with someone. In eighth grade, I went to see a counselor.

"Come back later," he said.

So I used the ploy learned from my parents: to get what you want, do something drastic. "But I'm on a hunger strike," I said.

"O.K. I'll see you."

When I told the counselor about Dad, he said, "Oh-h," leaned back and clammed up. Afterwards, he avoided me.

I never invited people over to my house, afraid Mom might be home. I didn't want her acting like a teeny bopper in front of my friends, when she was my mother, once a responsible adult. One day that spring, though, I decided to have three good friends over so I could tell them about my father.

As we munched chips on the porch, I said, "My dad is gay."

They were very quiet and then went home. They never mentioned it again. It was like the afternoon never happened. "This is something you avoid saying anything about," I thought, ashamed of my Abba.

I felt I was the only kid in the world in this position. When eighth grade ended, I really needed someone to talk about it to. Though scared, I called my best friend, confident she'd understand. I'd gone to her bah mitzvah and talked to her on the phone every night. "Ruth," I said as we talked that night, "I've got something very important to tell you. My father is gay."

"Why didn't you tell me before?" she said, annoyed.

" 'Cause I was scared, very scared."

She hung up. It was the last time we ever talked.

"Nobody is out there," I decided, "except my sister and me." And Tobie looked to me for support because I paid attention to what my parents were doing.

That fall I entered the High School of Arts and Sciences. One afternoon, going home on the bus, I was talking to this guy. Only one other person from school was aboard, a girl I barely knew.

All of a sudden the guy made the mistake of saying, "faggot," and I whisked around and slapped him. The guy just said, "What?" shocked, and we rode in silence the rest of the way. I was a little worried.

The next morning on the bus, the girl from the afternoon before leaned over my seat. "What was going on yesterday?" she whispered.

"My father is gay." It was the first time I'd said it to somebody face-to-face and hadn't freaked out.

"Oh." That was all.

A couple of class periods later, I realized, "She's going to spread it around the school. I'd better start telling people."

So for the rest of the day and week, every time I met people and started talking, I said, "My father's gay."

They'd go, "Oh," and that was it. Then I figured it out. The school had the top percent of kids in the city. They were interested in the idea of someone having a gay parent.

Many asked, "Well, how did you get here?"

I came up with snappy answers, like "Well, you know, the stork?"

From then on, I went around telling people about my father, acting like I was proud—though I wasn't. Lo and behold, reactions changed. "People are curious about something different," I thought, smiling.

I made some good friends that year. I also became militant. People couldn't make gay jokes around me or they'd be hit, especially if I felt they knew better.

At home, things got worse. Mom demanded more money and she and Dad fought about it. One night, they were downstairs yelling at each other. After an hour, Tobie came to my room, her face covered in tears. All I could do was hold her, because I was shaken myself.

I tried to keep up with what was going on and to calm my parents so they'd act human again. That role gave Mom somebody to vent on. I tried to ignore her, but it didn't work.

My one solace were my gerbils. Dear and sweet, I loved them. Mom thought differently. "Oh those gerbils," she commented one day. "They're horrible."

Just as Tobie hit puberty, Mom decided to go to college. To help pay tuition, she got some government aid. To Tobie and I, college was another way to ignore us. When Mom went up to study, we knew she could be interrupted, but you don't want to interrupt somebody studying. So, though in her room all the time, she wasn't really there at all.

To help pay for the tuition, Mom made plans to sue Dad to pay his "fair and full" share of child support. "Keep quiet about this," she told me. "I don't want your father to know." It wasn't the first of the secrets, but the main one.

The secrets, combined with not being able to get out of the situation, frustrated me. There wasn't anybody to take it out on and nobody I trusted enough to talk to. One night, I thought of just ending it all. Then I caught sight of my gerbils in the corner of my room. "No!" I cried. "What will happen to the poor little ones?" Recalling what Mom had said, I couldn't stand the thought they might get hurt.

School was how I coped after that. By joining clubs, I could stay at school as long as I wanted. At home, I locked myself in my room and did homework. There was lots of it.

The next year, they changed the school bus route, so Mom decided to drive me. Every morning, she had a new reason to go off about men. One day it was "Men are horrible and greedy." The next, it was "Men are irresponsible" or "inconsistent."

When Mom's lawsuit was filed, my father sat Tobie and I down and told us about it. That was stressful, because I knew what was going on.

The afternoon of the day my parents went to court, I telephoned them from the office of my music teacher. I called him "Pop" because I needed a parent who wasn't crazy.

"Nothing really happened," they said. But Mom didn't sound happy and I felt she'd be suing again.

Indeed, her Abba-bashing got worse. "It's absolutely wrong to vent on me," I kept thinking. "I feel a conflict of interests." Finally, I telephoned my father. "Abba, I'm moving in with you and Rob."

"You really can't do that with me so far away from your school. How about at the end of semester?"

"O.K."

There were more litigation and fights, but I knew I'd be moving out. "Just a little longer," I kept saying to myself.

My sister ignored everything. She went to school, came home, watched TV. In some ways, this worked, but she ended up cynical.

At the beginning of June, Mom really went off against Dad.

That night, I called him. "Abba, I'm moving in tonight."

"Please wait till Saturday, when I can come get you."

On Saturday, when Mom heard Dad come in, she called me upstairs. "Why is your father here?"

"O.K.," I said to myself and brought her down to the living room. She sat on the big chair, and my father, my sister and I sat on the couch opposite. "Mom, I'm moving out."

She was really unhappy and proceeded to tell me so, very loudly. Then World War III broke out: fighting and screaming on all sides. My mother accused my father of acting like his father, and he accused her of acting like her mother. For the first time, I saw a man cry, as Dad watched Mom and I looking at each other with straight faces, saying the worst things we ever said to each other.

For me, everything that had gone on over the four years since the divorce—all the secrets and lying, her immaturity—exploded.

Mom responded in kind. Finally she said, "O.K. Pack your things. Anything you leave is going to the Salvation Army."

I packed up everything I could but had to leave behind my Prom formal and two boxes of books. Leaving my precious books was why I sobbed as Dad drove me away.

The next weekend was a gathering of children of gay and lesbian parents that Dad helped organize. To meet forty kids, roughly my age, in my situation was the greatest. I also met my first boyfriend there. He walked up to me with a raspberry soda. "Here," he said. So sweet!

Living with my dad was great. I rode the train to school till the end of the year. Then we moved. Without dealing with Mom, I went to see Tobie, who begged to come live with us. Because of the location of her new school, there was no way she could.

Her school was homophobic. Without much of a minority population, the kids were close-minded hicks who refused to take in anything different. Tobie joined the ROTC, where she picked up more horrible attitudes. She told no one about Dad and began treating him like dirt.

When I went to Mom's house to see Tobie and Mom's parents were visiting, they wouldn't speak to me. Grandfather felt I'd hurt their little girl. They both hated Dad because he'd lied to their little girl, married her when he shouldn't have and then divorced her.

To Dad's parents, the divorce confirmed Mom wasn't good enough for him. Grandpa said, "I don't understand why your dad's the way he is, but I love him." Grandma asked if Rob was doing well but told me not to talk about Dad in front of her bridge club. That made me laugh because, by then, he was very "out" in the community.

For the last two years of high school, I joined after school clubs and stayed away from my parents—that is, my two fathers. Even before I moved in, I'd thought of Rob as my stepdad.

I loved my fathers. It was good to have parents that imposed restrictions, like a curfew. "I have somebody who cares about me now," I thought. They didn't demand things. It was "Keep your room clean or close the door." When I needed money, all I had to do was ask—though it cut down my allowance.

Mom wasn't in the picture at all. I couldn't stand talking with her. The Salvation Army comment hurt so. It was like she disowned me.

"If she could own up to it," I told Dad, "it'd be great."

When Mom called on my seventeenth birthday, I was polite but wanted her out of my face. She showed up at my high school graduation, a year later. Then, my first year away at college, we patched things up a little. Realizing she'd done what she felt was right at the time, I tried not to hold it against her.

Now, sophomore year, my father and I have grown apart, but that's natural. He is a very good, honest and honorable man. Anyone who's ashamed of him because he is gay has a lot more problems than him being "out."

This fall my seven-year depression suddenly has lifted, and I have a boyfriend. When I introduced him to Dad and Rob, they approved, and I burst with delight. "My fathers like him."

I'm happy with who I am. It was an interesting thing to live through. I'm very glad it's lived *through*.

Widening the Scope of Concern

"**P**arents are responsible for protecting the rights of their children," says Steve, nineteen. He has lived with his lesbian mother and her partner since her divorce when he was six. "Parents should protect children from any unnecessary interference with their growing up," he continued. "That's enough of a struggle."

Children's cognitive, social, psychological and moral development is their principal task in life. Families are the milieu in which their growth takes place. Straight spouses initially preoccupied with their own survival needs, often feel guilty that their struggle kept them from providing their children a more supportive family cocoon. Now, more self-confident, they can pay more attention to the condition of the cocoon and refocus on the needs of these youngsters at risk.

Although it is impossible to determine exact numbers, with estimated figures varying widely, most indicators suggest that there may be about 3,500,000 children, including adult children, of homosexual or bisexual parents in traditional marriages. Like their straight parents, most children do not know about the gay parent's orientation until the disclosure. Many never are told. Those who do find out go through their own coming-out stages as children of a gay, lesbian, or bi parent.

Children form the third wave of the family's coming out, following, first, their gay parent and, next, his or her straight spouse. Similar to both their parents, children need to reconcile the seeming contradiction of their mother or father being both gay and married.

Children's first reactions to the parents' disclosure are in constant flux, shifting from shock, anger, and distrust to relief and empathy.

Concurrent with these changing reactions is a cumulative buildup of concerns. Resolving them is a long process. Each child follows his or her own timetable which differs from an adult's sense of time. To a child, time stretches out forever. A period that seems short for adults, say a month, to a child may seem interminable.

Since the issues are complex and the children's development is gradual, most cannot resolve all their concerns fully until adulthood. Those who are teenagers when they find out that their parent is gay or lesbian experience the most severe problems but seem to come to terms with it by the time they leave home. Younger children, who accept the disclosure more easily, typically take longer to comprehend it because they have to reprocess the information during adolescence.

To understand the children's issues, it helps to consider their struggle in relation to the ordinary stages of growing up, from infant, preschool and school age, through preadolescent and adolescent, to adult.[1] Measuring what the children do and say against the normal growing-up work necessary for each age group provides clues as to what adjustments in the family support system might help them meet their needs more effectively.

Children are also affected by how their parents, brothers and sisters and other family members handle the parent's coming out and subsequent changes in family life—all within the context of prevailing attitudes of neighborhood, school and community.

Insights into the needs of children and the family are gained by:

- Discerning disclosure issues
- Tuning in to children's feelings about homosexuality, AIDS, and homophobia.
- Watching children cope within the family circle
- Hearing children's concerns about identity and isolation

Discerning Disclosure Issues

The parent's disclosure that he or she is gay, lesbian or bi triggers a roller coaster of reactions among children. By examining typical first reactions, spouses can pick up lost threads and create a more supportive environment for their children to deal with long-term issues.

Though some children figure out themselves or discover their parents are gay, most are told. Their age and the timing of the disclosure affect their immediate responses, which influence how they process the new information.

Preschoolers don't understand what "gay" means but may sense tension between Daddy and Mummy.

Preadolescents often accept the coming out with aplomb and relish continued contact with their gay parent even if the parents separate. Mark, eleven, able to visit his gay dad's twice a week, says, "It wasn't bad when Dad came out, just unusual. He's the same old Dad." He doesn't understand the concerns his older sister, Sarah, feels.

Sarah, fourteen, had overheard her mother talking about her dad's being gay but hoped it wasn't true. When he told them he was gay, Sarah retreated to her room in sobs and virtually stayed there for two months, hiding behind a book. "I kept telling myself he's going to be the same person. Nothing's going to change the father and daughter relationship." By keeping that in mind, she finally accepted the fact and ventured to visit him in his new apartment.

Adolescents like Sarah experience the most difficulty of all children as they try to reconcile the development of their own sexuality with the idea of the parent's attraction to the same gender. His or her disclosure challenges all concepts they have formed about gender, sexual identity and their future. Now, everything in their world seems suspect.

Some adult children, living or working away from home, disbelieve the disclosure and some try to understand how the father or mother could be gay. Others cut off the relationship or blame the straight parent for causing the changed orientation. Still others gradually respond to natural child-parent bonds and breach gaps in understanding.

Often, different reactions occur within one family, as in Effie's. In her twenties when she found out, she accepted her father's disclosure, while her older brother stopped seeing the father.

For children who find out when the parents married intend to stay, the disclosure nevertheless shocks them. It also makes them question their concept of marriage and the both-gay-and-married paradox.

Those who are told simultaneously that their parents plan to separate or divorce are doubly upset. The divorce news causes the greater pain but its effects intensify negative fallout from the coming out.

When a parent comes out after divorcing, children often feel relieved to know the real reason for the split. For many, it erases guilt that the breakup might have been their fault. For nineteen-year-old "Few," who couldn't understand why his parents divorced when they still had good times together and never fought, the disclosure clarified their situation. Sean was twenty-four when his sister told him. Finally he understood why, as a teenager, he couldn't bond with his dad. Such relief helps children accept the new information more readily.

If parents, still married, don't tell the children, they may sense it nonetheless. The secret long-term lesbian relationship of one mother in Kansas City may have been partially responsible for her daughter's eating disorder. The young girl's insides heard the family secret.

Most children, asked about ideal timing, advise, "The sooner, the better—so the parent-child trust is not broken." When kept in the dark, they feel the parents thought they weren't strong enough to take it. Amy, told when she was nineteen, a year after her father came out to her mother, adds, "If the gay parent doesn't want to tell the children, the spouse should say, 'If we don't tell them together or you alone, I will.' "

There is unanimous agreement that the younger children are when they are told, the easier it is for them. Having a gay parent becomes a given in their lives. Some children advise that it is better to let younger ones figure it out for themselves, with parents keeping the door open for them to ask questions. To discover their parents' homosexuality before they are ready is upsetting, as it was for Anne and Joan as well as Adrian.

Once the parent comes out, three questions arise in a child's mind: "What is my parent's homosexuality all about?"; "Will our lives change?"; and "What does it mean to be the child of a gay, bi, or lesbian parent?" Answering these questions typically uses up considerable emotional and mental energy until adulthood.

Tuning in to Children's Feelings about Homosexuality, AIDS and Homophobia

Children gradually discover what it means to have a gay parent as they encounter issues surrounding homosexuality, AIDS and homophobia.

Their feelings often reflect gender differences as well as stages of development. A lesbian mother in Florida, for example, came out to her seven children, aged sixteen to twenty-nine. Within the year, her conservative twenty-nine-year-old son went back to his psychiatrist, while two of his sisters, sixteen and twenty-four, visited their mom's new home and played with her partner's little granddaughters. They could do what comes naturally as women, while their brother had to deal with conflicts arising from a firmly established moral code.

Typically, elementary school children have some notion that gay persons exist, but that's all. "When I was ten," says Jo, now eleven, "I knew 'fag' wasn't a good thing to say about people, but I didn't know what it meant and never thought about meeting one."

If children have been brought up knowing gay and lesbian people among family friends, the parent's gayness is easier to understand than it is for those who have not met gay men or lesbians. Seven-year-old Adie, brought up that way, chirped as her lesbian mother came to breakfast, "What a cute little dyke you are!"

Children who haven't known gay persons often pick up misinformation from playmates and, if they ask their parents, learn the facts abruptly. Bobby, six, came home one day and asked, "Mom, what's a fag?" When she explained that it wasn't a nice term and that it means they like the same sex, he cried, "Yuck! *I* won't do that."

His sister, Lucy, eight, watching TV one night, saw a segment set in a bar where two men started dancing with each other cheek to cheek. "My daddy doesn't do those things," she shouted and ran to her room, where she thrashed on her bed, screaming over and over, "My daddy doesn't do those things." Again, her mother had to explain. "Yes, those men were gay, but you don't know what your daddy does."

Slightly older children generalize from their own experience, even if it hasn't been with gay people. Mark, the sixth grader, talks about his class project on slavery through which he and his classmates learned how to treat different people equally. "My friends will accept my Dad," he says. "Young people are more educated."

The idea of homosexuality seems to disturb children more strongly during adolescence and young adulthood. As boy-girl relationships begin to have sexual overtones, the idea that the parent is attracted to people of the same gender can be baffling. Confusion increases among children of the same gender as the gay or lesbian parent. For those with a bisexual parent, there is still an opposite sex attraction with which to identify.

At first, most teenagers can't formulate questions about their parent's orientation, but they yearn for information to help them integrate the parent's new identity into theirs. While all children value knowing that their parents are available to answer questions, teenagers especially want to know that the door is always open for intimate talk. When ready, they ask. Once that Sarah, fourteen, felt ready to ask her dad about his sexuality, she remembered his promise, "I'm only a phone call away." Only when he answered her questions did she feel ready to join her brother in spending Saturday nights at her dad's apartment.

Children's moral judgments about being gay usually differ according to age and gender. Elementary school youngsters are concerned about what is fair play. As they grow older, boys' standards of right and wrong begin to differ from those of girls. Boys generally stick to rules and abstract standards; most girls make exceptions to preserve relationships and take care of others' needs.[2] Hence, Adrian has no trouble judging his father's actions wrong.

In contrast, Rachel, twenty-two, respects her bi-straight parents' decision to stay together these past nine years for the sake of her and her sister, but she feels they should divorce so that each could be happier.

Sometimes age and gender make no difference. Three siblings, two girls and one boy, aged twelve to seventeen, did not like the fact that their mother discovered she was lesbian several years after divorcing. "We were a team, seeing Mom almost as the enemy, I hate to say," says Brian, now twenty. "I still don't agree with it. God meant men and women to be together, not women and women or men and men. We still love her, but I feel uncomfortable about it and pray that she might meet some man and remember what it used to be like."

Applying their values to their parents' lives sometimes changes children's moral views. Lou in "Fine Tuning" thought his mother should leave his bi dad because he wasn't monogamous. But when Lou saw his mother going over to his dad's apartment every weekend, he said, "You're over there all the time. You might as well move there!"

Similarly, Hugh, thirty, believes his mother's lesbianism goes against statements found in the Bible. But, concentrating on his love for her as his mother, says "God will forgive her just as he forgives me. We're all sinners."

Children more readily accept their parents' gayness if the parents are self-assured about their orientation, says Hope Berry, co-founder of Children of Lesbians and Gays Everywhere (COLAGE), the national children's network. (See Appendix B.) As Joan says, "If it isn't O.K. with Lil and Mom, it certainly is never going to be O.K. with me."

Children also like their parents to introduce them to their gay and lesbian friends from many walks of life so that they can realize they are no different from other adults in their lives.

Once young adults leave home for college or a job, their sexuality fairly well-established, having a gay or lesbian parent ceases to be a central issue. Cindy, twenty, for instance, jests with her dad about both of them noticing handsome young men on the street. For some adult children, gay concerns become the core of their careers or voluntary efforts, like the young men and women who run COLAGE.

Stereotypical behavior and details of the parent's sexual activities are more troublesome, especially to older children. Lynn's father's drunken antics with his lover, for example, embarrassed her, especially in front of her friend.

Just imagining the sexual activities of parents is difficult for any child. For those with gay, bi, or lesbian parents, it can be upsetting. Sarah, fourteen, asks, "Will it be different when Papa finds a lover and starts dating? It would be just weird. You see married couples hugging and kissing, but I can't imagine two men. It kind of sends a shiver down my spine." Similarly, Sean, thirty, accepts his father's being gay but doesn't like to imagine or hear about his same-sex activities.

Hearing details about their parents' gay activities or being present where gay or lesbian persons are openly demonstrative upsets most children. While young children can't put it in words, older children can express the discomfort they felt when younger. Courtney, from "Dad's Girl; Mom's Boy," now twenty-two, recalls "being exposed over my head at Dad's parties."

The biggest fear for children of bi and gay fathers is that they might become HIV-positive, contract AIDS, and die. Eight-year-old Adam, after seeing gay magazines around the house asked his mother why they were there. When she said his dad was gay, he confronted his father that night, yelling, "You need to go to a doctor right away!" and rampaging through the house.

At the 1993 COLAGE conference, some fifty children held a town meeting with their parents to express their fears about AIDS. They demanded that their fathers practice safe sex and not to resent that demand. "We have a right to make sure you stay alive," they chorused. They wanted their fears heard and honest answers given.[3]

AIDS is such a matter of life and death that a parent's silence about being HIV-positive can break children's trust. One gay father in Detroit, still married, promised nothing would be kept secret after he came out, but he didn't tell his three children for four years that he had tested HIV-positive. His broken promise caused one of his daughters, now twenty, to lose trust in him and everyone else in her life. Despite therapy and self-help efforts, her distrust prevails, paining her deeply.

Homophobia, a third issue connected with having a gay parent, raises fears among all children of gay, lesbian and bi parents, whether born in heterosexual marriages, born through artificial insemination, adopted or in foster homes. At one time or another all experience the pain of anti-gay verbal or non-verbal behavior directed at them or their parents at school, in their neighborhood or at church.

Terms like "gay" or "fag," used by school children to put down others, taint the children's parent—the model, anchor and source of comfort in their lives. The discrepancy causes shame and defensiveness to compete in their minds and hearts.

Often, children themselves become targets. Xan for example, lost a best friend in junior high. Courtney, in ninth grade, found "fag lover" written all over her locker. "I felt sad," she recalls, "at the ignorance that made that person hate so much."

As children get older and more confident, many stop fearing verbal attacks and learn to respond as did Mary, a college sophomore. Hearing some kids making snide remarks about gay men one day, she turned and said, "Gee, that doesn't sound like my gay father."

In schools, a sensitive teacher or counselor can educate students to respect differences and stop name-calling. Often parents provide a firsthand example of how normal a gay parent is, like Lois. She and her partner, also an African-American lesbian social welfare worker, have three adopted youngsters. One day, when their first grader told classmates about a Gay Parents picnic to which the family was going, one said, "Oh-oh, your mother's going to hell." The next day, when Lois was at school to drive for a trip, she went over to the little classmate and hugged him saying, "Oh, Tommy, I'm glad to meet you."

Incidents outside school can be resolved mainly within the family circle, as illustrated in "Two Minor Miracles." The youth minister's statement that all homosexuals will go to hell and the subsequent state-wide anti-gay rights campaign sent young Alex into hiding after school because of having a lesbian mother. Only after months of conversations with her and the gradual transformation of his parents' fights into renewed friendship was he able to resolve his doubts and shame.

A more dramatic turnaround occurred for Stefan, a Canadian teen-ager. A brick with "fag" written on it was thrown through the window of the dining room where he and his gay activist dad were eating dinner. He is now co-director of COLAGE.

Most children want to combat anti-gay behavior, but some fear being rejected or having the gay label applied to themselves. Seventh grader Raph, for instance, felt guilty that he didn't rebut schoolmates' gay jokes. His lesbian mom and straight dad explained that his silence was as good as rebutting. "Any gay person seeing you would know that you were for them," they reassured him. Older kids may become angry enough to object, as did Lynn in her psychology class.

Some children, fearing that their parents may be hurt by anti-gay attitudes, become so protective that they do not bring up concerns that might seem homophobic. Courtney, twenty-two, for example, has quietly listened to her father talk about his gay activities since she was eight, afraid that he, her idol, might abandon her if she objected. Now she can say, "I'm sick of hearing about his gay life," but not yet directly to him, anxious that he would feel insulted. Such unspoken discomfort that conflicts with a child's caring can breed further pain.

Adult children often feel more comfortable saying what they really think, because they can distinguish between the parent's gayness and the way he or she deals with it. Sean at thirty, for instance, can express anger over his dad's marrying his mother without telling her he was gay. At the same time, Sean accepts his dad's sexual orientation. "I'd much rather see you and Mama happy in our home in Columbus," he says, "but it can't be. So I'm happy you're both happier now."

Alongside stress, many children express pride in their parents for coming out in the face of homophobia. Lynn respects her father's courage and honesty, even as she fusses that he has less time for her. Xan, by acting proud when she tells her new friends about her father, loses her fears and honestly feels pride in her Abba.

Such experiences in school and community accelerate youngsters' own coming out as children of gay, lesbian, and bi parents. At home, the process involves more subtle changes.

Watching Children Cope within the Family Circle

How families carry out their business varies widely; each family creates its own constantly changing world. One person's actions, no matter how small or hidden, affect everyone else's. To children the family seems to revolve around them as they go about their work of growing up. Everything that happens is seen as being "done to us."

When a parent comes out, family interactions, established over the years, change. For children whose parents divorce—the majority—the family breakup usually causes more disruption to family dynamics than the disclosure does. Effects of the divorce and the coming out are so closely linked, however, that the parent's gayness often becomes the scapegoat for the chaos resulting from the divorce. It may be argued that all the problems, like a line of dominos, result from the parent's disclosure. But the two events are uniquely different, even though they operate together in the family's life. Discerning what divorce does, as distinct from effects of the parent's being gay, helps heal the wounds caused by the coming out.

Just the idea of divorce sets some children into a panic. "I don't want to be a suitcase kid," wailed Raph, twelve, when his parents told him and his sister that their mother was lesbian rather than bisexual and that they would no longer be living together.

When Pamela, exhausted from raising three young children as her gay husband absented himself more often to be with gay friends, moved out, her nine-year-old begged her to come back. "Mum, just try harder," he pleaded. She heard his pain, came back, and tried harder for another eighteen years.

If parents decide to divorce, the announcement raises children's fears of abandonment, insecurity, distrust and conflicting loyalties.

Custody negotiations become hurtful for the children if the gay factor becomes an issue. Some straight fathers, for instance, initially balk at allowing the lesbian mother to assume primary care, though they eventually realize that sexual orientation has nothing to do with parenting skills.

Court disputes and quarrels over visitation rights usually arise when straight parents and judges operate on misinformation and define the gay parent only by the sexual behavior in which he or she engages for just a small percentage of time. In reality, most gay and lesbian parents do not expose their children to sexual activities any more than straight parents invite the children into their bedrooms.

Stereotypical thinking on the part of professionals, too, can operate against the children's welfare. A counselor in Ohio, believing that straight husbands tend to abuse their lesbian wives, told her lesbian client not to be in the house alone with her husband to work out custody details. It was the one time left to clear up several problems before going to court. The parents didn't meet and arrangements for the children remained ambiguous, increasing their insecurity.

Children who become pawns in such disagreements between their parents, suffer for the long term. One child, who ten years ago, had to appear in court twice when her gay father's visitation rights had been violated, recalls nothing of that period. The fun she had on those visitations is obliterated along with the difficulties.

As any child feels in a divorce, these youngsters feel bereft of a two-parent home and the family unit. Though generous visitations and flexible custody arrangements may be planned, youngsters feel the loss of the other parent when they are with the one. Cliff and Pris worked out such a schedule for their adopted Korean son, Curt. But, whenever Cliff came to get Curt on weekend evenings when Pris went out with her lesbian friends, Curt said, "I hate you. I want my mommy. You're not my friend. It's not fair." The best times were when the three of them ate at Cliff's apartment and Pris took Curt home. Then he asked, "Dad, why don't you come stay with us?"

Since custody is more commonly granted to the mother, most children spend less time with their fathers, straight or gay. Both are short changed. Most children therefore welcome being with their fathers often and treasure an open sharing of feelings as well as tender loving care that includes hugs given to both sons and daughters.

A number of gay fathers lose all contact with their children because of the straight parents' negative attitudes toward their orientation. As shown in "I love You, Peggy and Jeff," the loss deprives children of a personal support system known since birth.

Custodial mothers also may not be as available as before, if they have to go to school or work to achieve financial security. Like Xan and Lynn, children resent their parents not being there for them as they used to be. Legitimate as the parents' reasons are for not being home as much, they cannot make up for the loss children feel. Children therefore rejoice when parents limit their social and work-related time to be available. "I've really become a recluse," Mark's and Sarah's mother says with a chuckle.

Children feel abandoned even more when either parent starts to date seriously, the gay parent to act fully on his or her liberated sexuality or the straight parent to validate his or her sexuality.

Youngsters may connect the gay parent's new sexual identity with their feelings of abandonment since it is that parent's coming out that usually causes the family breakup and the parent who often becomes involved in outside gay social or political activities more quickly.

Children react to the perceived loss in different ways according to their age. Bobby, five-years-old, for example, sings over and over in the car and his bedroom, "My daddy left and I miss him. I miss him so much. Why did my daddy have to be gay?"

Eight to thirteen-year-olds seem to have the hardest time. Jo, eleven, feels trapped when she is in one or the other parent's home, without the other one close by when a different approach is needed. Some nine-to-ten year old boys have a particularly rough time and become suicidal. Possible reasons include: the need to become competent in dealing with the world; sensitivity to family dynamics combined with reluctance to verbalize feelings and conflicting emotions about an absent father and an imminent break with the mother. Boys of this age need a variety of outlets for physical activity and opportunities to share concerns with their parents or some adult.

Surprisingly, college age kids suffer, too. Divorce removes the stable home which they need as a safety net when taking their first steps toward an independent life. As a result, reported in *Adult Children of Divorce Speak Out*, their confidence, self concept, trust and ability to relate to others may become damaged.[4]

Typical of all children of divorce, some youngsters blame themselves for the breakup and try singlehandedly to bring family back together or to make the family function with less pain. Courtney, in "Mom's Girl and Dad's Boy," tried to be as good as she could be from age eight through eighteen as a way to reunite the family. Tackling such a task, of course, is fruitless. Frustration lessens when parents tell children explicitly that the divorce was not their fault and that nothing anyone can do will bring the family back together.

Changes in living arrangements trigger uneasiness and resentment for some children and surprise and enjoyment for others. Young kids often find going to the new house of the non-custodial parent to be an adventure. Mark loves the fact that he and his dad play games. "We never did that here," he explains. Older children like his sister, Sarah, find it more difficult. "To go from learning Papa's gay to spending the night at his house is a big jump," she says. "I took another step only when it was comfortable."

As the non-custodial gay, bi, or straight father develops his new life, the mother becomes the children's last connection to "how it used to be." Even this tie often begins to fray, however, if money problems resulting from split assets impose limitations on activities family members used to do, such as eating out, taking trips, and buying clothes.

Soon the children's shuttling between houses, schools, friends, and homes becomes a way of life and feelings of uncertainty increase. There's a new bedroom and new friends in the new place or places, but they miss a single home base. Jo, eleven, bridges the gap by telling the story of her father's coming out over and over to her cat in his house and to her stuffed animals at her mother's. Her younger brother, when they're at their father's home, dresses up his teddy bear to represent his mother whom he misses.

When children grow older and develop distance from the trauma, many joke about having two houses. As one child said, "In Mom's house, we ate out of the refrigerator and in Dad's, we ate breakfast off china and sterling in the dining room."

New partners of either parent add another threat to the child-parent relationship. Frequently, it is the gay or lesbian parent who first introduces new persons into the children's lives. A number of lesbian mothers have lovers before the divorce or shortly afterwards. Some gay fathers have partners also, and others have a series of special friends as well as a growing friendship circle. Their children therefore must develop new adult relationships. To do this, while trying to integrate the parent's gay dimension into their understanding, is hard.

Negative concerns about the new partner may go unheard. Sis, eleven, told her mother that she didn't want to visit her house when her lover was there. The mother's therapist then said it would be good for Sis to do so, "to get used to the situation." Forcing such changes on a child before she or he has come to terms with the immediate effects of the divorce and coming out may become counterproductive.

In many instances, new partners become sources of joy and stability as adult friends and mentors. This turned out to be the case for Anne and Joan with their mother's lover and for Xan with her father's.

Children feel grateful for meeting gay and lesbian adults through their parents and for joining in gay and lesbian community activities like child-parent picnics. Meg, sixteen, says, "As a six-year-old I loved having all those daddies. I cherish knowing gay men and lesbians. I attribute my not being prejudiced to knowing such diverse people."

Conflicting loyalties to the two parents is a another common fall out from divorce. As Mark says, "I'm so like Mom, I feel guilty being happy with Dad while she's crying her eyes out."

Children's relationship with each parent is frequently fueled by one overriding emotion, such as fear, guilt, trust or anger. The post-divorce tug-of-war toward and against each parent often feeds into these feelings. Seven-year-old Lucy suffered increased migraines after her gay father left, but turns on her mother, complaining, "You never told me that there was such a thing as divorce."

Adolescence, a time of rebellion, is often the battleground for divided loyalties. Steve, when sixteen, left his lesbian mother to live with his straight father and stepmother. The move backfired when he found his father's household was rigidly homophobic. His mother insisted that he finish out his year's commitment, as a lesson in taking responsibility for one's decisions. He rejoiced when he returned to the stability of her home as well as to the counsel of her partner, who had become his mentor.

Stability is not always permanent in second homes. Like Dan and Sally's daughters in "Not Enough of A Man," Joan and Anne suffered a second divorce when their mom and Lil broke up. Some children experience third and fourth divorces in the course of growing up.

Conflicting loyalties easily become gay versus straight issues unless parents clarify the nature of problems that arise. Common problems include financial problems connected with the divorce; developmental issues concerning the children, such as hypersensitivity to sexual information during their puberty; and social questions like the children's participation in gay activities like gay pride events.

When straight parents speak honestly about their own feelings regarding the gay parent, the child's sense of parental conflict is minimized. The mother of Bobby and Lucy, tells them, "This is how I feel about Daddy, but I want you to make up your own mind."

As family arrangements change, children are given or take on new roles in the old home and assume new roles in the new home. One child may begin to express everyone's feelings, another, like Xan, may keep track of what's happening to the family and a third will organize family events.

Some roles are less constructive than others. The mediator and maternal roles that Xan played became so much of a burden that she wanted to end her life. Her life might have been made easier had her mother been able to see what her daughters needed and kept her divorce problems to herself.

A number of high school girls who take on the role of mediator or observer become suicidal. Among possible reasons for such despair could be the tendency of girls, sensitive to relationships, to keep track of family interactions. This task is too much for any teenager. As Lynn watches the comings and goings of her brothers and parents, her anger deepens because she cannot control what they do. Instead, she strikes out at herself with scissors.

Such anger, if not released through therapy, reflection or constructive activities, may gnaw at the children for many years until, as adults, they are able to forgive their parents and achieve their own peace.[5]

Taking on the family's problems makes many children feel forced to grow up too fast. Children need and want a balance of work and play, of both serious and lighthearted times. They need time for daydreaming, creating, and just plain growing—and time to be silly, even if the dishes aren't done one night. At the same time, they also want rules, like curfews, to give order to their lives and to demonstrate that the parents care what happens to them.

Grandparents often play important roles in the family, such as being a listening ear for the grandchildren or offering them respite from the home front. Though many youngsters don't talk about their parent's gayness to their grandparents and many grandparents are not told about it, a number seek support in dealing with the aftermath of their parents' disclosure. One grandmother who recently attended a panel of children of gay and lesbian parents, aged five to seventeen, asked them, "What should I do for my grandchildren?" One after one, they said, "Be a grandmother! There's no need to take sides or take a stand. Just be there for your grandchild."

Lynn's paternal grandmother illustrates the helpful grandparent. Knowing that Lynn's brother, Andy, is loath to talk about his dad, she asks him to do chores at her house where, as he works, he shares his concerns about his dad and his own sexuality. "I have him over," she says, "to give him that opportunity." For the sake of all the grandchildren and their mother, with whom she sympathizes, she invites everyone to family gatherings: the grandchildren, their father and his partner, their mother and her boyfriend, as well as other relatives. "I don't want those children to be hurt in any way," she explains.

Similarly, Frank's mother in "I Love You, Peggy and Jeff," has kept communication lines open with the grandchildren. As a result, Jeff visited her twice since he graduated from college. Such contacts help grandchildren keep in touch with family from whom they might otherwise have thought they were cut off forever.

A different reaction was encountered by a lesbian daughter, whose divorced mother came out after raising her and her sister and whose gay father died of AIDS. Her maternal grandparents stopped sending cards and gifts after her father came out, since he had hurt their daughter. After his death, they said to the granddaughter, "It's time for you to put this behind you."

Some grandparents, by denying the problem, keep the parents from meeting the family needs satisfactorily. Pamela's parents, for example, thought she was crazy to say Craig was gay, discounted her desire to divorce and refused to probe reasons for his absences. She therefore had to keep the family together all alone. How much better it would have been for everyone had the family secret been faced honestly. Then all members could have pitched in to help make the family work.

Other relatives' reactions often confuse children and, if not supportive of the gay parent, provoke deep anger. Amy, twenty-six, meeting an aunt for the first time, hoped the experience would enrich her picture of the family. Instead, her aunt asked if her gay dad had ever molested her brother. "Of course not!" Amy said, disappointed.

In the context of such diverse family interactions, children go about their business, carrying their suitcases and knapsacks back and forth between the two parents' homes. At each site, they cope in different ways with the changes. Xan loses herself in books, and Sarah listens to music that matches her moods. "I involved myself in clubs and sports," says Courtney, "to fill the emptiness. I smiled a lot, too. After a horrible day, I'd say, 'Well, tomorrow will be better.' "

In Ling's family in "What the Buddha Said," Lionel never talked about his father and as a teenager, acted out. His sister, by contrast, shared her feelings in a support group and wrote poems about her AIDS-stricken father. She later read one at his memorial service.

Each child develops a coping strategy that feels comfortable and safe for controlling what is happening to them. These behaviors, however, conceal deeper issues with which they are wrestling. That is why children tell parents, "Be there for us."

"Be there for us," according to children of all ages, means: Be honest and open and available as much as possible even if you are ignored. Just watch and wait. Bring the subject up when you can, but not too much. Keep asking if we want to talk but don't force us to express our feelings. Give us time to process information and let us take baby steps. Once we start talking, let us talk as long as we want. That's how we think things through. And listen to our feelings, whether you like them or not. Don't judge or be defensive.

Children want respect given them and all family members. They want their parents to accept differences among the siblings and to honor each one's privacy. While not all parents can become huggers, youngsters appreciate efforts to demonstrate love and caring in any form. Also welcomed are calmness and humor when resolving conflicts.

These requests sound simple but are difficult to fill. It means parents need courage to listen without becoming defensive, to admit mistakes and to change. The interaction of Joan and her mother illustrates the rewards that can accrue to both child and parent and also to the relationship when they are open and honest with one another.

Children's requests are but surface waves of an undercurrent of concerns about themselves. From their perspective, the effects of the coming out and divorce destroy three constructs of how the world and their lives are supposed to work: marriages last forever; men and women fall in love and get married; my gender and sexuality are like my same-gender parent. Some see the destruction as a triple death.

Hearing Children's Concerns about Identity and Isolation

With the loss of their assumptions about marriage, love, and gender, two issues become increasingly worrisome: identity and isolation. The children's views of their gay parent, of the family world and of themselves have been drastically changed, leaving them without reference points by which to measure themselves. In their minds, they no longer have a normal family or a normal parent. They themselves are no longer normal. As far as they know, no other kids do not have gay or lesbian parents. They are alone and different.

Among all adolescents, the question of "Who am I?" becomes paramount. They must not only establish their sexual identity but also form a clear, integrated sense of self and the life they want to lead. For teenagers with bi, lesbian or gay parents, stress from both the parent's coming out and for most, the divorce interferes with this developmental process and may promote instead what psychologist David Elkind, Ph.D., calls "the patchwork self."[6]

As teenagers work on establishing who they are, they begin to identify more with their peers, all of whom are struggling with their identities and puberty also. Neither boys nor girls, during this sensitive period, want to be or to appear to be unlike classmates. Having a gay parent adds one more factor that might make these children appear different to their peers.[7]

Comparing the sexuality of the gay or lesbian parent with their own burgeoning feelings, many teenagers become confused. Sue, seventeen, says, "I get turned on when I see a girl walk by and when I see a boy walking by." Lynn, unsure of her future as a woman, confides, "I don't want to marry and I don't want children."

In the last years of high school, children look to older mentors, such as teachers, counselors or friends of their parents, as they form a coherent self-image that can withstand outside stresses. Therapist Patricia Stark, Ph.D., calls the process the building of their inner house. "If you can build your self inside," she counsels teenagers, including those in this situation, "you'll always be at home, no matter where you are."[8]

Young adults, after their self-identity is in place, sometimes find that questions about their sexuality come up again when they exchange family information with new friends. Thinking through the question once more only clarifies their sexual identity. "It always comes out the same," says Sean, thirty. "I like women too much to be gay. If I am, I am, but I wouldn't want to give up women."

The feeling of being all alone in the world because of the parent's being gay is the most common concern voiced by children of all ages. The social stigma attached to homosexuality is now attached to the child as well as to their parent. Stigmatization and the need to protect the parent by keeping his or her gayness a secret push children into their own closet. The danger of being isolated within psychological walls is that it may prevent the children from developing the capacity to relate intimately with other people.

For many, seeing themselves as children of a gay, bi or lesbian parent becomes so fearsome that they share the secret with only a chosen few or no one. They constantly fear that the wrong person might find out and they would lose friends or the parent might lose his or her job. Their world begins to revolve around the question of whether or not to tell anyone and, if so, who and what might be their reactions.

Young children and preadolescents often see no reason to tell anyone. If they do share the information, most friends accept it without judgment. For adolescents, telling becomes a major concern and the feeling of being the only one in this situation reaches its height.

Most teenagers learn, almost by instinct, how to tell which friends are tolerant and who might be negative about gays. When adolescents enter high school, some, like Xan, become bolder. Meg, sixteen, daughter of a bi-straight couple, enjoys telling everyone her married dad is gay. "It shows I'm trustworthy and tests them. If I can tell them this, they know they can trust me with their secrets," she explains.

Other children, particularly those who were young when their parents came out, never talk about their parents' being gay since it has been part of their lives for so long. Nevertheless, the burden of not talking about it may become too much. Renee's dad came out when she was seven. Because she deeply missed the daily routines they once had enjoyed doing as father and daughter, her parents took her to a therapist. While he asked questions, she played with the toys and said nothing. Now at seventeen, she exclaims, "I want so badly to talk with somebody. My feelings are ready to burst out and I'm afraid what I'll find."

Other children, like Anne and Joan, are told not to tell anyone in order to protect the parent or the partner. Such forced secrecy makes it harder for children to develop trust, not to mention intimacy. Anne and Joan were fortunate to have each other for support, illustrating how important siblings are to each other.

Keeping the secret may make children feel embarrassed about their parent as well as themselves for being the child of a gay parent. Shame fades when parents clarify the difference between secrecy and privacy: "This is a private family matter, not a secret we're ashamed of."

The problem of not telling seems to affect girls and boys differently. While girls want to protect their parent and themselves from homophobic taunts, they suffer from having to keep the secret. Remaining silent about it in girl-to-girl confidences limits the fulfillment of their need to form relationships.

Boys, too, don't talk about their parents' homosexuality as a protection strategy. "Few," for example, doesn't want his pals to change their picture of his gay father as the wonderful, muscular guy they all adore. Boys also don't want to besmirch their own image as a macho guy among their friends.

To boys, having to keep the secret is of less consequence than it is to girls. Boys' relationships with their buddies rely less on sharing intimate personal facts. Peer esteem comes from being one of the guys, not from telling each other secrets. Thus, Lynn's brother goes off to play basketball rather than discuss feelings about his father.

Isolation cuts teenagers off from peer support just at the time when friends are sorely needed in the struggle to be independent of the family and to form a sense of who they are. Even the few friends who know the secret cannot conceive fully what it means. Little by little, many children find themselves coping with their deepest concerns alone.

What children need most now is support from other children in this situation. Those who find the few existing support groups, like Anne and Joan, speak unanimously of "an immediate bonding." Some groups are led by therapists, but possibly the most effective are run by young adults who are children of gays, bisexuals and lesbians, like COLAGE groups. Peer leadership frees children to say what they feel and to have as listeners only people who have been there themselves.

Many children find at least one trusted person—a parent, relative or teacher—to whom to talk. Such mentors act as a sounding board and listen to their fears, worries and anger without judgment.

Once in the work force or college, separated somewhat from family and community, adult children feel freer to talk or not to talk about their gay or lesbian parent. Cindy, away from her gay dad who is still married to her mom, hardly thinks about it and only shares when gay subjects come up with her friends. Adrian doesn't feel a need to tell anyone. "They're not mature enough," he says. "Besides, it's family business." Others, like Sean, enjoy telling acquaintances who ask about his family. "My dad is gay and my sister is a lesbian" he says, with the idea people need to be more aware of this topic.

Through coping with these complex issues, largely alone, the children come to know themselves well. They can pinpoint their tolerance limits, such as how much they can take of one parent's dumping on them about the other. They set boundaries for how much intimate information they are willing to listen to before silencing the parent.

Most older children say that the experience made them grow up more quickly than their friends, "too quickly," many add, because it robbed them of their childhood. Adolescent girls find that the forced growing up made them more mature. Teenage boys think that it gave them more responsibilities, which some see as negative and others as positive. Adrian thinks that becoming the man of the house "sucks," probably because he thinks his dad shirked his responsibility. "Few" thinks it's great to have taken over for his dad whom he admires.

Eventually, most children find their own inner strength. As they leave high school, they are clearer about their identity. Many have formed intimate friendships and, some, sexual relationships. Some young adults, however, still struggle with trust, commitment and intimacy issues. A number still do not accept the coming out on moral grounds, and others remain angry about the hurt. Many value individuals for who they are inside and welcome the diversity of people. While recognizing their parents' limitations as persons and parents, most respect and love them and value their relationship with them.

Out of this chorus of children's voices emerges common themes: a cry for honesty and open communication, distress from hiding the secret, fear of AIDS, stress from feeling alone, confusion about identity and the future, divided loyalties and desire for a stable home and parents who are there for them. While each family is different, the common purpose is to help the children transform such feelings into compassion, understanding and confidence.

How can straight spouses meet the children's needs and also continue their own recovery? Whether the parents are still together, separated or divorced, the family concept can still be central in decision-making on the part of the parents.

Two goals take precedence: reducing the harm already incurred and increasing the likelihood that the children become confident, sensitive and responsible adults. Achieving these goals involves both sacrifice and pleasure.

As the children struggle with their issues, the closest adults in the children's lives—the parents—can provide a model of transformation for them to mirror as they grow into adulthood. Part Seven explores that process, tracing how straight spouses break out of old patterns and transform their lives within the marriage or after divorce.

seven

BREAKING THE MOLD

TRANSFORMATION OF SHATTERED BELIEF SYSTEM

Turning the coming-out crisis into an opportunity to create a new life with new purpose, outside or within the marriage, is the last challenge on the long road to recovery. Even after restoring self-identity and integrity, many spouses find themselves without direction. To find meaning and hope for the future, they are challenged to shift roles from victim to victor and to overcome difficult circumstances in their lives.

For most people, it is easier to cling to a familiar way of life than to plunge toward an unknown future. The spouse needs to make a quantum leap in perception in order to let go of the past as well as transcend any blame, guilt and regret that may linger. This may require forgiving partner, society, oneself and sometimes God for the pain so that energy can be freed up for new growth.

Transformation generally begins during the third year after the coming out, and only after practical and personal issues have been resolved. The first step, abandoning the past, brings grief and emptiness. The second step, typical of anyone in crisis, requires that the spouse come to terms with his or her pain. To achieve this many spouses find it helpful to view their crisis from a larger perspective. In this context the pain no longer seems unique and can be seen as an example of the suffering inherent in the human condition. Spouses are not alone in their hurt. Unrequited love and betrayal fill the pages of history.

The goal is to stop seeing the coming-out trauma as a gay versus straight conflict but rather as a universal paradox. The truth that frees one person may hurt the other. Hurt and love coexist in life.

When this broader philosophy is grounded in the belief that positive values do exist and constructive change is possible, spouses can make a breakthrough in their lives. The recognition of even the slightest glimmer of beauty, joy or love in everyday experience helps create the seeds of a new belief system. Many spouses also seek something beyond themselves to bring meaning into their lives. This can be a sense of nature, the cosmos, a divine being or a deep individual spirituality. Such faith expands the possibility of transformation. Once a belief-centered philosophy is established, hope and purpose return and a new future seems possible.

The following stories depict the transformations of one married and two divorced spouses. The final story recapitulates all of the issues straight spouses typically face in their struggle toward transformation. The concluding analysis examines the crisis of faith spouses face, along with strategies for creating a new belief system through which they can break the mold and transform their lives.

Personal Stories

The Joy of Openness
Jim

In the old days homosexuals were "fags" and "queers," people you pointed at and made fun of. No way could I connect that image with Janie! She wasn't any of those terrible things. So obviously she wasn't homosexual.

Before we married in the mid-sixties, she'd referred vaguely to intense friendships with women in high school and college. Later she disclosed that some of these had been physical.

"What's she talking about?" I thought. "Girls dance with each other and hold hands and hug and even kiss all the time."

"I'm not out molesting young people, Jim," she said, "doing what the far right portrays gays and lesbians as doing. I don't desire that. So I'm not lesbian. I just love women."

Curious, I began to read everything on homosexuality that I could lay my hands on during my business trips as a fairly high-powered executive on the East Coast.

Most of the considerable amount of literature on homosexuality wasn't very positive. Slowly over a two-year period, I found that most of my knowledge about it was inaccurate, the result of being fearful and ignorant. As I learned more, I kept comparing the information to what I knew about Janie until one day I said to myself, "She *is* a lesbian! The definition we've been using is wrong."

She and I talked about it constantly, though never using the words "lesbian" or "homosexual." Every now and then Janie said "gay," but it was like choking to get it out.

Meanwhile, while we had some lovely sexual experiences in private, whenever I came into the kitchen and started caressing Janie, she moved away. Yet when we went out, she held me and squeezed my hand as the loving wife. Alone with me, she backed off.

For eight years I travelled all over the country very impressed with myself and my company perks. Meanwhile, Janie gave birth to two sons, Jimmy and Chet, went through the seminary and was ordained as a minister. In 1972, I realized something was missing. At that time, middle managers in companies like mine were being jailed for illegal pricing. Two years later, not wanting to be the fall guy for my firm, I left to manage a book company in San Francisco. It was our tenth move since we had married. Once there, Janie looked up an old friend, Jackie, to assist me.

Four years later I became active in our Presbyterian Church at a time when people were confused over what was happening in the gay world. Use of the word "homosexual" had the same effect on the congregation as a four-letter word. The vote of the Presbyterian General Assembly which I attended that year was on whether or not to ordain gays as ministers or to the offices of deacon, elder and teaching elder.

The committee who had investigated the issue for two years had made a majority report approving ordination. The conservative members of the church then successfully organized a lobby to elect people to express *their* point of view. A new majority opinion was drafted stating that practicing homosexuals were ineligible for ordination to any of the offices. This was the issue to be voted on at the assembly.

"You know this violates the church government," I said to Janie as I prepared to go. "The sole authority for ordaining ministers is the local presbytery. The sole authority for ordaining elders and deacons is the church unless two-thirds vote of all the presbyteries in the nation change the rule."

It was late afternoon when I arrived at the assembly. By the door a diminutive man was handing out brochures and all the people recessing to go to supper were giving him a wide berth. "What's going on?" I asked someone.

"Oh, he's the one who wants to be ordained."

Hearing that the Presbyterians for Gay Concerns (PGC) were holding an agape feast in the basement of a nearby church, I joined the group going to it which included the outgoing and incoming moderators of the assembly and a bunch of other powerful folks.

There we were, 120 of us having communion, singing and full of joy, yet on the verge of experiencing a monumental setback. During all this love and singing, I suddenly was overcome by something powerful inside me. "Here are 120 people aligned against 4,000 over there," I thought. "How can they be so thankful they've come this far!" My antennae were tuned to the energy in the room, especially from the people I knew were gay, the closeted ones who were trying to give support but not be found out. I was moved to tears.

Once my eyes were opened to the religious truth of this agape experience, I couldn't close them to it again. "If they can fight, so can I," I said to myself on the way home.

Once home, I started a PGC chapter in our church. We had no real idea of what we wanted to do or how to begin. Though my involvement was sporadic, Jackie, by then financial secretary of the church where Janie was assistant pastor, came down to work regularly in the chapter.

Through my sales visits to libraries up and down the coast, I continued reading about homosexuality. One day I discovered Don Clark's *Loving Someone Gay*, published just after the American Psychiatric Association declared that homosexuality was no longer a psychiatric disease—thus curing it by writ.

"This is the most straight-forward, honest book I've discovered!" I told Janie, handing it to her as I left on another book-selling trip.

When Janie finished reading the book, she went to see Don Clark in Palo Alto. Next, she saw Bill Johnson, a gay minister who, along with a woman, had been ordained in the United Church of Christ.

On the way home from my trip the next day, I stopped at a pay phone to tell Janie when I'd be home. When she answered I heard tears in her voice. "What happened?" I asked.

"I met with Bill Johnson. Jim, I'm definitely a lesbian."

"Oh, Janie!" That was it. I knew that her admitting her homosexuality meant there was no question about it. Every bisexual person I knew was just afraid to be gay. Once gays discovered that they weren't awful people, they gave up masquerading as also being straight.

Back in the car, I drove down the freeway sobbing. "I've finally won the argument," I thought. "Janie agrees that she's gay."

Within days we sat down at the kitchen table with Jimmy, nine, and Chet, seven. "Daddy's heterosexual and Mommy's homosexual," we told them, "and it doesn't work. We've been trying, but it just doesn't work."

Then the four of us sat there and cried.

When we stopped crying, the boys asked, "What does that mean? What are you going to do? Don't you love each other?"

"Yes, we love each other. We don't know what we'll do. Probably we won't stay together."

By the end of the week, we saw divorce as the only thing to do. On our thirteenth wedding anniversary, Janie moved to a condominium she'd bought and I to an apartment I'd rented.

Soon afterwards I said to her, "We can't have an ugly falling out. I love you too much."

"And I love you. I don't want to give up the family."

"Janie," I said, "divorced or not, you're family. And as for the kids, I already lost them for nine years of their lives through mismanaging my time. I'm not going to lose them for their last nine years at home like other divorced men I know. Why don't the boys spend half the time with you and half with me?"

"I'm for it."

My schedule didn't lend itself easily to the arrangement nor did Janie's. Now a minister in a church that served the poor in downtown Oakland, she and her lover moved across the bay and bought a house in the hills.

About that time California State Proposition 13 was passed, killing my business as every library in the state cancelled all orders. I sold the company and got into life insurance, which allowed me to work from home and spend time with my boys.

Since Janie wasn't "out" yet, I couldn't tell people why we'd split. It was hard explaining how we loved and respected each other but were no longer married. Actually, people in our church thought I was the gay one. First, women aren't "queer," only men. Second, it couldn't be Janie, an ordained minister. Third, I'd been up to my ears in all those gay rights activities.

My "coming out" like this was kind of fun at first, finding out what it was like to be in the closet. People crossed the street to avoid meeting me. People I thought loved Janie and me changed their seats when I sat down in a pew. "Who are my friends?" I wondered.

One night I thought, "This hurts, but I have an advantage over gays or lesbians. If I get too scared, I can run away saying, 'O.K., you guys, I'm straight.' "

Yet friends' reactions hurt so much that, in my first love affair, I modified everything I said to my lover in support of gay persons until I wasn't me anymore. Realizing that, I ended the relationship, vowing, "I'll never adjust my behavior to fit into somebody else's life again even if it's His Holiness, the Pope!"

About three years after Janie left me, the head of her church telephoned her to say, "We want to talk about your 'lifestyle.' "

Telling me about the call, Janie said, "It must relate to my downtown ministry and my house in the hills. It doesn't look good to live in a rich white area and work with poor blacks."

"Naive Janie!" I thought and then said, "No, they want to talk about your lover. The word is out. They're coming after you."

They came and forced her out, the lesbian minister who'd been doing an incredible job for many years. "This is what you do when you hate gays and lesbians," I told myself. "You punish this one woman for no good reason."

It was now 1981. Many gay people were being fired. Most of them went quietly away so that the "sin" of whatever had occurred wouldn't be known. Each time it happened, I said to myself, "Come on, you guys, fight!"

When Janie was fired, she came out of the closet. I took the responsibility for the local news stories on it, especially the article for our county paper assigned to a somewhat homophobic woman reporter.

The night before the article was to appear, the boys were staying with me. Calling them into the living room, I said, "There's going to be a story in tomorrow's paper about Mommy. They may even have her picture."

Jimmy, twelve, sat crying in the corner, still feeling the peer pressure from school where the word was already out.

Chet, barely ten, looked up at me and said, "Hey Dad. Somebody's got to be the first to use the 'Whites Only' fountain and ride in the front of the bus."

Then it was my turn to cry.

In the days that followed, I gave up worrying about what people thought. Remembering the agape feast, I told myself, "If you're going to be friends with gay and lesbian people, you'd better be ready to deal with the negative stuff."

Soon I found my conversations couldn't go on for three minutes without my saying, "gay" or "lesbian." It was now such a part of my life that it just came out.

I became the "gay day parade" type, celebrating the community feeling of the minority, the joy of openness. It did a whole lot for my soul and was an outlet for a lot of poison in my life.

Each time I celebrated that joy in my church by talking about homosexual concerns, it offended half the members. "Who wants to be a trouble maker?" I finally said. "I'm not going there any more."

When straight friends spoke with prejudice about gays, I corrected them until I got tired of both the hurt and the effort to correct them. After I stopped feeling hurt, I thought, "They're dumb when it comes to homosexuality. I don't want to be with such ignorant people." So I dropped most of those friends.

It was different when I met closeted homosexuals. "I'm happy you're gay," I'd say right away.

That mesmerized them. It was often the first time that anyone had said that to them and had identified with them as being truly oppressed. "Don't you see," a gay friend explained. "I've lived all of my life afraid of people. When you treated me with the same respect you'd give any human being, it had a profound impact on me."

The first time I acknowledged a gay person, it was as if a door had been opened. I had a sense that he cared about me too. Over time I found that if you do anything positive such as treating gays and lesbians as being part of God's natural order, they become your friends no matter who you are. Seeing people as human beings who also happened to be gay created a spiritual bond between us.

Gradually I came to live pretty much in the gay world with Janie and Jackie. Jackie was one of the few people who appreciated our relationship. Her friendship with Janie had begun long before I'd met either of them. My coming into the picture, loving and being loved by Janie, hadn't altered their friendship. Jackie had left a twenty-five-year-long marriage. She knew the people she wanted to be with and why.

After the newspaper article appeared, the three of us went around speaking to students at local high schools. We called it "The Jim, Janie and Jackie Pony Show." At the start of each session, the students expressed great curiosity about seeing a real, honest-to-God lesbian.

They always asked, "What were your kids' reactions?"

"Well," one of us would say, "Jimmy, the older son, is the more open. Janie was assistant pastor at our church when he was growing up and youth minister for a group that included him and all his friends. They loved her, 'queer' or not, giving Jimmy strength not to fear being identified with a gay mother."

"Chet's situation is different," another of us would say next. "He hesitates to be open because of pressure from his friends who were too young to understand why Janie was fired at the time." Then we'd describe Chet's incredible reaction, "Someone has to be first." That always got the students' attention.

Four years after our divorce, I married Jackie. Janie was the one who married us, adding another topic to our pony show. The kids always asked Jackie, "How can you sit beside your husband's ex-wife? Aren't you jealous?"

"We were friends," she said, "before Jim knew either of us."

After our wedding, Jackie became my business partner. We worked out of the house I'd bought. When her father died, her mother moved from her quiet little town to live with her only daughter, now married to a gay rights activist. Although she had never known a gay person before, she went to functions with us and in the process shared our friends, by then mostly gay. Some became more her friends than ours.

Three years later Janie split with her lover, left their house and came directly to ours. Jackie's mother, the only one home at the time, invited her to live with us. When Jackie and I got home that night, there was my ex-wife with my ex-dog and my mother-in-law having a great time.

Valium kept me going for a week before I could take it all in. When I calmed down a bit, I told myself, "Janie's just a friend. I can give up the past. Everything's going to be normal."

That decision worked with twenty to thirty Valium a week plus sitting down for spells. Yet soon I settled down, drug free, to live with my wife and ex-wife.

For two months it was dynamite. The boys lived at our house full time, no more back and forth. Then Janie found another lover and moved out.

About this time, the first diagnosed AIDS patient died and the insurance industry began to wonder about honoring these claims .

The gay community was screaming, "Discrimination. You can't trust an insurance company. They're all crooks."

The insurance companies were screaming, "You can't trust gays!" For the first time, I had an insurance claim rescinded.

In September I read that the Concerned Insurance Professionals for Human Rights were holding a meeting in Los Angeles. I flew down to discover that the group shared my view that an AIDS claim could be honored on legitimate policies.

Although most members weren't life and disability brokers like I was, the group became my beacon. When a question came up, I could call several of them to ask, "Hey, is this homophobic or is it the appropriate thing to do?" Together we explored the larger question, "Is insurance by nature discriminatory since it separates everyone, not just gays, based on criteria?"

We got information as needed out to hundreds of thousands of agents in language their communities could understand. Gradually we made an impact on the industry.

Then my seventy-six-year-old father, a vital man who grew and canned his own vegetables and fruit, made furniture and toys and shoveled everybody's walk, got a melanoma and died. It was my first taste of death.

Though grief counseling helped, I wasn't doing well at all. My panic and fear were channeled into working with the insurance group until September 1985, when I became emotionally paralyzed. By January our business had declined by four million dollars because of AIDS cases. To salvage what we had, I declared bankruptcy and sold our house.

Jackie insisted that we go to counseling. Having been in therapy all my life since my mother was an alcoholic, I fought it. Finally I agreed.

Had we not gone, I couldn't have told this story now. Even so, I was out of business for several months and only medication allowed me to handle the peaks and valleys.

Meanwhile Janie became involved in the Ministry of Light, an outgrowth of the Presbyterians for Gay Concerns. This group became responsible for Birthright, Parents and Friends of Lesbians and Gays, a gay youth program and a county AIDS support network. They also opened up a San Francisco chapter, which has had great impact on the church and our old presbytery. At each monthly meeting, the Ministry of Light gives its report. No one is offended by the word, "homosexual," any more.

What I do now in my life follows my own agenda, not just "the cause." Out of the openness of agape, I now have a string of friends and relationships which will last a lifetime. Doing things for these people I love gives me pleasure.

Yet the sum of all of my efforts is focused on my family. Last Christmas, seated around our dining room table were Jimmy and Chet, Jackie's mother, Jackie's son and his wife, my grandfather, Janie, her mother and father and her lover—all of us getting along fantastically.

No matter what I think or don't think, Janie is always going to be a lesbian and the mother of my two boys. We remain very close friends, arm in arm for such a long time.

We Don't Fit the Script
Barbara

Everyone knew Josh was gay—family, friends and people at work. In fact, few of his friends were straight. He'd been in Manhattan fourteen years when we met at work.

When I first saw this tall blond, my immediate thought was, "This man is gay." If you're a woman living in Manhattan, you learn to recognize gay men and stay away from them unless you have a propensity for suffering, which I didn't. Besides, I was dating lots of other men. My mid-twenties was a time to have fun.

After we met, Josh smiled whenever our paths crossed. One morning, he asked, "Hey, Barbara. What about lunch today?"

"Wait a minute," I thought. "This man's making advances. There's sexual energy here. If a man's gay, he's gay with none of the energy this one gives off."

After lunch at a sandwich place around the corner, he told me he volunteered in a gay rights organization.

"Well," I thought, "that sort of settles it."

Yet he kept flirting with me over the next few weeks, making me wonder, "This is very strange. This is a shy man, not the type who flirts with everyone he knows."

One afternoon a few weeks later, I announced to my co-workers, "I feel like going out for a drink after work. Anyone interested?" Josh, of course, was my target.

"Sure!" he said.

One other person joined us as we left for the bar down the street. Josh and I kept ordering until we drank her under the table. Once she left, it felt as if we were on a first date—awkward with each other—quite out of character for me.

After we finished our drinks, we walked toward my apartment, where I lived with three other women. "Want to come up?" I asked.

"O.K., but why not go to my place? It's closer."

I agreed and that night we made love. Though stilted, it seemed to be a serious thing. It wasn't as if I were an anonymous woman Josh had bumped into, but instead someone he knew and wanted a relationship with. As for him, I didn't know what his gayness meant, whether he'd had sex with a couple of men or with one lover only or many.

During our next night of lovemaking Josh said passionately, "The only time I've ever been this excited is with a man."

The comment stayed in my mind for weeks. "What sparked this passion?" I wondered. "How was our lovemaking like that of men?"

One evening I asked Josh what he'd meant. He couldn't answer. As our relationship continued, I realized he wasn't being evasive. The problem had to do with language, with not being able to describe such a feeling.

By then we were going out a lot and, without much ado, Josh told me about the one long male relationship he'd had and his many "tricks." "But I'm not interested in the gay life any longer," he said. "I got tired of the scene six months ago and had three casual affairs with women. I want a real relationship with a woman," he added, "but not because I want to settle down with a family."

I was dating several other men at the time. When one of them came down with crabs, I was beside myself and called Josh. "Can I come over? I want to talk to you about something."

Once at his apartment, I told him flat out.

Well," he said, "get some Quell and we'll wash. Let me know if it works." All matter of fact. His easygoing attitude about sex attracted me.

At this time, which was a period of experimentation for me, I was also having a relationship with a woman.

When I told Josh, he said, "Well, you know, honey, just because you have sex with a woman doesn't mean you're a lesbian. But if you are, you are. There's nothing you can do about it."

With that reassurance I got the feeling, "No matter what happens, I can talk to this man about it and gain some satisfaction."

This was very different from my first long-term relationship in college, who never let me rest if I did anything with another man. Without let up, he would keep insulting me to remind me of it.

One day Josh said, "I think we're seeing each other too much. Let's cut down to weekends and once during the week."

We followed this schedule until we had a little fight and he walked out. A day later at work he acted furious.

After everybody else went home, I said, "All right, now, what's this?"

"I'm mad at you, Barb, because I went out and tricked. Then I felt guilty for the first time in my life."

I looked at him. "You felt guilty? Why?" We were only dating. The relationship wasn't going to last.

"Because of you."

"Why me?"

"I don't know. I just did. Somehow you're to blame."

I laughed at this comment. Though it didn't make sense, I liked him enough to keep dating. We had fun and were comfortable together, yet he wasn't a man I could commit my life to.

I also kept watching for signs that he was gay. "When is he going to change back? Is he just running away from it like other men I know? But who would he be running from? His parents know. The gay group he's working for knows. Who else?"

For Josh, the issues were settled. No running away. No more questions. His seeking a woman wasn't an accident. One evening he asked, "How would you like to live with me, Barbara?"

"I'll have to think about it." I'd never lived with a man.

As I thought, what struck me the most about Josh was his comfort level with sex, perhaps stemming from having had sex with so many people. He was comfortable being naked and seeing me naked. No big deal.

After two weeks I said, "O.K., I want to live with you."

"Well, if your decision took this long, we shouldn't do it."

Several months later he said he wanted to move back to Chicago where he'd gone to graduate school and where my family lived.

"Well, I'm not ready to."

"O.K." he said.

While he made plans to move over the next year, our relationship continued. Then I got sick of my job. "Josh," I said one night, "I want to go to Chicago too."

"Fine," he said. "We'll move in together."

We arrived in Chicago with only the hope of finding jobs. Josh was hired right away by an architectural firm. It was harder for me to find a job in my field of sociology. Then through Josh's gay friends from prior political activities, we located an apartment in a four-unit building. Gay men occupied the others.

In the late seventies, a gay man living with a woman was enough to intimidate these men as well as his former gay friends. Their reaction to Josh in essence was, "What do we have to talk to you about?" Despite his many calls to them, none kept up the friendships. They didn't like to know about people like Josh, who had broken the unspoken rules. We weren't following the script.

In our new life together, Josh and I didn't talk about marriage but we did discuss children. "I'm too selfish to be a father," he said one day "I want to be free and independent."

Independence was a problem area for us. Josh had gone from living alone to living with someone else. I'd changed from living with three other people to living with only him. For me, the problem was that I was alone all day. When Josh came home I would lunge at him. But he needed space and time for himself.

In our second year in Chicago an agency job opened up for me. The personnel officer there suggested that I go to graduate school to be assured of continued employment through funded grants. About a week before Northwestern was due to send out letters of acceptance or rejection, my doctor told me I was pregnant.

Telling Josh that night, I said, "I just know it's going to be a girl, but I'm not sure I want to keep it." It was a big issue for me, a pro-choice person.

I thought about it for a long time, but not about the moral issue about whether or not to have a child. I wanted the baby, but not to carry it by myself. My question was, "Does Josh want to be a father?" If he didn't want to share parenting, I'd decide to have an abortion.

For days Josh thought about why he didn't want to be a father. After he thought, we talked and then he thought again and we talked some more. By the end of the month he said, "I'd like to be a father after all, Barb. I love you and we've been together almost two years."

Keeping the baby meant that marriage was a strong possibility. That raised the gay issue again in my consciousness. The question sent me to Gladys, a marriage counselor who'd been my mentor from college days.

After telling her the details, I asked, "So, what do you think? Should I marry the guy with his history?"

"Well," she said in her no-nonsense way, "if you're concerned about him cheating on you, straight men cheat on their wives too— fifty percent of them, one study shows. If it's a question of whether or not it will work, you can never can tell. The oddest people who shouldn't be together stay together. Relationships which seem made in heaven, aren't. Do you love him?"

"Yes."

"Do you get along with him?"

"Yes."

"Then go for it."

Yet the gay issue stayed in my mind. "How can he be gay and want to marry?" I kept asking myself. "If he does, can it work?"

I discussed each question with Josh, bringing his gayness back into his mind. One night while we did the dishes, I asked, "Don't you ever think about going out with men?"

"No. I don't want to."

"Why not?"

"It makes me feel too guilty, Barb. I'm with you. I'm in love with you. I'm involved with you."

I kept on reading all the books and research articles in the graduate school library, comparing that information to my experiences with Josh and wondering, "How can he be a legitimate gay man if he doesn't fit any of these things?"

One night I asked, "How come you don't go to the baths?"

"I don't want to go."

Another time I asked, "What do you fantasize about?"

"Barb," he said, "I really don't like being your guinea pig."

"I know. I'm sorry. I just want to sort it all out."

"Well, sometimes I fantasize about men and sometimes women."

Then rereading the books and articles, I'd think, "Wait! This doesn't apply to Josh." It got to the point where I asked myself, "Why am I plying this theme? Do I want him to go out to seek a relationship with a man just so he'll fit in with the scene? He's decided to live a straight life. What am I doing?"

That was the end of that, but the question of marriage remained. "The outside world won't consider our relationship valid, married or not," I told Josh one weekend. "It doesn't match their expectations about gay men. Also, the research says marriages between straight women and gay men are doomed to fail in several years."

At that time our sex wasn't as frequent as we wanted and sometimes our interest in making love didn't coincide any more. When I was interested during semester breaks, he wasn't. Other times when he was interested, I wasn't.

One day I suggested we both see Gladys about the gay-straight issue. "With her experience with couples, she might have some answers. Our sex life's been a bit unsettled lately anyway."

"Sure. Let's go."

Once we were in Gladys' office, I told her our concerns about getting married.

"Well, I can't help you with that, but let's work on the things I know," she said quietly, "the relationship issues." So we talked about Josh's wanting independence, my loneliness and our unsettled sex. Gladys pointed out how our different work schedules might be affecting our sexual drives. Then she said, "Barbara, your loneliness probably comes from your dependency on Josh, which in turn affects his need for independence."

That helped, but it didn't answer my questions. My girl friends couldn't answer them either. They knew less than I did about how gay-straight marriages work. So Josh and I talked again.

"I don't know, Barb. I love you. I want to be with you and marry you and don't want sex with men. That's all I can say. I can't give you any definitive answers to refute the research."

So simple and clear. Our relationship had internal validity regardless of outside standards. I knew it would be long-term too in view of Josh's long, monogamous relationship with his lover before. "That's his nature," I thought.

Our wedding was a small gathering. It including my parents, who didn't know about Josh's past lifestyle.

"Why must they know?" I commented. "It would only be a reason to object." Then I chuckled. "It would certainly shake them up!"

Once we were married, it suddenly hit me that Josh wasn't going to wake up some morning and say, "By the way, Barb, this has been fun, but I'm a homosexual. See you later." I was in the bedroom looking in the mirror at the time. I just sat there, brown eyes twinkling as I thought, "This is going to be an enduring relationship!"

Later that day I reflected, "Gayness is part of Josh, but it's part of his history. Right now he's heterosexual. His straight lifestyle is his identity. Just because I've had sex with two women," I smiled, "I don't perceive myself as lesbian."

That convinced me to stop prodding Josh about his gay lifestyle. Then I wondered, "Did my probing encourage him to act on what isn't his style anymore?"

Once Josh mentioned a married gay man that he'd met. "Do you know he has sex with boys, brings them home and has them there for breakfast with the wife and child?"

"Good Lord! That would go against my grain too much. He'd be out on his ear," I said.

"I couldn't tolerate it either," Josh said in his quiet way.

Rachel was born that spring. We found a house to rent in a working class neighborhood and began a new life. Josh helped take care of the baby along with housework and laundry, as he'd always done. If anything, he did more housekeeping than I did because he was the neat one. Comparing notes with my girl friends about who did domestic chores in their households, I saw we had more equality than any of them.

When Rachel was two I returned to graduate school. If anything can kill your sexual desire it's graduate work. Constantly exhausted and preoccupied, I sometimes found myself finishing a term paper in my head as we made love. "Now that paper on...if I just added a quotation from...." Afterward I felt horrible about it. Then there were the surprises when sex improved during semester breaks.

Other times Josh rebuffed me because he was tired. If this happened three times in a row, the gay issue popped up again in my head, "That's why he doesn't desire me any more."

Then I'd quickly ask, "Is it because you're homosexual?"

"Of course not." It wasn't his nature to question why he thought or did what he did.

Whatever Josh answered gave me more to think about. Then I talked with him some more and thought some more. It was tough exploring the gray areas in what seemed like a very black and white issue. Yet each time we did, we worked through our problems a little more and made further resolutions about our relationship.

Nobody else knew as much about us as we did. The support group I tried was of no help. Since most of the women had just found out that their husbands were gay, their issue was betrayal, which didn't apply to me. "They're angry too," I thought, "something I don't feel at all."

Josh was unhappy with his career at that time, while I was going through the ups and downs of graduate school. We were both taking care of Rachel and getting her to child care while working on housekeeping and cooking issues, as well as worrying about our sex life. For months there was never a stable period.

Every now and then on a Saturday night, I went out with my girl friends while Josh stayed with Rachel. He didn't like that much. Not that he wanted to go with me. He just wasn't having fun at the same time.

Then four years after we married, I dated another man. He was aggressive and married. One night as we kissed and embraced, I remarked, "Josh doesn't react to me this passionately!"

"I can't believe anybody wouldn't desire you the way I do," he said in his baritone voice.

Flattered as that made me feel, we didn't have intercourse. Back home as I lay in bed with Josh about to make love, guilt and thoughts of the other man's desire and his flattery obsessed me.

"Am I attracted to him because Josh isn't that passionate?" I wondered. "Does the fact that Josh doesn't act as delighted with me as this man mean that he's gay after all? If I had an affair, would that make Josh go out and have sex with other men?"

As old doubts were triggered, I sat up in bed and cried, "Josh, I can't make love till I tell you about tonight."

When I finished, Josh said, "I know the man and don't like the idea that you went out with him, Barb. Are you going to again?"

"Oh, no! I don't have any desire for him."

For two hours we talked it out, how I felt, how he felt and how an outside relationship couldn't be kept going without affecting ours.

By the time we finished talking, I thought, "Why would I pursue a relationship with this other man when I have intimacy with Josh? If his wife had done what I did, he wouldn't have dealt with it as casually as Josh did. What I have here is more precious than sex with that man. Here's trust, perhaps more so than in any straight relationship I know."

Yet the gay issue lurked below the surface. Whenever anything went wrong in our lovemaking, it was so easy to say, "See, it's him!" It became a defense by making Josh the issue rather than the relationship.

Occasionally I compared married sex to my fervent experiences as a single woman. The contrast was hard to accept until I remembered that I had been in my twenties, without a child or the responsibilities of married life. "Besides," I thought, "I don't masturbate that often anymore either."

Over the next two years, Rachel started school, I finished my doctorate and Josh developed his own architectural project which he pursued more aggressively than anything before. Sex remained an important part of our life, something neither of us could live without.

Gradually the challenge became, "How intimate can I get with Josh?" It's much more difficult to have both an emotional and an erotic relationship than it is to have just casual intercourse. Since I had experienced both, there was no need to see if sex might be different elsewhere.

"I want to be the one bringing my husband to orgasm," I said to myself one night. "I want him to think about me when he thinks about sex because I'm the one who can please him. If he slept with a walrus," I thought, grinning, "I'd be jealous because he'd be reaching heights of intimacy without me."

It took a while for us to write this script for ourselves. We've survived seven years of marriage by tolerating the ambivalence of what we are and the uncertainty of what could happen. It has always come back to our ability to communicate expectations and what our relationship means to us. When I have doubts or fears, I just tell Josh with no assumptions, no judgments, only the belief that he'll help. In turn, he has become less shy about sharing his fears and thoughts.

If Josh came to me now and said, "I've decided I want to have sex with a man," would that mean the end of the relationship? No. In addition to a nice life and all of the reasons anyone would stay in a marriage, I love him. He's the one I like to be with and want to be married to. Besides, I don't think that sex with a man would be a meaningful emotional experience for him now.

If Josh decides some day that he doesn't want to be married, would I say that I made a foolish error? No. We have a life together. He's the father of my child. My time with him is now.

❦   ❦   ❦   ❦   ❦

Two years later Josh and Barbara decided that they wanted a second child and Barbara began to study Josh's religion, Judaism, to provide deeper roots for her family.

Coming of Age
Kirstin

Friends called us a "storybook family." Living in our old-fashioned house outside of Houston, Paul and I and our children, Karl and Heidi, did everything together, home projects, city explorations, weekend excursions and vacations.

Paul and I met at a party in the fifties. When a friend introduced me to this chestnut-haired man, his lively conversation impressed me. He was thirty, four years older than I, and he'd just moved to Houston to work for the state. I'd left Minneapolis several years before to be an assistant editor in a publishing house.

Several weeks after the party, I called him on an impulse.

"I remember you," he said. "How about meeting for a drink?"

Our drink extended to dinner and an evening of intense conversation and much laughter. From then on for two months, we saw each other as often as possible to picnic on the Gulf, dine and dance, go to films and galleries and hold deep discussions about many topics, especially our shared liberal political views. Yet coming from conservative families, we had an unspoken agreement to forego premarital sex.

Despite my sexual reserve, I was prone to outbursts of hugging and kissing, to which Paul, like previous boyfriends, responded in kind.

When my company transferred me back to Minneapolis, I thought constantly of Paul but heard nothing from him. After three months I began to date. That fall, two men proposed. One was a charming man with a history of depressions for which he'd been hospitalized. I told him, "No." Marriage alone was challenge enough without possible depressive behavior.

When my doctor friend proposed, I said, "Yes." He seemed perfect, intelligent, passionate, desirous of having many children, supportive of my career and part of a large circle of friends. But after one too many arguments with him over my belief in spiritual values, I broke the engagement.

"I love you," I said, "but marriage shouldn't start with disagreement on basics."

My mother, concerned that I wasn't married yet, suggested writing Paul about the breakup.

He telephoned at once. "I'd heard you were engaged, but I knew it wouldn't last," he said. "I knew you'd marry me."

"So how come you didn't write?"

"I thought you knew how I felt," he explained. "Anyway, let's pick up where we left off."

For months Paul courted me by letter and phone, sent tokens of his affection and then invited me to Houston for the Fourth of July weekend. When I saw him at the gate, his face hidden behind a bouquet of yellow chrysanthemums, I threw my arms around him saying, "Yes!"—without realizing he hadn't asked the question that was between the lines of his letters. "I mean," I stammered, nodding my blond head, "Of course I'll marry you."

The next three days together were nonstop activities, dancing, picnicking, going to galleries and walking everywhere. The few hours left of the last night were spent in his apartment rather than at my friend's place where I was staying. Exhausted, we slept side by side fully clothed. More ardor would have been welcome, but Paul's reserve was a relief. I was determined to wait for sex until marriage.

The wedding was in Minneapolis that winter in the church where I'd gone as a child. A church ceremony was important to me, symbolizing my belief that marriage was a spiritual as well as a physical commitment.

On our wedding night, undressing for bed, I was somewhat nervous until Paul said, "Come on in! The water's fine!"

Laughing, I slipped into bed with him and let myself go at last! It was wonderful being spontaneously responsive and expressive, skin touching skin. Making love was even more exciting.

Once in Houston again, I volunteered in community organizations and took some classes. At home Paul and I shared everything from his career problems to joint investment projects. We had luncheon dates, went to cultural events, partied with friends and travelled in the States and Latin America. Our friends were mostly my old friends, now married—his were still single—and new ones made through my volunteer work. As we circulated together at gatherings, Paul would say, "There's no one here as interesting as you."

After two years, my optimism about getting pregnant began to wane. We'd been trying from the start. My irregular periods didn't allow conception to be planned with any certainty despite faithful charting of my cycle. Then one day out of the blue, the doctor said I was two months pregnant.

After a shaky first trimester, I blossomed. "Oh, Paul!" I said one day with a radiant smile from the sensual pleasure I felt as the baby grew, "This is so great!"

Heidi was born in December. Nursing, not a common practice at the time, was a delight. As the baby grew, Paul and I kept exchanging astonished glances each time she did anything remarkable, like learning to sit up.

A year later we moved to the suburbs. When Heidi was three, I discovered to my surprise that I was pregnant again. Karl arrived that summer. For two more years, except for community work, motherly duties and pleasures absorbed my hours.

One night Paul said, "Why don't you go back to work, Kirstin? It's more rewarding, dear, than volunteer activities."

The publishing house rehired me for a different department. Whenever work made me late, Paul made dinner. Otherwise, while I cooked, he read to Heidi and Karl. On weekends we four went to parks, museums, the movies or our favorite corners of the city.

One night Paul brought up the idea of not having more children. "I don't have enough emotional energy," he said.

Never having thought of limiting our family, I spent weeks mulling over what that would mean. Our children gave me tremendous pleasure, yet Paul had a point.

"He's over forty and I'm in my late thirties," I thought. "We'll be in our fifties and sixties when any new children would be teenagers! Could we give them the same level of support we give these two?"

I finally agreed reluctantly. The next question was how to achieve our objective of no more children. Paul didn't approve of vasectomy and my doctor had cautioned me, "The birth-control pill or any mechanical or surgical contraceptive method is too risky for you, Kirstin."

After two other doctors confirmed his judgment, our old "taking my temperature" method seemed to be the only option.

When I told Paul, he said, "Charting didn't work when we were trying to have children. It won't be reliable to prevent it."

The ultimate choice therefore was either no sex or taking a chance on having more children.

Whether or not to stop our sex life during my childbearing years preoccupied me for weeks. "Paul shows his love in so many other ways!" I argued with myself. "He hugs and kisses me whenever I want. He's always saying how much he loves me and what a wonderful wife and mother I am. What would it be like without the most intimate aspect of marriage?"

I went back and forth in my mind with the problem. "I'd hate not having sex!" I told myself, thinking of our warm moments together. "But I don't want Paul to get angry if I get pregnant either. Besides it's only a postponement of pleasure till menopause." A Depression child, I knew how to "make do."

Eventually I agreed to give up sex in order not to have any more children. It was back to premarital days, waiting to make love again. Menopause became the light at the end of the tunnel.

Then I thought, "Paul will have a harder time with this since men have the more powerful sex drive. I don't want to tempt him any more than necessary." So I stopped wearing perfume to bed and rarely undressed in front of him.

For a number of years, Paul stayed as demonstrative as ever. We hugged and kissed every chance we got. In the meantime, art projects, guitar, tennis and my now full-time job diverted my sexual energy.

During this time Paul was promoted and the children did well in school. As our investments grew, we moved to a bigger house where we continued to entertain. Family trips took us to Latin America and we each travelled for our jobs. Paul seemed to thrive on travel, saying it made him feel like a different person, "almost flamboyant!" Our life was wonderful and friends accused me of wearing rose-colored glasses.

As Heidi entered her teenage years, a crack appeared in my rosy outlook. One vacation when I had to handle some business by phone, Paul said, "We might just as well have stayed home."

"Oh," I thought. "Doesn't he understand that work isn't on my mind except for this call that so much depends on?"

Several months after I stopped working during vacations, Paul said, "Kirstin, your job makes me jealous."

Even when I cut back overtime hours and forbade home calls from clients, something still felt amiss. Then as Heidi began coming home late and going to wild parties—no longer our exemplary daughter—Paul stopped doing chores around the house and suggested that we stop giving our annual fall party.

One Saturday as I was mending socks, Paul came into the bedroom. Startled to see this grim man seating himself on our lounge chair, I put down my darning to give him full attention.

"Kirstin," he said, his face colorless, "I've changed as much as I can. All I want now is peace."

My insides froze. "He wants a divorce!" flashed across my mind. Suspecting that he was referring to the family stress that Heidi's new behavior had caused, I thought, "This is another of his one-liners, said after exhausting all other solutions. It sounds like an ultimatum."

After a minute I said, "All right, Paul. I'll take care of keeping the peace."

From then on the children's problems and disruptive behavior became my concern. Karl, who was entering his preadolescent identity struggle, contributed to family changes as his grades began to fall. Week after week I resolved potential catastrophes before they reached Paul's notice. Playing the go-between, I explained the children's moods to him and Paul's needs to them, hoping that their mutual understanding might lend some peace to the household.

Then all of a sudden, anger seemed to be brewing just below Paul's control. I heard him shout angrily at others in business dealings and I didn't want the children or me to be his target. Once, trying to diffuse his potential fury after Karl had done something annoying, I said, "Karl's just trying to figure out who he is, Paul. It's typical. He'll grow out of this phase."

"You sound like a tigress protecting her young!" Paul snapped at me. He no longer said, "You're such a wonderful mother."

Before long there were no more surprise gifts, no more luncheon dates and only a rare "I love you!" My emotions were called superficial. When Paul began to eat dinner before I came home, many of my evenings were spent alone in front of the television experiencing unexpected bursts of pleasure from paltry love scenes.

I kept checking with my doctor, knowing that some women in their late forties get pregnant when they think childbearing is over. When he finally said, "No way can you can get pregnant now," I could hardly wait to tell Paul. Sex at last!

When Paul heard the news, he looked across the table at me and shook his head. "I don't think I can," he said.

I was speechless. Days passed before his statement sank in. Eventually I decided, "If he can't or thinks he can't, then he can't. It would be fruitless to try to persuade him."

When I confided what had happened to a professional friend one day, she said, "Well, take a lover."

"Oh, no!" I said. "I'm not about to commit adultery!"

Over the next months the friendly hugs of male friends and colleagues sustained me, though they were unaware of how much their male responses meant to me.

A year or so later, browsing in a city gallery, I came upon etchings from Picasso's *Erotica*. I returned again and again to see them, so often that a curator approached me one afternoon convinced that I was a serious buyer.

Heidi was off at college by then and Karl was struggling through his junior year of high school. That spring, one Saturday after our twenty-first anniversary, Paul and I were lingering with our wine after lunch. For a brief moment his green eyes twinkled, a look which, though rare now, always prompted a surge of love. As I rushed to hug him, he turned away as he'd done for some time.

"Paul, why do you duck when I kiss you?"

His answer came quickly. "Oh," he said in a calm tone, "I'm not into marriage any longer."

At that my world fell apart. All the negatives of the preceding three years tumbled into my lap. Since Paul never wasted words, I knew the truth was out there on the table and I'd have to deal with it.

As we talked into the late afternoon, I cried often into my wine, which I kept replenishing. At one point I said, "I'd like more affection, something physical between us."

"There are other couples our age who don't have sex," Paul replied. "It isn't unusual."

"But, we're not 'other couples'!" I said and then asked, "Am I a burden to you, Paul? Do I keep you from expanding?"

"No." After a pause he asked, "Do you want a divorce?"

"We can't decide that now. That takes time."

As I arose, weak and nauseous, Paul came over, arms outstretched to embrace me. "Kirstin, you're still the most wonderful person I've ever known," he said, holding me. "I'm just complicated." Then he went upstairs.

I stood there dumbstruck and confused. Here was my husband no longer "into" marriage, yet saying that I was still the most wonderful person in the world. He'd just mentioned divorce and then hugged me as never before. I was too exhausted to figure out what had happened or what it meant. It took another three years to do so.

Over the next few weeks, I took down all photographs of myself from the family room, put away mementos of our trips and slept as far over on my side of the bed as I could.

Next I invited old friends to lunch or for a glass of wine after work, both women and men. Many I hadn't seen for years. I needed them to affirm me, whoever I was. I no longer knew.

Both at home and while commuting to work, I reviewed the preceding twenty-one years to see what I'd done to make Paul feel he was out of the marriage. Wine became a way to relieve tension and deaden sensitivity. With a glass by my side, whether I was in the kitchen or in hotel lounges after meetings, I jotted down all aspects of our marriage and ways to improve our relationship. To understand why I'd married Paul, I listed his best qualities. To figure out who I was, I listed my strengths and failings, likes and dislikes, as well as goals.

Reading books on psychology and marriage, often devoured on the run in city or airport bookstores, my goals shifted from trying to prove I was right to trying to work it out.

After six months of this turmoil, I was down to ninety-two pounds, "looking like an old lady of 110!" a friend said later. I couldn't talk to friends without bursting into tears.

One friend insisted that I see her therapist, Frances. At the end of the first session in which I did all of the talking, Frances commented, "You're an articulate, intelligent professional, but you don't seem to have any idea of what your feelings are."

For months Frances listened and clarified, helping me identify my feelings. At home I tried out the new skills I'd learned from her. One Saturday morning as I was about to drive Karl to some project he was starting, Paul said, "Let him take the bus. You spoil him!"

"That hurts, Paul!" I said and as he kept implying that I was a bad parent, I repeated it over and over.

"But I'm right, aren't I? That isn't the thing to do."

"That's not the point," I insisted. "What you said hurts."

Later that month Paul tripped on an oriental rug in the hall. Running out from the kitchen, I found him sprawled on the floor and took him in my arms for the first time in years. When he came to, he pushed me aside and stumbled away. I didn't move from where he left me, unable to express so deep a hurt.

Then I discovered *Love is Letting Go of Fear*, by Gerald Jampolsky. "Aha!" I thought, reading it, "Personal attacks are signs of the attacker's inner pain, not an actual assault."

Trying to figure out what was bothering him, I asked Paul one night, "What are your plans when you stop working?"

"To find happiness. I didn't find it in marriage or the family."

I gasped silently. "But Paul," I continued, remembering Jampolsky's theory, "you're not going to find happiness outside of yourself. It's *within you*."

That fall Paul took a leave of absence and began to explore sports activities he'd missed as a boy. Then a freak accident to his lower back made him stop all of them. Five different specialists, varied exercises, exotic medicines and a cumbersome brace did not ease the pain.

Each night when I came home, he was bundled up in a wool jacket reading in his den. Before eating my dinner, I played the therapist, listening hard to discover a clue to his misery. Night after night he aged before my eyes.

Like a yo-yo, I alternated between being my spontaneous self, who wanted to share my natural euphoria with Paul, and being a submissive woman who expected to be rejected. Holding myself back to avoid rejection made me feel deprived. But if my *joie de vivre* bubbled over, it turned to pain when he didn't respond.

Trying to get through to him, I used his favorite perfume once again and wore sexy clothes around the house. While he read in the bedroom, I undressed in front of him. He never noticed.

As the aura of rejection pervaded the house, I realized that the Kirstin whom Paul had chosen to marry had disappeared under layers of accommodation. "Is there anything left to change?" I thought.

To keep my sanity, I played my guitar, worked in the garden and bought a bound journal for composing my thoughts. Reading it regularly like a book, I saw that my feelings were beginning to focus on what I wanted rather than on what I didn't have.

One night after musing about how much happier he was before marriage, Paul commented, "I feel imprisoned by responsibility."

All of a sudden a way to free him flashed in my head. "Why not take a trip, Paul?" I suggested, remembering how he thrived on travel. "Stay as long as you want. We'll be here when you get back." My thought was, "He'll come home his ebullient self. We'll have fun again and stay together as a family."

That weekend Paul said, "All right, Kirstin. I'll leave. But I'll wait till Karl takes off for college."

"I didn't say 'Leave'!" I shouted in alarm.

When my emotions settled down, I wrote Paul a note explaining that a trip would be a chance for him to be happy. To make sure my words wouldn't be twisted again, I added, "Whatever you decide, do it on the basis of what you want for yourself not on what you think I want."

Nothing more was said on either side.

For the next three months, I went on with work and family life like a perfect wife, ignoring the possibility that Paul would actually leave. I tried to be the perfect parent too, telling Paul and the children to work out their persistent animosity themselves. "I'm not going to be the go-between any longer," I told each of them.

One day after Paul had ignored Heidi when she came home from college, making her cry bitterly, I decided that he had to know that she felt hurt. As we talked about it, remembering his negative feelings toward his mother, I said, "You know, I think you hate women!"

Paul said nothing.

Our twenty-third anniversary came the next week. After thanking me in the morning for the hanging I'd made for his den, Paul didn't mention the anniversary again.

That night I thought, "I can't take this slap in the face silently, even if speaking up means the end of the marriage."

The next night I forced myself to enter the den where Paul was writing letters. "Paul, I want to talk about something."

Sitting down, I began what I'd rehearsed all day. "I noticed you didn't say anything about our anniversary yesterday other than 'Thank you.' "

"Why celebrate a marriage that doesn't exist?"

"Oh!" I said, startled. For several moments I said nothing, formulating what I needed to express out of my pain of the preceding five years. "Well," I continued in a quiet voice, "I can't go on any longer without any emotional or physical interaction."

Another long pause.

"I'll be moving out," Paul finally said.

"I could go back to the city," I said. "I wouldn't mind."

"No, the husband always moves."

We stayed where we were in silence for several minutes as twilight darkened the room. Even now I can see Paul sitting in the shadows, motionless. He didn't say that he'd try to be more responsive. I didn't say, "Don't go." In that silence the final decision was made.

In the emotional vacuum of the next few months, Paul and I play-acted at being married. I hated it and didn't want to feel that hatred. It wasn't part of the Kirstin I knew.

While I was deciding when we'd discuss how to tell the children he was leaving, Paul told Karl who told Heidi. Home for mid-semester break, she came to me very upset. "Why didn't you tell me? Is it because of me?"

"Of course it isn't because of you!" I said, putting my arms around her. "It's a matter between Dad and me." I didn't tell her I was flabbergasted that for the first time, Paul and I hadn't jointly decided a family affair.

Paul moved out in June. As I left for work I kissed him good-bye, saying, "I hope you find the happiness you want." Then I went out to the car knowing that he and whatever furniture he'd chosen would be gone when I returned that evening.

There was a sense of peace without Paul in the house that night. There was also a sense of new life which contrasted with the morgue-like emptiness that had pervaded the house when he had been there. Over the following weeks, I opened the blinds to the trees and blue sky, put a bright-colored comforter on the bed and bought more lamps. The photographs of me went back into the family room.

For the next five months, Paul and I did things together in Houston, often at his apartment complex where he introduced me as his wife. Although he no longer wore his wedding ring, I still wore mine.

"He looks so much happier and younger!" I told a friend one evening. "His pain has disappeared!"

"Kirstin," she asked, "Why are you doing so much with Paul? What about your own life?"

Realizing that my involvement with him used up time I should be spending on my life, I took Paul out to lunch at our favorite spot the following Sunday to suggest that we see less of each other.

Tears ran down his cheeks. "You mean you're going to take away my best friend on top of making me leave!"

I couldn't believe my ears. "That's not true," I said. "I didn't make you leave. I suggested that you take a trip."

Then the conversation somehow turned to the end of our sex life years before. "Oh," Paul said, "I suggested it because you were frigid."

"Frigid!" I exploded. "You said it was because you didn't want any more children. You mean you covered up your real reason?" Clear white anger filled my being. I was ready to scream, to throttle him in front of the other patrons.

He continued, "I didn't know what else to do and you didn't like sex anyway."

"I loved sex! Why didn't you check it out with me?"

I was seething that he had deceived me about a major decision in my life. Not wanting to make a scene in public, I called for the check and invited myself back to his apartment.

For five hours I screamed and yelled. "How dare you assume what I think? What else have you assumed? What else haven't you checked out with me? I feel so betrayed!"...and on and on.

As my fury abated I said, "Intimacy meant so much to me! I looked forward so much to having sex again."

"I don't know, Kirstin," Paul said. "Maybe I just burned out. I did all I could."

Then I described my deep sexual feelings and how men had found me sexually attractive over the years, although nothing had ever come of it.

"They didn't have to live with you," Paul replied.

I couldn't take any more. Driving home, my anger spent, I wondered what Paul thought of my outburst. Shortly before we separated he'd said, "Kirstin, it's so frustrating the way you don't ever get angry!"

The impact of the episode diminished over the months as I struggled to survive each day and keep family communication going. I was waffling between hating Paul's behavior and wanting to save our marriage. Then Paul had minor surgery. The day after the operation, I visited him in the hospital with some investment papers to be signed, a bouquet of flowers and a bottle of wine.

He was sitting up in a chair, dressed in his lounging robe and still under medication. Once the papers were signed, we chatted about mutual friends as he drank a soft drink and I some wine.

After half an hour he said, "I've got something to tell you."

"I think I know what it is," I murmured without thinking, somehow wanting to make it easier for him to tell me whatever it was and to prepare myself for something I suspected he might say. A hunch about his lack of responsiveness had floated briefly across my mind a year before we separated.

"You do?"

I nodded.

"I'm gay!"

I smiled slightly.

"How did you know?"

"I didn't, really," I said. "But as you became more withdrawn and unhappy and didn't respond to my wiles, it seemed possible that you might be a latent homosexual and not know it."

It was more than that. For an hour Paul described his first explosive homosexual experience before he'd met me, his lover before our marriage and his gay lifestyle since our separation. "I was never active," he reassured me, "while we lived together."

As Paul recounted each detail, his medication acting like truth serum, his words transported me into an unreal world. At times we both broke into laughter, saying, "It's better than a soap opera!"

Astonished at the revealed chapters of his life, I thought, "This is the man I lived with for over twenty-three years, the man I tried to re-attract for so long!"

"My love for you was so strong," Paul went on, "that I thought that although it wouldn't change me, it would overpower the homosexual drive. I often wanted to be killed in a crash so I'd never have to tell you."

I sat mesmerized. "This man sitting here, presumably my husband but now a stranger, held this secret inside him all this time, a secret which profoundly affected me," I thought. "He's still the same person I laugh and talk with, but in a new body unknown to me, in a world completely separate from mine."

At the same time I felt a new closeness to Paul since I now shared his secret self. All of him was available to me for the first time. "Here's the vibrant man I married," I thought, "plus a new joy of his own that is no longer repressed."

Sitting in shock, I seemed to be acting out a part someone else had written for this ludicrous scene, Paul in his robe and me in my tailored dress, the sterile hospital room serving as backdrop for the climactic moment.

That night I wrote in my journal:

All has fallen into place. Now I must absorb this new side of him, though he's still the same Paul. But my struggle is over. So is my slim hope that we could reunite. Yet who knows? I can't give us up especially since he's more expressive now.

My struggle was nowhere near over. I didn't give up hope for over a year. It took fifteen months to admit that there was a wall between us, impossible to penetrate, to scale or to break.

The morning after Paul told me the truth, I went off to work carrying his secret which I'd agreed not to tell to our mutual friends. Since my close colleague didn't fit that category, I told her.

"So what else is new?" she said.

I gulped.

"My husband picked it up when they met that one time."

Her words made me blush. I felt foolish that her husband, a stranger, had figured it out while I hadn't.

For weeks my emotions contradicted one another as I immersed myself in Paul's new life and went on with my own. From moment to moment, I felt relieved or sad, happy or hurt, amazed or angry.

Tremendous relief came from knowing the real reason why Paul had changed so drastically during our last years together. "Now I have the key to what locked him away from me," I thought. "It wasn't anything I or the children did or didn't do."

When I told Frances that Paul had come out, I smiled wistfully at having continued to try to attract him and sighed, "How ironic!"

"Poignant," she said.

"Well, it certainly explains why he found me frigid."

I was also deeply sad about how Paul had suffered from hiding his gayness. "It nearly crucified me, Kirstin," he commented a few days after he came out.

Then I read *Now That You Know*, written by parents of gays and lesbians, which made me view Paul as a parent might. My sorrow about his prior suffering turned to joy that, "complete" at last, he could be who he really was and express his true nature.

Reading everything available on married gay men, I became an instant expert. As the bias of other people's opinions became more evident, I decided it was more reliable and more fun to do things with Paul in his gay world and find out for myself what gay men were like.

Paul was eager to have me meet his friends. "After all," he chuckled, "you like men."

His friends were of all ages and physiques, some previously married, others single, some with their lovers. They included a travel agent, a computer programmer, an architect, an investment broker, a former athlete, an ex-priest. Some were attractive, some not. They were open, sensitive and knowledgeable in many areas.

In contrast to the last cold years Paul and I had lived together, he was now openly affectionate with me.

"Why couldn't you have just hugged and kissed me like this?" I asked him one evening. "That would have been enough."

"It would have been misleading."

"No it wouldn't," I thought. "We could have set limits."

Sometimes we went out with his preferred friend at the time. Walking down the street between two handsome, attentive men, I fantasized about the three of us living together.

Despite such delightful times with the revived Paul and his friends, I felt empty and alone once I returned home. I was "in the closet" now, forced by Paul's secret to deal with my sorrow without support from friends who had helped me before.

Fortunately I had a network of professional friends across the country. On my first business trip after Paul told me his secret, I dragged my closest colleague to a private spot on the conference grounds. As I told her, deep sobs shook my body. For the first time I felt like the victim of a long cruel plot.

When I mentioned my fantasy of a *menage à trois* with Paul and his friend, she queried, "How would you like to have Paul making love with a man upstairs in your house?"

"Oh-h-h," I groaned, "I hadn't thought of that."

Back in Houston the negative aspects of a threesome were forgotten as I continued to search for a way to live happily ever after with Paul. "What about a *menage à trois*?" I asked him.

"No," he said emphatically, "I'm too monogamous."

That night I wrote in my journal, "Literal monogamy is more important to him than acting like a real monogamous husband who cherishes his wife."

The next day I thought, "But I'm no longer his real wife!" Off went my wedding band for good.

Soon I noticed that each time we dined in a gay restaurant, Paul would look around to spot attractive men —he who had always found me the most interesting person in a room. Besides feeling horribly insulted, I felt defeated. "By competing with these strangers for his sexual attention, I'm the loser," I thought. "With women I'd have a fighting chance."

It also hurt to see Paul glow when he looked at gay friends. To watch him embrace them with obvious pleasure became torture even though I knew it was important for gays, as "misunderstood people," to demonstrate mutual support.

Yet he kept embracing me, too. One night I wrote:

Irony! He wants to kiss, hug, express love for me as a 'total person' but not as a man to woman. And I can't respond to him sexually, knowing it can't be consummated. I yearn for a man who loves me as a woman.

A few months later I realized that Paul's world was as separate from me as mine was from him. "He's in good company," I thought, "but it's a dead end for me in the romance department."

Yet I couldn't envision life without Paul. It would have no meaning. Even as the reality of his gayness poked holes in my fantasy of living happily ever after, I wondered, "Could we resurrect our marital bond as it was, outside of his gay world?" The idea went in and out of my journal ad nauseam.

He acts so much like the man I first fell in love with, the person who was lost for so long!

Then a few days later I wrote, "I have to remind myself of how awful it was before he came out, when he was miserable in his prison."

Paul didn't remember his withdrawn state before he'd come out. "Everything was fine," he said one day. "I could have gone on forever like that. You're the one who broke the marriage vows."

I broke the marriage vows? My rage boiled up. "What vows?" I thought, feeling too weak to confront him directly. "Vows not to have sex? By imprisoning himself from men, he'd locked me out too. Didn't that break the vows?"

For months when least expected, Paul made digs at me mid-conversation. One night he said, "You made me go out into the world I didn't want."

Anger rose up the back of my neck. "Now he's blaming me for living a gay lifestyle," I thought bitterly. Taking a deep breath, I repeated what I'd said so often. "I didn't make you go. I suggested that you take a trip."

Eventually I blotted out Paul's accusations, thinking, "How pained he must still feel to be doing this!"

By this time I'd started to go to a spouses of gays support group suggested by Paul. Most of the other women were attractive and articulate, between twenty-five to fifty years old and still lived with their husbands. They were models of how we too might work it out. They also helped me face my growing awareness of hurt and anger.

When they heard how Paul had said that I'd made him leave, one woman made a fist, shouting, "I'd like to sock him in the nose!"

Then the group leader said, "People with low self-esteem tend not to own up to what they've done. Instead they blame others."

"Aha!" I thought. "Another reason for Paul's blaming!"

Spurred on by my reading and my support group, I finally asked Paul directly if he thought we could get back together.

He shook his head. "No, I'd probably end up the same way as before."

That was when I saw the bittersweet paradox: his coming out released the man I wanted to find again but made him unavailable as a husband. With that loss of hope came great sorrow.

There was also deep anger. Most of my rage had been spent over Paul's accusation that I was frigid, the unspoken reason why he'd suggested we end our sex life. My anger now was at another level. Out there in the world were gay men for me and other women to fall in love with unknowingly and with expectations that could never be met.

Yet I still felt compassion for the agony Paul had felt from repressing his homosexuality in order to live in a society which said he didn't belong if he were gay.

"It's tragic!" I said to a former colleague. "Paul believed he'd find happiness by doing 'the right thing.'"

She nodded. "Yes, I've seen you support people at work like this, people who have hurt you gravely. It's a bit unreal, you know."

Many friends felt uncomfortable with my compassion as if it invalidated their anger. Some of them had figured out what had happened. Others I'd told after Paul had come out publicly. Several pressed me, hoping to rouse some rage.

"Of course I'm angry at what Paul did," I explained, "but not at him! He thought that he was making the right decision in marrying me. I resent not being part of a decision which determined my life for twenty-four years and I'm furious at being deprived of sex for so long. But he didn't hurt me on purpose. His own pain blinded him to mine."

That fall I went to Brazil for a conference and decided to stay longer. Sitting on the beach or in cafés, reminiscing about visits there with Paul, I began to wonder what I could have done differently so that things wouldn't have turned out as they did.

Gradually my sanity seemed to slip away. I couldn't buy a railway ticket without anxiety. Finally solace came in old churches, where their coolness refreshed me in the heat of Rio. As I prayed I felt that God understood what was going on in my life. I wasn't absolutely alone. I wasn't crazy.

Back home I reflected in my journal:

> I cry easily and can't rejoice about my superb vacation. Aloneness is so overpowering that I can't be assertive. I don't care about anything enough to have a preference. I'm stuck in a place I thought I'd left behind. My past is a distant motion picture. I feel empty, a non-woman. Can I resume response to anyone?

A year after Paul had come out, I finally said to myself, "Cut the shackles. Stop using your energy on the relationship." Yet I clung to it as a drowning person grabs a splinter to keep afloat.

Then one day I realized, "Paul is having his cake and eating it too. I have neither a sex life nor him as a husband."

Something had to be done, but I was too weak to do anything beyond surviving in my hectic work schedule. One morning, weeping, I telephoned an old friend in Minneapolis. "My dream is dead," I mourned, seeking sympathy.

"Well, create another!" he replied simply and sharply.

There it was. It was pointless to think any more about whether or not I'd failed in my marriage or given up the fight to save it. It was time to work on a new life. Known for creative problem-solving, I knew I could do it.

Yet starting a new dream required many risks for a woman in her mid-fifties. Although half our assets and my salary would provide enough financial support, could lost time be made up by forming relationships with straight men? I prayed for insight to figure out what to do and the courage to do it.

It was clear that only divorce would reflect the reality of our relationship. It was a matter of integrity. The following Saturday I told Paul my decision.

Once I had decided, the need to "get on with it" drove me forward. Friends encouraged me, saying, "Leave Paul to his life and start the rest of yours." Yet cutting our bond was hard.

> I don't like the tension that accompanies the drive toward the divorce. This isn't Kirstin, the person who cares and listens and reflects. Will I surrender to the uncried tears, the unscreamed anger, the stiffened muscles, the barren heart?

Breaking what was by now a twenty-five-year habit, I no longer referred to "us." Paul was no longer "my husband." I called him less often and turned down joint activities that I'd have enjoyed. When he brought up gay topics, I changed the subject.

Then Paul began to give me surprise presents as he had early on in our marriage. They didn't dissuade me from moving on. "Doors are ajar," I wrote. "I have the choice to close them."

In May I saw a divorce lawyer although Paul and I planned to work out our own terms. Propelled by a sense of adventure, I travelled more in my job, changed my hairstyle, bought some new clothes, negotiated with Paul and went out with male friends.

Soon I realized that my men friends weren't romantic prospects. "I've got to do something to find real dates," I decided. "Men aren't going to come looking for me."

After finding no prospects in the several night classes I was taking or the political group I'd joined, I placed a "personal" ad in a metropolitan weekly. This and later ads opened up a treasure chest of men of all ages, occupations and objectives for this inexperienced, fifty-five-year-old woman.

One of the first persons to answer was a younger man, an artist and ex-military psychiatric social worker. His invitation to make love a few weekends after we met startled and scared me.

"Give me a minute to think about it," I said. In that minute I said to myself, "Kirstin, if you don't do it now, you never will. You'll always have an excuse."

I said, "Why not?" Holding my breath, I led the way to the bedroom with an armful of candles he had me gather. After lighting them all and placing them around the room, we proceeded to make love.

Gently and patiently he introduced me step by step to basic sexual experiences to arouse me. "You're like a seventeen-year-old virgin," he whispered with a smile.

I smiled too, thinking, "I'm not frigid at all. Inexperienced, yes, but clearly responsive."

On the second evening at my house, he remarked, "You're so playful and giving!"

Astounded to find out that partners need to help each other in order for lovemaking to give pleasure to both, I saw how my ignorance and Paul's silence had worked together to deprive me.

That concern went out the window in my delight with my lover-teacher-healer, who introduced me to a realm I hadn't known. Then he left for Mexico to paint for an unspecified time.

I contacted Frances, my counselor, to help me handle the turbulent feelings unleashed with my sexuality. My opening-up revealed the weak, vulnerable faults that I'd carefully controlled over the years in order to be "perfect" and avoid criticism, my own as well as others', especially Paul's. A whole, imperfect Kirstin faced me for the first time. I didn't want to see her.

Listening to my sobs alternated with laughter, Frances said quietly, "You're experiencing a rebirth of Kirstin!"

As I talked with her over the next weeks, I remembered the waves of attraction I'd felt toward Paul, but no particular passion from him toward me. "I never felt desired as a woman with Paul," I said with some bitterness. "I never heard 'I love your body.' "

Before long a sense of betrayal inflamed me. "My God! My sexuality was sacrificed for Paul's secret!" I told a friend.

A broken wrist and sprained knee indicated that I should slow down and use my limited strength wisely. Something had to be done about the scraps of the old dream which kept floating in and out of my consciousness and distracting me from my resolve.

I must use all available energies to get on with my own life and to become the person I'm supposed to be. It's self-defeating to spend it on a story that's over.

Soon after my home reflected a new lightheartedness as I entertained more and rediscovered the nesting instinct, adding pillows, an easy chair, more lamps and plants. Karl and Heidi remarked on my new strength. At work I held my own in a beleaguered situation. New men came and went, some from ads, others from organizations I joined. I took an AIDS test to allay any fears men might have, even though there was no possibility I'd been infected. I expected the new men to take AIDS tests also, to protect us both. I was on my own, not having sought Frances' counsel for some time.

That fall I planned a two-day "transition" rite. It was to take place at an inn on the Gulf, where I'd sit before a fire all night to let thoughts and emotions freely flow to create a new perception of me and my life and to leave the old one in the ashes.

Instead the ritual took place in a hospital, where I was taken with a severe case of pneumonia brought on by exhaustion. During the months of recovery at home, I read voraciously. Several men I'd dated had introduced me to writers of non-Western spiritual philosophies I didn't know, like Hesse and Gurdjieff. These readings led to others, rekindling a dormant interest in the spiritual realm.

As I was unable to work, I had hours to reflect upon and incorporate many of these ideas into my view of life. By the time I returned to my job, part time, "living" and "loving" meant something broader and deeper than achievement and romance. A new Kirstin had been molded, no longer connected with Paul.

When the divorce became final that summer, I didn't cry much although I wrote in my journal, "I'm sad that my former life is over."

A year later, the family gathered for Christmas as usual—Paul from the city and Heidi and Karl from inland towns where they worked and lived. After gift-opening, we laughed over family stories as we enjoyed a leisurely feast in the house we'd once shared.

As Paul left he hugged me, saying, "The children become nicer every year. You were a wonderful mother!" We had come full circle to years before as if nothing had happened in between.

I responded to his embrace as a "family" gesture, not a sexual experience. Only the bonds of shared history and parenthood remained for me. The passage of time had created a healing distance from the hurt and left but a sad reflection of what we'd endured.

While I was still anxious that too much time had been lost in my sexual life for any straight male to want me as a lifelong mate, a new bond was developing with a caring, accepting, spiritual lover who made me feel fulfilled as a complete woman, faults and all.

That Christmas night, I wrote in my journal:

Whatever uncertainties of life lie ahead for me in the New Year, I feel confident that I can meet and overcome any obstacle or challenge in my path.

In my fifty-seventh year I had come of age.

Creating a New Belief System

Breaking loose from timeworn patterns to form a new life is the final hurdle for the straight spouse. Shattered beliefs and assumptions must be incorporated into a new belief system. Then spouses can move forward into what is for many the most rewarding period of their lives, with or without their partners.

Examples of such transformations appear throughout this book: Jane regained her womanhood and entered the ministry; Siri asserted herself to create a new marriage form with Jerry; Grant became an active, caring father for Heather; Wes worked through his homophobia and found he still loved Milly as a friend and co-parent; and Kirstin fulfilled her potential sexually, psychologically and spiritually.

Dramatic and profound change cannot be realized through impulsive decisions made out of shock or anger felt in the early months. True transformation comes only after all issues have been resolved: damaged sexuality, altered relationship, conflicting parental-spousal concerns, destroyed identity, confused morality and fragmented belief system.

Once autonomy and integrity have been restored a sense of restlessness or dissatisfaction often begins the spouse's transformation. Almost overnight there is a subtle shift in how everything is viewed—partner or ex-partner, family, job, present circumstances. Reality no longer seems so fearsome or overwhelming. Threats to autonomy can be countered. The spouse no longer feels so vulnerable to other people's actions.

While natural regeneration and the passage of time assist the process of change, there also needs to be an explicit affirmation on the part of the spouse that change is possible. Yet for the spouse whose former beliefs lie in fragments, the mere thought of moving into a new realm can be terrifying.

Many spouses have overcome such fear to create a new life. Through willpower, inner work, persistence and sometimes prayer, they have broken the bonds to their past to effect change. Seven strategies enable transformation to occur.

- Letting go of the past
- Learning to forgive
- Coming to terms with loss
- Reformulating a philosophy of life
- Reestablishing a belief system
- Creating a new dream
- Taking the first step as a new person

The more focused the process of transformation is, the more assured the progress will be. For this reason, it is vital to have a confidante, professional counselor or journal for reflecting upon the journey.

Letting Go of the Past

Before change can begin, the spouse needs to clear away any leftover feelings that could impede growth. If any denial of pain, dependency, residual anger or self-pity remains, chances for a breakthrough are diminished. Feelings of insecurity, such as "You can't do it. You'll fail again" need to be left behind. Letting go of such impediments from the past is the first and possibly most difficult challenge of transformation.

Yet endings are part of the natural cycle of life. As William Bridges, Ph.D., explains, "New growth cannot take root on ground still covered with the old, and endings are the clearing process."[1] Yet just because something ceases to exist doesn't mean that it has ended. The spouse's shattered life cannot be resuscitated but it can be recast.

To do so requires a conscious decision to leave the painful past behind, but it can be and has been done.

It also takes time for spouses to break free from their former lives, which may or may not include their partners. Jim was prepared intellectually for Janie's coming out and consequent ending of the marriage. Yet until she actually did, he put off dealing with the emotional loss involved. When she finally came out, he broke into sobs. He then carefully organized equal parenting time and mediated Janie's public coming out. He didn't acknowledge the "end" of their life together until he remarried a few years later.

Although the passage of time weakens past ties, the deliberate act of cutting them, like pruning, hastens regrowth. Talking about what it meant to be the ex-spouse of a lesbian to high school students helped Jim give up the "wife" image of Janie and form a "family" connection with her.

It is common for spouses to hang onto the old relationship for months even if separated or divorced. Often a wife clings to her husband for security. Admitting that the bond has ended would mean being cut adrift. She may wonder, "What would I have left? What would give meaning to my life?" Kirstin, for instance, while knowing her storybook dream was dead, still couldn't cut the connection to Paul.

Then something happens to impel the spouse to finally break the ties. A friend may say out of exasperation, "It's over! Cut bait!" Or the partner may do something that excludes the spouse from his or her gay world. At that moment the ending is crystal clear. It can seem like awakening from a prolonged nightmare to find that one is really alive and the sun is out.

Learning to Forgive

Despite the sense of liberation the spouse feels, anger towards the partner may linger. Anger is as much a bond as love and must also be left behind. While it is a normal reaction, it can drag a person down in its whirlpool of negativity.

The most effective resolution of anger is forgiveness. This enables the spouse to switch roles from that of judge to disengaged observer. To forgive the partner for all of the pain suffered from the coming out is one of the hardest but most powerful turning points of the transformation process. The aim of this second task of establishing a new belief system is to replace emotional turmoil with peace of mind.

In this stage anger is often expressed as general negativity about the entire situation and the partner is cast in the role of "the enemy." Such an adversarial view is counterproductive. Angry thoughts reinforce the bond to the partner and limit the expression of more positive emotions, such as compassion, needed for transformation.

Perpetuating an adversarial relationship makes reconciliation increasingly difficult. After Patty heard that Frank had AIDS, in "I Love You, Jeff and Peggy" of Part Three, she telephoned him, whispering, "I wish I could be there to hold you." But by the next day her anger had resurfaced.

Persistent resentment may blind the spouse to aspects of the situation that could be changed for the better, such as her or his own fear, vindictiveness or dependency. Focusing on what can't be changed, such as the partner's new sexuality, goes against the guiding principles of the most effective recovery program.

Anger comes from judging the partner as uncaring, deceitful or hurtful because of the painful consequences of the coming out. Yet who has the right to judge another? Who knows the myraid motives of others? The complexity of the partner's motives cannot be reduced to one single reason. Many factors that even the partner may not be aware of operate in the coming-out process.

The act of forgiving the partner frees the spouse from judging and from feeling responsible for the partner's actions. Forgiveness allows the spouse to cease struggling to change the unchangeable. Forgiveness reopens the door to the partner's side of the closet. The spouse can then accept the partner as a fellow human rather than as the oppressor.

For forgiveness to be a sincere rather than a mechanical exercise, spouses need to consider all aspects of the harm they feel their partners have done, deliberate or not and then forgive them. Spouses may need to forgive themselves too for whatever role they may have played in the situation.

It isn't easy to surrender the false sense of power that comes from judging. Tremendous humility is needed to give up the right to "pardon." Remembering that the goal is peace of mind will lessen the urge to punish or get even.

Forgiveness may be done anywhere and in any way as long as there is sufficient time to do it. Walking in the park, sitting on the beach or lying in bed; anywhere is fine provided there are no distractions. It helps to write down what needs to be forgiven in a journal or talk with a close friend, counselor or spiritual advisor. By discussing forgiveness with someone else, troublesome feelings that arise, such as the natural urge to vindicate oneself, can be put into perspective.

The act of forgiving is simple. The spouse simply acknowledges what was done and then, no matter how horrendous or painful, lets go of it. While the statement of forgiveness may be made in any form, it needs to be deliberate, explicit and heartfelt. It doesn't even have to be said face-to-face to the partner. A simple, "I forgive him (or her) for what was done," will suffice. The sole aim is to accept and forgive.

Some spouses forgive through prayer, turning over painful memories to God or some other spiritual being to be healed.[2]

The rewards of forgiving compensate for the pain it evokes. A middle-aged professional in San Diego, for instance, guided through the forgiving process by her parish priest, remarked, "As I forgave Ron unconditionally, I was in tears, exhausted but cleansed."

Forgiving doesn't mean forgetting what happened nor the lessons learned from it. To maintain a sense of self and to revive purpose in life, it is critical to maintain continuity with the past. True forgiveness brings a balanced picture of the marriage into focus, which includes the partner's admirable qualities and happy times together.

Three years after Moira's story, "Brainwashed" in Part One was told, she was able to write, "The anger that engulfed me is no longer there. I am grateful for that new peace as I can now really enjoy family events with Tim. I realize that to get on with my life I have to release the past."

Coming to Terms with Loss

Cutting the last ties to the past causes a profound sense of loss. This act is the reprise of all the phases of the coming-out struggle. Though similar to the loss of a husband or wife by death or divorce, the loss felt by spouses of gay or lesbian partners is unique. Widows and widowers mourn grievously, but don't have the tangible presence of their partners to fan passion and remind them of their pain. Straight spouses often remain vulnerable to powerful feelings through continued contact with their partners, such as Jim who had to take Valium to cope when Janie moved in with him and his new wife. In contrast to divorced heterosexuals, where the possibility may exist of rekindling a sexual response from the ex-partner should they desire it, most straight spouses of gays and lesbians know that their sexual relationship with their partner is over forever.

This sense of loss is probably the most profound feeling of the coming-out crisis. Recently a multiracial group of wives and former wives, ranging in age from early twenties to late fifties and coping at different stages of recovery, all agreed that loss—whether of their partner, marriage, personal identity, or hope—was the cause of their greatest pain.

This overpowering grief can be turned around by viewing the loss as a doorway into a new life. Some spouses find it beneficial to mark the ending of the past with a formal "commencement" celebration. Cutting the cord thereby becomes a rite of growth, unleashing energy for new life.

Such a ritual can be done in many ways, but most spouses do it alone. Methods vary from removing all traces of past pain from the home to reflecting upon the end in a private hideaway. The rite can be conducted in nature, in one's bedroom or at a retreat house. Although Kirstin's illness kept her from performing a transition rite in the inn as planned, her hospital stay turned out to be an appropriate place and time. Wherever it happens and whatever the ritual, the culminating effect for many spouses is a feeling of empowerment.

When the past is finally released, there is often a sense of disorientation, but it differs from the confusion felt after the coming out. Although the spouse is still on unfamiliar ground, he or she now has a stronger sense of self and of personal values. The idea of forging a path through the unknown doesn't seem so daunting.

Some spouses may not have sufficient physical or emotional strength to take immediate action. There may be only enough energy to reaffirm the desire for change. Current circumstances such as children to be nurtured, work to be done or bills to be paid may also pose a barrier too strong to overcome. Yet as spouses cope with these problems, the seeds of the next step are germinating.

Reformulating a Philosophy of Life

To forge a new path, spouses need to have a clear vision of the direction in which they want to go. To achieve this goal, their views of life, in many cases turned upside down by the coming out, need to be reformulated. Creating a new philosophy, the fourth task of this stage of recovery, begins with reflection upon the larger meaning of the coming-out trauma.

Until this point spouses tend to see their devastation as unique, crying, "No one who hasn't been here can understand!" With their self-confidence restored and no longer controlled by the past, they can now begin to view their individual crises from a broader perspective. To do so, they might ask themselves, for example, "Can I get anything positive out of my experience? What would Shakespeare say? How would a TV sitcom handle it, or a documentary? What can my experience teach me?"

It is hard for many spouses to look at the crisis from a different perspective because of the intense suffering it engendered. They typically wonder, "How come this happened to me?" as if the trauma were an unmerited punishment. This feeling comes from viewing suffering, which is an inherent condition of life, as something voluntary.

Professor Elaine Pagels, Ph.D., explains that because people think suffering is related to voluntary behavior, they see it as a sign that they have lost control of the moral quality of their lives. Consequently, they feel guilty about feeling such pain. Believing that "This is punishment for doing something wrong," makes them feel in control.[3] In reality, no one decides when or if he or she will experience suffering. It is involuntary and a necessary part of the human condition.

By reflecting on their pain, many spouses eventually come to understand the universality of suffering despite unique circumstances. Sooner or later everyone suffers pain and dies. No one is exempt. The only choice is in how to handle it.

Another pitfall of the coming-out crisis is the temptation to view everything in either straight or gay terms. Transcending such polarized ways of thinking enables the spouse to formulate a more encompassing viewpoint on the situation. Developing a broader view is fundamental in creating a new philosophy of life.

An effective strategy for overcoming straight-or-gay thinking is to see human sexuality as a continually shifting spectrum. Few people are totally "straight" or "gay" in all thoughts, fantasies and behavior throughout their lives no matter where their basic orientation falls on the scale. Does having the occasional same-sex fantasy, desires, one or two random gay experiences make a person a dyed-in-the-wool homosexual or bisexual? These are the questions Barbara asked at first. The more significant question to consider is the quality of the total person, not his or her sexual orientation.

Many aspects of homosexuality are also presented in either-or terms such as the debate over whether homosexuality is the result of choice or destiny, biology or environment. It is far more enlightening to consider such issues from the viewpoint of a both-and relationship. Both free will *and* destiny operate in life. Prenatal *and* environmental factors exert a major influence on how all people turn out. Through both-and thinking, what may have seemed like a divisive issue can be seen as reflecting the puzzling nature of the human condition in general.[4]

Unifying concepts underlie many of the paradoxes of the coming out. By reflecting on the contradictory aspects of their situation, spouses may be enlightened about life in general. For example:

- The partner's deceit, originating from a wish to avoid hurting the spouse, hurts her or him.
- The coming out of the closet for the partner is often the going into the closet for the spouse.
- The partner's liberation is the spouse's devastation.

All three paradoxes illustrate a universal fact of life: In any situation, what's good for one person may be bad for another. The question is, "Is there a middle ground or a long-range good for both?"

In examining the love-hurt dilemma in the coming out, spouses may reflect upon the fact that love and hurt coexist in all aspects of life. Life is neither all happy nor all hurtful, but a mixture. The essential point is what can be learned from it. As a monk advised one spouse, "Ask, 'For what aspect of this painful experience will I be grateful some day?' "

As spouses become aware of the universal meaning in their individual crises, their trauma no longer seems so unique or overwhelming. The devastation can now be viewed with some dispassion. For example, a wife's futile attempts to seduce her husband may take on a bittersweet irony. Such a woman in Indiana, three years after her husband came out, shared the following vignette with her support group:

Wife: (sighing, after months of rejection and trying to entice her husband) "Well, is there another woman?"

Husband: "No, dear. I never look at other women."

She might not have been able to tell the story earlier without blame and self-pity. Now it's an inside joke, a sign that she's left the gay-straight closet. Having transcended the pain, the spouse may be able to laugh at the incongruities in life, to see that the world is a funny as well as a serious place. With this view, a new philosophy emerges.

Reestablishing a Belief System

For transformation to take place, the spouse's philosophy of life needs to be grounded in belief. This is the fifth task of this stage of recovery. The most valuable of the spouse's shattered beliefs need to be regenerated, new ones discovered and both sets integrated into a cohesive blueprint for living.

The spouse may need to do some soul searching in order to find old beliefs that still seem valid. Discoveries can be made through talking with others whose points of view are respected, reading meaningful literature, observing what others learn from crises or writing in a journal. Sometimes reflection is enhanced by engaging in a dialogue with oneself, a spiritual being or unseen force.[5]

In this search for new meaning, insights may seem to come out of nowhere. Realizations may pop up amidst everyday events: a cloud over a sunset, the look on a child's face, a phrase in a book, a theme in some music, a prayer in a church service, a scene on television, the comment of a friend, an image while jogging. According to an ancient Sufi teacher, "For him who has perception, a mere sign is enough. For him who does not really heed, a thousand explanations are not enough."[6]

However small, the insight or revelation may fill the void in the spouse's life. Kirstin, feeling abandoned, found a whisper of faith in the empty church she entered to cool off on a hot afternoon in Brazil. In the emptiness, she sensed that someone was aware of her pain. That someone was God. Just as instantaneous was Jim's experience at the Presbyterian assembly before Janie came out. Participating with the supporters of gay deacons in an agape celebration being held despite the expectation of being outvoted, he felt a rush of joy.

Such glimmers of meaning are the seeds of a new belief system. Many spouses do not see the meaning in their lives until the emptiness and hunger characteristic of this period impel them to look for it.

Forming a personal connection to some intangible being or force beyond themselves provides an anchor for many spouses. The spiritual dimension has been a critical part of transformation for a number of spouses studied for this book. Kirstin, for example, introduced to spiritual philosophies by men she dated, devoured metaphysical books during her hospital stay. Others have increased their spiritual awareness through retreats, workshops, nature walks or meditation.

The reflective process cannot be hurried. It requires patience on the part of friends and family who may be exasperated by the spouse's seeming lack of progress. They may need to be reminded that the spouse's confusion or indecision hides considerable internal activity that will eventually produce profound change.

Slowly but surely through many possible avenues, a belief-centered philosophy can be formed. Then spouses may at last feel that their lives have meaning and purpose. Jim's spontaneous experience of agape, love that gives more than receives, became his keystone for life, empowering him to be open to gays.

Lynn Conley, founder of the National Support Organization for Spouses of Gays and Lesbians (no longer in existence), stayed in constant dialogue with a higher being while recovering from her coming-out crisis. "I never thought the pain would go," she said. "Now I'm glad I went through it. It taught me a lot. I'm very different. I'm sure of myself and love myself."[7] Such assuredness is the mark of a strong belief system. With it returns the hope that was missing for so long. Now nothing seems impossible.

Creating a New Dream

When Kirstin wept that her dream was dead, a friend said, "Well, dream another." There are always new dreams to be dreamed. This time around the spouse can base these dreams on reality. Creating a new dream may be the boldest decision of the spouse's life as she or he must break out of a lifelong mold of habits. In fashioning a new dream, the sixth task of transformation, the focus shifts from the present to the future.

Through the processes of releasing the past and creating a new belief system, the spouse has already broken down many former patterns of thinking about the world, marriage, partner, family and self. For some spouses, such changes provide sufficient peace of mind.

Others feel compelled to make radical changes in their behavior or environment. Their goals are to pursue individual convictions and passions, to ensure continued individual growth, as well as to challenge their unique potential to reach its full realization.

The dream can be realized inside the marriage as well as after separation or divorce. Spouses still married need to take into account whether their partners respect their beliefs and goals. A compromise may have to be reached so that the dream will not be negated by opposing factors or lack of support.

If the positive factors in the marriage such as love, security and emotional satisfaction outweigh sexual frustration or destructive relationship patterns, the spouse's dream may be to create a more reciprocal relationship. However, the partner's cooperation has to be ensured in order for such a plan to be realistic. As the stories illustrate, only a minority of spouses feel that the marriage is an integral part of their growth. Barbara is among them, having chosen life with Josh as part of her dream.

The more common situation is that in which gay-related goals of the partner run counter to the imperatives of the spouse's new belief system. Once the spouse is confident that all has been done to keep the marriage going, she or he may have to stop trying to make the marriage work and instead concentrate on making her or his own life work. Most often the decision is to divorce or separate.

In envisioning separation, spouses need to be aware that parts of their new lives will be linked to their old lives. Resuming old habits may become tempting. Therefore they need to examine carefully any aspect of separation which might keep them from being consistent with their new belief systems.

The vision of a new life separate from the partner differs from individual to individual. Jim sought the joy of openness and passion for gay advocacy, while Kirstin wanted fulfillment of her psychological, spiritual and sexual identity.

Many spouses are already divorced when they reach this stage. Though being unattached is lonely and painful, divorced spouses have endless possibilities to envision. One woman in her twenties, Anne, realizing that family tradition and stereotypes about women's roles had kept her from pursuing a childhood dream to be a business woman, made that her new goal.

Dreaming and actually making it come true require different skills. Waffling over what to do or hesitating from fear of failure won't bring the new dream to life. Such delays are unnecessary because there's really nothing to fear. With everything in place for a new life to begin, a great leap forward is possible.

Taking the First Step as a New Person

Bolstered by courage and faith, the spouse is now ready to take the first step toward the new goal. A sense of adventure and mystery impels many spouses forward. Nothing can block the way to making the dream a reality. Though the path may not be smooth, each step will take the spouse further ahead in the chosen direction.

The journey will not be as difficult if some of its pitfalls are anticipated. With each new step, the spouse will experience some feelings of insecurity. Echoes of fear, self-pity, frustration, blame and guilt may be heard, requiring willpower to ignore them. Such emotional changes can make each step feel like a giant leap upward, requiring rest and reflection to absorb the significance of it. Energy may slacken and spirits falter, making it crucial to call upon partner, friends, family, therapist and support groups for help.

Spouses who choose transformation within the marriage find it a harder task than expected. Those who succeed discover that individual goals need not be sacrificed for the couple bond to grow stronger. The two are not at cross purposes but complementary if beliefs are constantly reinforced and not abandoned for the sake of the relationship. This is why Barbara continually questioned and talked with Josh as they rewrote their script.

Most spouses who stay married, usually straight wives, find a way to maintain the relationship without compromising beliefs. Along with the personal qualities defined in Part Two, flexibility, openness, honesty and humor; commitment to something beyond themselves seems to help many spouses resolve problems. Barbara focused on positive qualities in the relationship and on Josh as a total person rather than on personal concerns regarding the gay issue. Eventually rising above the gay-straight dilemma, she reached a deeper level of understanding. To strengthen her belief in family values, she decided to adopt the Jewish faith.

It is crucial that partners support their spouses in their transformation. Josh's willingness to listen to Barbara's concerns and to express his own was critical in shaping her development from a twenty-five year old who saw gay men and marriage as mutually exclusive to a non-judgmental, loving and autonomous wife of thirty-five.

Other resources are available to help wives change themselves within the marriage including psychotherapy, marriage counseling, sex therapy, communication workshops and self-help books such as those listed in Appendix A.

The majority of spouses achieve transformation through separation or divorce. For each spouse the breakthrough is different and occurs at different rates. Divorce results in the most abrupt change yet its pain provides energy for moving ahead. For example, Jim's pain from the break up, mixed with the joy of his agape experience, propelled him to create a new life. Once remarried he included his sons, mother and mother-in-law, Janie and Janie's lover and even the dog into one big family. His work, social life and family activities revolved around issues of oppressed gays. The transformation of this corporate businessman into a gay advocate was strikingly different from Janie's reluctant coming out.

Similarly, Anne, who became a businesswoman, was driven by the devastation of cutting ties to her husband upon whom she had depended for everything. She entered the business world "like a steamroller," opened a service shop and in a few years opened a second. Next, she adopted a daughter.

Whether divorced, separated or married, each spouse must forge his or her own path from trauma to transformation. Though none can be duplicated and each has its unique lesson, there is a typical process that spouses undergo that can serve as a guideline for others. Kirstin's story recapitulates the common sequence:

- Paul withdraws and Kirstin suffers an identity crisis.
- When Paul moves out, Kirstin feels new life enter their home.
- Kirstin becomes angry when Paul says she was frigid.
- Paul comes out and Kirstin, though relieved, is in shock.
- Feeling closer to Paul, Kirstin supports his gay activities.
- Feeling excluded from Paul's gay world, she becomes enraged both at his deception and the homophobia in society.
- She rebuilds her self-concept and no longer sees herself as a wife.
- She falls into severe depression and finds spiritual support.
- She clings to the relationship.
- She finally decides that getting a divorce will best reflect the reality of her situation.
- She begins a frantic schedule of work and social activities.
- Through dating she discovers that she's a fully sexual woman after all.

- She explores new spiritual theories while ill.
- She remains friends with Paul and holds family gatherings.
- She is promoted at work and enters into a heterosexual relationship.
- Her divorce final, she believes she can overcome any challenge.

As in real life, Kirstin's transformation does not follow a logical order. Yet there is an overall forward thrust to her journey. Other spouses tell of similar crisscrossings through darkness to final breakthrough. Although the path is uphill, all spouses can reach the summit given courage, awareness and faith in their capabilities.

The journey of transformation is never finished. There is a human need to continue to explore and expand one's potential. Although the devastation that precipitates the straight spouse's recovery isn't to be wished on anyone, the process of resolving it mirrors the struggles of many heroes and heroines in myth and history.

The journey of transformation is ultimately a quest for meaning and transcendence. As psychiatrist Jean Shinoda Bolen comments, in a statement applicable to anyone—man and woman alike—"Travelling this path, the heroine may find, lose and rediscover what has meaning to her until she holds on to these values in all kinds of circumstances that test her...until finally the danger of losing her selfhood is over."[8]

afterword

BEYOND THE CLOSET

Like parables, the straight spouses' stories reveal larger meanings in life. Collectively they depict the emotional suffering that results when rights and responsibilities are abrogated. They caution us about people who feel forced to be less than they can be and people who unknowingly enter into damaging situations. They warn about a society which is deprived of the contribution of all its members. Encapsulated in these stories is the universal dilemma of individual freedom versus social accountability.

The straight spouses' experience affords us a look behind the headlines that too often present gay rights issues in pro- or anti-gay extremes. As members of the mainstream who are also intimately involved with gay, lesbian or bisexual partners, spouses know firsthand both sides of the controversy, from militant gay activism to oppressive homophobia. In coping with the problems posed by a mixed-orientation relationship, spouses forge a middle ground between the two extremes. Their intimate understanding of sexuality and family issues provides a unique perspective for comprehending what may be one of the most significant societal-political-moral changes of this century.

As the partner's disclosed sexual orientation threatens the stability of the family, the straight spouse is forced to examine nearly every issue our society faces from privacy to prejudice. Major questions include "What is the full range of human sexuality? Who is my husband or wife as a total person? What are a parent's socio-moral responsibilities to ensure the children's security in the family? What are my rights to fulfill my own needs and potential?" Exploration of this wide range of profound questions results in a comprehensive view of homosexual behavior in relation to the total dynamic of both the family and the community.

In contrast, public discourse most often approaches gay-straight affairs as either-or issues. This position is either pro-gay or pro-straight. A person's sexual orientation determines whether his or her actions are applauded or denigrated regardless of the consequences. Harm inflicted on homosexual and bisexual persons solely because they differ from the norm impels many of them to hide, flaunt or fight for their freedom to be who they are. A vicious cycle of attack and counterattack is thereby perpetuated.

Having created such conditions of fear and hate, our society can reverse them by ceasing to view homosexual behavior in stereotypical terms of abnormality or immorality. A realistic view of homosexuality and bisexuality as natural variations of sexual orientation that have existed throughout history needs to be formulated.

Just as the heterosexual majority needs to look beyond homophobic labels, so homosexual and bisexual individuals need to look beyond their closet. Many tend to view all straight persons through heterophobic lenses without seeing them as individuals with specific needs. A seemingly anti-gay viewpoint may, with closer scrutiny, turn out to be a legitimate concern about a specific hurt to someone or a thoughtful question about broader principles of which the gay issue is but one part.

In seeking civil rights, gay and lesbian groups have a responsibility to respect the rights of others and to consider the possible consequences of their actions on all concerned. Although it is tempting to ignore the needs of others when fighting for freedoms denied by years of oppression, liberation won't be complete until other people's concerns are honored as well.

As we move ahead into the next century, facing the complex demands of an increasingly diverse society, a comprehensive view of the polarized gay-straight controversy is sorely needed to heal the wounds and to integrate the two camps into a complementary relationship. All sides of the issue need to be considered in the media, research, social theory and religious thought. Only then can equitable solutions be found for a problem societies have grappled with for thousands of years.

As in most controversies, the more realistic and constructive solutions to the gay-straight dilemma will be found between the extreme positions. To formulate public policy that ensures an equitable balance between civil rights and conventional precedents, we need: social realists to affirm society's need for stability by exploring alternative marriage and family arrangements and sexual realists to point out the diversity of sexual orientations as part of the natural order and but one aspect of the individuals who make up society.

Through a balanced approach to the gay-straight conflict, sexual orientation will no longer be used as a measure of personal worth. Individual character will replace irrelevant labels. No one will be prevented from contributing his or her gifts to society. Homosexual and bisexual men and women will no longer be unjustly deprived of their rights and in turn will feel less pressure to hide or to fight back.

To implement such a transformation, we need leaders, legislators and jurists who will consider the full range of concerns intrinsic to gay-straight issues including legitimate rationales at both extremes. We need communities and schools to take concrete steps towards ending ignorance and prejudice. We need individuals who can see beyond personal interest to determine the common good.

Respect for individual differences and rights, as well as the espousal of social responsibility by all members of society—gay, lesbian, bisexual and straight—is the ultimate goal. Honesty can become the cornerstone of social relations. Social justice can prevail. Liberation and responsibility can go hand in hand. With the elimination of divisive labels, we may move beyond a closet mentality to enter the new century, the new millennium, as an inclusive society of fully contributing members.

appendix a

ADDITIONAL READINGS

Understanding Homosexuality and Bisexuality

Barrett, Martha Barro. *Invisible Lives: The Truth About Millions of Women Loving Women*. New York: William Morrow and Company, 1989.

Bell, Alan P., Martin Weinberg, and Sue Kiefer. *Sexual Preference and Its Development in Men and Women*. Bloomington, IN: Indiana University, 1981.

Bi Any Other Name: Bisexual People Speak Out, edit. by Loraine Hutchins and Lani Kaahumanu. Boston: Alyson Publications, Inc., 1991.

Bisexuality: A Reader and Source Book, edit. by Thomas Geller. Ojai, CA: Times Change Press, 1990.

Blumstein, Philip and Pepper Schwartz. *American Couples: Money, Work, Sex*. New York: William Morrow, 1983.

Bode, Janet. *View From Another Closet: Exploring Bisexuality in Women*. New York, Pocket Books, 1977.

Clark, Donald Henry. *The New Loving Someone Gay*, rev. and updated. Berkeley: Celestial Arts, 1987.

Faderman, Lillian. *Odd Girls and Twilight Lovers: A History of Lesbian Life in Twentieth Century America*. New York: Columbia University Press, 1991.

Fairchild, Betty and Nancy Hayward. *Now That You Know: What Every Parent Should Know About Homosexuality*. New York: Harcourt Brace, Jovanovich, 1979.

Homosexuality: Research Implications for Public Policy, edit. by John C. Gonsiorek and James D. Weinrich. Newbury Park, CA: Sage Publications, 1991.

Jones, Clinton, R. *Understanding Gay Relatives and Friends*. New York: The Seabury Press, 1978.

Katz, Jonathan Ned. *Gay American History: Lesbians and Gay Men in the USA*, rev. edit. New York: Meridan Books, 1992.

Marmor, Judd. *Gay, Straight, and In-Between: the Sexology of Erotic Orientation*. New York: Oxford University Press, 1988.

Martin, Del and Phyllis Lyon. *Lesbian Women*, rev. and enl. Volcano, CA: Volcano Press, 1991.

McWhirter, David P. and Andrew M. Mattison. *The Male Couple: How Relationships Develop*. Englewood Cliffs, New Jersey: Prentice-Hall, 1984.

Reinhardt, Regina U. "Bisexual Women in Heterosexual Relationships: Study of Psychological and Sociological Patterns," dissertation published in Research Abstracts International, Fall 1986.

Tripp, Martin. *The Homosexual Matrix*. New York: Mcgraw-Hill Book Co., 1975.

Two Lives to Lead: Bisexuality in Men and Women, edit. by Fritz Klein and Timothy C. Wolf. New York: Harrington Park Press, 1985.

Weinberg, Martin S., Colin J. Williams and Douglas Pryor. *Dual Attraction: Bisexuality in the Age of AIDS*. New York: Oxford University Press, 1994.

Wolff, Charlotte. *Bisexuality: Theory and Research*. New York: Quartet Books, 1979.

Sexual Healing

Barbach, Lonnie. *For Yourself*. Garden City, New York: Anchor Books, 1975.

———. *For Each Other: Sharing Sexual Intimacy*. Garden City, NY: Anchor Books, 1982.

Gochros, Harvey and J. Fischer. *Treat Yourself To A Better Sex Life*. Englewood Cliffs, NJ: Prentice-Hall, 1980.

The Complete Guide to Safe Sex, edit. by Ted McIlvenna. San Francisco: Institute for the Advanced Study of Human Sexuality, 1987.

Kitzinger, Sheila. *Woman's Experience of Sex*. New York: G. P. Putnam's Sons, 1983 (reprint, Penguin Books, 1985)

Money, John and Patricia Tucker. *Sexual Signatures on Being a Man or Woman*. Boston: Little Brown, and Company, 1975.

Strong, Bryan and Rebecca Reynolds. *Understanding Our Sexuality*. New York: West Publishing Company, 1982.

Spousal and Couple Issues

AIDS: A Self-Care Manual: AIDS Project Los Angeles, edit. by BettyClare Moffatt, Judith Spiegel, Steve Parrish, and Michael Helquist. Santa Monica, CA: IBS Press, 1989.

Higham, Charles. *Charles Laughton.* London: W. H. Allen and Co., 1976.

Malone, John. *Straight Women, Gay Men.* New York: Dial Press, 1980.

Nicolson, Nigel. *Portrait of a Marriage.* New York: Atheneum, 1973.

Rubin, Lillian B. *Just Friends: The Role of Friendship in Our Lives.* New York: Harper and Row, Publishers, 1985.

Schneider, Jennifer and Burt Schneider. *Sex, Lies, and Forgiveness: Couples Speak Out on Healing from Sexual Addiction.* Center City, MN: Hazeldon Educational Materials, 1991.

Tannen, Deborah. *You Just Don't Understand.* New York: Ballantine Books, 1990.

The Bisexual Spouse, edit. by Ivan Hill. McLean, VA: Barlina Books, Inc., 1987.

Two Lives to Lead: Bisexuality in Men and Women, edit. by Fritz Klein and Timothy C. Wolf. New York: Harrington Park Press, 1985.

Parental Concerns

Corley, Andre (Rip). *The Final Closet: The Gay Parents Guide for Coming Out to Their Chidren.* Miami: Editech Press, 1990.

Gay and Lesbian Parents, edit. by Frederick W. Bozett. New York, Praeger, 1987.

Gay Fathers of Toronto. *Gay Fathers: Some of Their Stories, Experience, and Advice.* Toronto, Canada: Gay Fathers of Toronto, 1981. (Box F, 730 Bathurst St., Toronto M552R4, Canada).

Schulenburg, Joy A. *Gay Parenting.* Garden City, NY: Anchor Press/Doubleday, 1985.

There's Something I've Been Meaning to Tell You, edit. by Loralee MacPike. Tallahassee, FL: Naiad, 1989.

Rebuilding Identity

Beesing, Maria O.P., Robert J. Nogosek, C.S. C., and Patrick H. O'Leary, , S.J. *The Enneagram: A Journey of Self Discovery.* Denville, NJ: Dimension Books, Inc., 1984.

Bolen, Jean Shinoda. *Gods in Everyman: A New Psychology of Men's Lives & Loves*. San Francisco: Harper & Row Publishers, 1989.

Gawan, Shakti. *Creative Visualization*. New York: Bantam Books, 1978.

Johnson, Robert A. *Inner Work: Using Dreams and Active Imagination for Personal Growth*. San Francisco: Harper and Row, Publishers, 1986.

Keirsey, David and Marilyn Bates. *Please Understand Me: Character and Temperament Types*. Gnosology Books, 1984. (Distributor, Prometheus Nemisis Book Company, Box 2082, Del Mar, CA., 92014).

Norwood, Robin. *Women Who Love Too Much: When You Keep Wishing and Hoping He'll Change*. Los Angeles: Jeremy P. Tarcher, Inc. 1985.

St. Teresa of Avila. *Interior Castle*, transl. and edit. by E. Allison Peers. New York: Doubleday (Image), 1989.

Schaef, Anne Wilson. *Codependence: Misunderstood—Mistreated*. San Francisco: Harper and Row Publishers, 1986.

Tao Te Ching, trans. by Stephen Mitchell. New York: Harper Perennial, 1988.

Resolving Moral Dilemmas

Boswell, John. *Christianity, Social Tolerance and Homosexuality*. Chicago: The University of Chicago Press, 1980.

Fortunato, John E. *AIDS, the Spiritual Dilemma*. San Francisco: Harper and Row, 1987.

Nelson, James. Embodiment: *An Approach to Sexuality and Christian Theology*. Minneapolis: Augsburg Publishing House, 1978.

McNeill, John J. *The Church and the Homosexual*. Kansas City: Sheed, Andrews, and McMeel, 1976.

Spong, John Shelby. *Living in Sin: A Bishop Rethinks Human Sexuality*. San Francisco: Harper and Row, Publishers, 1990.

Woods, Richard. *Another Kind of Love: Homosexuality and Spirituality*, 4th edition. Fort Wayne, IN: Knoll Publishing Co., 1988.

Children and Family Issues

Deevey, Sharon. "When Mom or Dad Comes Out: Helping Adolescents Cope; with Homophobia," *Journal of Psychosocial Nursing and Mental Health Services* 1989, 27:10, pp. 33-36.

Different Mothers: Sons and Daughters Talk About Themselves, edit. by Louise Rafkin. San Francisco: Cleis Press, 1990.

Dodson, Fitzhugh. *How to Grandparent.* New York: Harper and Row, 1981.

Gantz, Joe. *Whose Child Cries: Children of Gay Parents Talk About Their Lives.* Rolling Hills Estates, CA: Jalmar Press, 1983.

Patterson, Charlotte J. "Children of Lesbian and Gay Parents," *Child Development*, November 1992, pp. 1025–1042.

Webster, Harriet. *Family Secrets: How Telling and Not Telling Affects Our Children, Our Relationships, and Our Lives.* New York: Addison-Wesley, 1991.

Personal Transformation

An Interrupted Life: The Diaries of Etty Hillesum 1941-43. New York: Pocket Books, 1981.

Campbell, Joseph. *Myths to Live By.* New York: Bantam Books, 1973.

Eisler, Riane. *The Chalice and the Blade: Our History, Our Future.* San Francisco: Harper and Row, 1988.

Frankel, Viktor E. *Man's Search for Meaning*, rev. and updated. New York: Washington Square Press, 1984.

Huxley, Aldous. *The Perennial Philosophy.* New York: Harper and Row, Publishers, 1944.

Krantzler, Mel. *Creative Divorce: A New Opportunity for Personal Growth.* Philadelphia: J. B. Lippincott, Co., 1973.

Lerner, Harriet Golhor. *The Dance of Anger.* New York: Harper and Row, Publishers, 1989.

Smith, Huston. *The World's Religions.* San Francisco: Harper San Francisco, Publishers, 1991.

appendix b

INTERNATIONAL RESOURCES

United States

Bay Area Bisexual Network, 2404 California Street, San Francisco, CA 94115.
 Information and magazine, *Anything That Moves: Beyond the Myths of Bisexuality.*

Bisexual Information and Counseling Services, 599 West End, New York, NY, 10024.
 Information and counseling for individuals and couples.

Bisexual National Network of the United States (BiNet), P.O. Box 772, Washington, DC 20044.
 Information.

Children of Lesbians and Gays Everywhere (COLAGE). 3543 18th St. #17, San Francisco, CA 94110 415-861-KIDS, Email: Colage@Colage.org
 Network of children of gay, lesbian, bisexual, or transgendered parents. Chapters, newsletter, annual conference.

East Coast Bisexual Network (ECBN), P.O. Box 639, Cambridge, MA 02140.
 Pamphlets, the International Archives on Bisexuality and the annual *International Directory of Bisexual Groups.*

Family Pride Coalition (formerly, Gay and Lesbian Parents Coalition, International) (FPC). P.O. Box 34337, San Diego, CA 92163, 619-296-0199. Email: director@familypride.org, web: www.familypride.org.
 Newsletter, chapters, conferences, resources on parenting for gay, lesbian, bisexual and transgendered parents

Gay and Married Men's Association (GAMMA), P.O. Box 28317, Washington, DC, 20038.
 Support group and contact for GAMMA Wives. Information about GAMMA groups as well as LAMMA—lesbian wives and their families.

Gay Switchboard—in most large cities.
 Information on local resources. If there is no local Switchboard, contact *The National Gay and Lesbian Task Force* (listed on next page).

Institute for Advanced Study of Human Sexuality, 1523 Franklin Street, San Francisco, California, 94109.
 Workshops and graduate courses, library and information.

Institute of Sexual Behavior, 4545 Park Blvd., Suite 207, San Diego, California, 92116.
> Information and counseling services.

International Directory of Bisexual Groups, annual directory, compiled by Robyn Ochs and published by ECBN.
> Lists several hundred resources in the United States, Europe, Asia and Africa. Available for $5.00 from ECBN, (address on previous page).

National AIDS Information Hot Line, 1-(800) 342-AIDS.

National Gay and Lesbian Task Force. 1734 Fourteenth Street NW, Washington, DC 20009-4309. (202) 332-6483.
> Information on homosexuality, events and resources.

Parents, Families and Friends of Lesbians and Gays (PFLAG), 1101 Fourteenth Street, NW, Suite 1030, Washington, DC 20005. 202-638-4200. Email: info@pflag, web www.pflag.org
> Pamphlets, newsletter, bibliographics, conferences, resources related to gay, lesbian, bisexual, and transgendered youth and adult children.

Straight Spouse Network (SSN). International network of heterosexual spouses and partners, current or former, of gay, lesbian, bisexual or transgendered mates. Newsletter, support groups, state and country contacts, articles, research papers. 8215 Terrace Drive, El Cerrito, CA 94530-3058. 510-525-0200, Email: dir@ssnetwk.org. web: www.ssnetwk.org.

Australia

AIDS Council of New South Wales, Inc. (ACON), P.O. Box 350 Darlinghurst NSW 2010 Australia. Information, counseling and support groups for women whose partners are HIV-positive or infected with AIDS.

England

Contact through US-based Straight Spouse Network, (listed above).

Germany

Bine - Bisexulles Netzwerk e. V, Postfach 1134, 0-1136, Berlin.

New Zealand

Wellington Bisexual Women's Group and Wellington Bi Men's Group, P.O. Box 5145, Wellington, Aotearoa/New Zealand.

The Netherlands

Orpheus, Postbus 14121 3508 SE, Utrecht, Holland Telephonic help and meetings for mixed-orientation couples. Correspondence network with Belgium, Germany, Switzerland and Spain.

ENDNOTES

Introduction: Coming Out in Marriage

1. This is a modest estimate based on the 1991 United States Census figures of 90,052,000 men eighteen and over and 97,491,000 women eighteen and over; commonly accepted research estimates as well as recent, much lower survey estimates of homosexual behavior and commonly accepted percentages of married gay men and lesbians. Figures from studies beginning with Kinsey's 1948 and 1953 reports and including more recent surveys range from two to ten percent of adult males reporting more or less exclusively same-sex activities over a three year period and lower percentages among women. Variations among studies stem from differences in terminology, methodology, time period covered in questions, geographic location of respondents, composition of the sample, rate of response and base population used. For example, using the total United States population that includes children under eighteen skews estimates of the number of married gay adults.

    The 2,000,000 figure is derived from a conservative estimate of the incidence of more or less homosexual behavior (a mid-range figure of four percent among adult men and half as much among adult women), generally accepted percentages of gay men who marry (twenty percent) and of lesbians who marry (eighteen to thirty-five percent), the percentage of bisexual men and women (at least twice as many as homosexuals) and the percentage of married bisexual persons (undetermined). See Alan P. Bell and Martin Weinberg in *Homosexualities: A Study of Diversity Among Men and Women* (New York: Simon & Schuster, 1978); Tom W. Smith, "Adult Sexual Behavior in 1989: Number of Partners, Frequency of Intercourse, and Risk of AIDS, *Family Planning Perspectives*, 23 (3): 102–107, May/June 1991; Samuel S. and Cynthia L. Janus, *The Janus Report on Sexual Behavior* (New York: John Wiley & Sons, 1993) and Morton Hunt, *Sexual Behavior in the 1970's* (New York: Dell, 1974). See also Notes 3 and 4.

2. This is a reasonably safe estimate of the number of children produced by homosexual or bisexual parents in traditional marriages. The 3,500,000 figure is based on the 1989 average birth rate of 1.75 children for women 44 and under and the estimated number of married or once married gay, lesbian, and bisexual adults. See Note 1, explaining variations among reported figures.

3. Alfred C. Kinsey et al, *Sexual Behavior in the Human Male* (Philadelphia: W. B. Saunders, 1948) and *Sexual Behavior in the Human Female* (Philadelphia: W. B. Saunders, 1953). Charles F. Turner, primary author, *AIDS, Sexual Behavior, and Intravenous Drugs* (Washington, D.C.: National Academy of Sciences Press, 1989), based on a study of 1450 men in 1970 and 638 in 1988, confirms Kinsey's four percent figure but suggests slightly lower percentages for adult males reporting occasional or frequent homosexual contact leading to orgasm. More recent studies report even lower percentages.

4. Figures vary with composition of groups, research method, and indicators of homosexuality. See, Bell and Weinberg, *op. cit.* A summary of research and discussion of many dimensions of sexual orientation is found in Fritz Klein, *The Bisexual Option*, second edition (New York: The Harrington Park Press, 1993).

5. Twenty-one dimensions form the Klein Sexual Orientation Grid. See *Ibid.*, Ch. 2.

6. This is a commonly accepted percentage among the diverse findings. The most thorough study is Michael Ross, *The Married Homosexual Man* (Boston, Routledge and Kegan Paul, 1983).

7. *Ibid.*, pp. 142-51.

8. *Tearoom Trade: Impersonal Sex in Public Places* (New York: Aldine Publishing Company, 1975).

Part One: Sexual Mix-match

1. Unpublished essay on spouses' sexuality, May 2, 1986, p. 2.

2. See Sandra Auerback and Charles Moser, "Groups for the Wives of Gays and Bisexual Men, " *Social Work*, 1987. pp. 321–25 and Jean Schaar Gochros, *When Husbands Come Out of the Closet*, (New York: Harrington Park Press, 1989). These findings along with author's contradict earlier descriptions, such as the five neurotic wives of husbands in therapy to change their homosexuality reported by Myra Hatterer, "Problems of Women Married to Homosexual Men," *American Journal of Psychiatry*, 131(3), 1974, pp. 275-58 and descriptions of wives in Brenda Maddox, *Married and Gay*, (New York: Harcort Brace Jovanovich, Publishers, 1982).

3. Interview, May 23, 1986.

4. Dorothea Hays and Aurele Samuels, Abstract of "Grief Reactions of Heterosexual Wives Who Have Learned That Their Husbands are Homosexually Active," paper presented at symposium on unsanctioned and un-

recognized grief, sponsored by Foundation of Thanatology and Columbia University, April 1987. See also Hays and Samuels, "Heterosexual Women's Perceptions of Their Marriages to Homosexual or Bisexual Men," *Journal of Homosexuality*, 17(3/4) 1988, pp. 81–100.

5. "Abstract" cited in Note 4.
6. Gochros, *op. cit.*, Chs. 5 and 10.
7. *Coming Out: An Act of Love* (New York: Dutton, 1990) Chs. 6-8 and pp. 161–70.
8. *The Joy of Sex: A Cordon Bleu Guide to Love Making, revised* (New York: Pocket Books, 1989).
9. *Radical Love: An Approach to Sexual Spirituality* (P.O. Box 3216, Fremont, CA 94539: Dharma Cloud Press, 1993).

Part Two: Trial and Error

1. Auerback and Moser, *op. cit.*, p, 323.
2. Gochros, *op. cit.*, pp. 193–216.
3. Brian Miller, "Women Who Marry Gay Men," *The Advocate*, (April 25, 1989), pp. 22–30.
4. *Goodbye, I Love You* (New York: Jove, 1989).
5. "An Investigation of Sexual Behaviors in Mixed Sexual Orientation Couples: Gay Husband and Straight Wives," Institute for The Advanced Study of Human Sexuality, San Francisco, June 1987, pp. 31, 39–40.
6. See David R. Matteson, "Married and Gay," *Changing Men*, Spring-Summer 1988, pp. 14–16, 45. Matteson also discusses lesbian wives.
7. Deabill, *op. cit.*, pp. 41–42.
8. Susan Gerrard and James Halpin, "The Risky Business of Bisexual Love," *Cosmopolitan*, (September 1989), p. 204.
9. Deabill, *op. cit.*, p. 40.
10. See Melody Beattie, *Codependent No More: How to Stop Controlling Others and Start Caring for Yourself* (New York: Harper and Row, 1987).
11. Interview, October 10, 1990. Matteson, *op. cit.*, discusses how gay or bi husbands help keep their marriages working.
12. See Dennis Wholey, *The Courage To Change* (Boston: Warner Books Edition Houghton Miflin Company, 1984), pp. 138–151.
13. Unpublished essay on gay-straight couples, April 5, 1990, p. 2.
14. *Ibid.*
15. Barry Kohn and Alice Matusow, *Barry and Alice: Portrait of a Bisexual Marriage* (Englewood Cliffs, NJ: Prentice Hall, Inc., 1980).
16. *The New Couple: Woman and Gay Men* (New York: Seaview Books, 1979).
17. *Uncommon Lives: Gay Men and Straight Women* (New York: New American Library, 1990).
18. Nahos and Turley, *op. cit.*, p. 12.
19. *The Road Less Traveled* (New York: Simon and Schuster, 1978).

20. Deabill, *op. cit.*, pp. 41–42.
21. *The Art of Intimacy* (New York: Prentice-Hall Press, 1987), p. 73. See also "Participation," p. 269.
22. See Timothy Wolf, "Selected Psychological and Sociological Aspects of Male Homosexual Behavior in Marriage," Graduate Faculty, School of Human Behavior, U. S. International University, San Diego, CA., 1982, (University Microfilms International No. DA 83131477).

Part Three: Growing Pains

1. Full Frame Products, San Francisco.
2. "Growing Up With a Gay, Lesbian, or Bisexual Parent: An Expoloratory Study of Experiences and Perceptions," Unpublished Dissertation, University of California, Berkeley, 1986.
3. *Homosexuality and Family Relations* (New York: Harrington Park Press, 1990).
4. Judith Wallerstein with John Berlin Kelly, *Surviving the Breakup: How Children and Prents Cope with Divorce* (New York: Basic Books, Inc, Publishers, 1980).
5. Paul, *op. cit.*, p. 77.
6. Janet Ghent, "When Mom or Dad is Gay," *Oakland* (CA) *Tribune*, January 29, 1987, p. C-2.
7. Paul, *op. cit.*, p. 93.
8. *Ibid.*, p. 89.
9. *Ibid.*, p. 80. Sons' concerns may relate to the "fragility of the masculine role" in our society, in contrast to the strong feminist model to which many daughters are currently exposed.
10. Peck, *op. cit.*, pp. 120–130.
11. *Mothers and Divorce: Legal, Economic, and Social Dilemmas* (Berkeley: University of California Press, 1986), p. 100.
12. Paul, *op. cit.*, p. 93.
13. Unpublished "Letter to the Editor," January 14, 1987.
14. Judith Wallerstein with Sandra Blakeslee, *Second Chances: Men, Women and Children a Decade After Divorce; Who Wins, Who Loses and Why* (New York: Ticknor and Fields, 1989).
15. Paul, *op. cit.*, p. 93.

Part Four: What About Me?

1. Unpublished commentary, February 7, 1990.
2. Says the *Dhammapada*, transl. by Eknath Easwaran (Petaluma, CA: Nilgiri Press, 1985).

3. Suggested readings include Indries Shah, *The Way of The Sufi* (New York: E. P. Dutton, 1970); *The Song of God: Bhagavad-Gita,* transl. by Swami Prabhavananda and Christopher Isherwood (New York: The New American Library, Mentor, 1951); Gerald Hausman, *Meditations with the Navajo* (Santa Fe: Bear and Co., 1987); and *The Old Testament, The New English Bible with the Aprocrypha,* Oxford Study Edition (New York: Oxford University Press, 1976), pp. 569–674.
4. *The Message of the Psalms: A Theological Commentary* (Minneapolis: Augsburg Publishing House, 1984), p. 54.
5. Interview, February 23, 1990.
6. Auerback and Moser, *op. cit.,* p. 232.
7. *Talking to Yourself: Learning the Language of Self-Support,* (New York: Harper & Row, Publishers, 1981), p. 1.
8. *How to Survive the Loss of a Love* (New York: Bantam Books, 1977).
9. Wolf, op. cit., pp. 109–10.
10. *Love Is Letting Go of Fear* (New York: Bantam Books, 1970).

Part Five: Power of the Lie

1. Interview, May 28, 1986.
2. *Lying: Moral Choice in Public and Private Life,* (New York: Pantheon Press, 1978), p. xvii.
3. See *Anger: How to Live With and Without It,* (Secaucus, NJ: Citadel Press, 1977).
4. *Uncoupling: Turning Points in Intimate Relationships* (New York: Oxford University Press, 1986), p. 193.
5. Bok, *op. cit.,* p. 74.
6. Vaughan, *op. cit.,* p. 26.
7. Unpublished essay on deception, November 16, 1987, p. 4.
8. *Shattered Secrets* (Los Angeles: Libbe HaLevy, 1990).
9. *Is the Homosexual My Neighbor? Another Christian View* (San Francisco: Harper & Row, Publishers, 1978), p. 121.
10. Interview, November 8, 1990.
11. Scanzoni and Mollenkott, *op. cit.,* p. 12.
12. "An Open Letter to Gay and Bi-sexual Men," (P.O. Box 6692, Philadelphia, PA 19149).

Part Six: Family Voices

1. See Erik Erikson, *The Life Cycle Completed: A Review* (New York: W.W. Norton, 1982). Of particular interest is the chart of developmental challenges, pp. 32–33.

2. See Carol Gilligan, *In a Different Voice: Psychological Theory and Women's Development*. (Cambridge: Harvard University Press, 1993).

3. Excellent discussion of children's concerns about AIDS can be found in Stefan Lynch, "Fags, Dykes, and Kids: A guidebook for Daughters and Sons of Lesbians and Gay Men," unpublished Senior thesis, Social Science Faculty (Great Barrington, MA: Simon's Rock College of Bard, Great Barrington, MA, 1993).

4. Berman, Claire, *Adult Children of Divorce Speak Out: About Growing Up With—and Moving Beyond—Parental Divorce*, (New York: Simon and Schuster, 1991), *passim*.

5. *Ibid.*

6. *All Grown Up & Nowhere to Go: Teenagers in Crisis*, (Menlo Park, CA: Addison-Wesley Publishing Company, 1984).

7. Interview, psychologist Michael Cohen, professional consultant for COLAGE, at their 1993 Annual Conference, Orlando, July 4, 1993.

8. Interview, October 15, 1993.

Part Seven: Breaking the Mold

1. *Transitions* (Menlo Park, CA: Addison Wesley, 1980) p. 91.

2. See, for example, Matthew L. and D. Linn, *The Healing of Memories: Prayers and Confession—Steps to Inner Healing* (Mahwah, NJ: Paulist Press, 1974.

3. *Adam, Eve, and the Serpent* (New York: Random House, 1988), p. 18.

4. Another way of putting it is to develop tolerance for apparent ambiguity. Such non-dichotomous thinking about sexual identity can be found in Ronald C. Fox, "Bisexual Identies," in *Lesbian, Gay and Bisexual Identities*, edit. by A. R. Augelli and C. J. Patterson (New York: Oxford University Press, in press).

5. "When I go down into myself, I discover the universalities." "Conversations with Howard Thurman," Video series, for private home use only (San Francisco: Howard Thurman Educational Trust, Inc., 2018 Stockton St., San Francisco, CA 94133, 1987).

6. Idries Shah, *op. cit.*, p. 222.

7. Interview, January 15, 1990.

8. *Goddesses in Every Woman: A New Psychology of Women* (San Francisco: Harper and Row Publishers, 1984), p. 293.